Handbook for Psychiatric Trainees

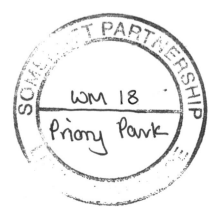

Handbook for Psychiatric Trainees

Edited by Dinesh Bhugra and Oliver Howes

RCPsych Publications

RCPsych Publications is an imprint of the Royal College of Psychiatrists,
17 Belgrave Square, London SW1X 8PG
http://www.rcpsych.ac.uk

British Library Cataloguing-in-Publication Data.
A catalogue record for this book is available from the British Library.
ISBN 978 1 904671 34 3

Distributed in North America by Balogh International Inc.

The views presented in this book do not necessarily reflect those of the Royal College of Psychiatrists, and the publishers are not responsible for any error of omission or fact.

Printed by Bell & Bain Limited, Glasgow, UK.

Contents

Tables, boxes and figures

Contributors

Gwen Adshead Consultant Forensic Psychotherapist, Dadd Centre, Broadmoor Hospital, Crowthorne

Martin Baggaley Medical Director and Consultant Psychiatrist, South London and Maudsley NHS Foundation Trust HQ, Maudsley Hospital, London

Sube Banerjee Professor of Mental Health and Ageing, The Institute of Psychiatry, King's College London

Dinesh Bhugra Professor of Mental Health and Cultural Psychiatry, Institute of Psychiatry, London

Jonathan Bindman Clinical Director, Lambeth Adult Mental Health Services, South London and Maudsley NHS Foundation Trust, Lambeth Hospital, London

Joe Bouch Consultant Psychiatrist, Gartnavel Royal Hospital, Goldenhill Resource Centre, Clydebank, Glasgow; former Director of CPD Online for the Royal College of Psychiatrists, London

Alistair Burns Professor of Old Age Psychiatry, University of Manchester, Manchester

Vanessa Cameron Chief Executive, Royal College of Psychiatrists, London

Jerome Carson Consultant Clinical Psychologist, Lambeth Community Mental Health Services, South London and Maudsley NHS Foundation Trust, London

Eleanor Cole Consultant Psychiatrist, South London and Maudsley NHS Foundation Trust, London

Anne Farmer Professor of Psychiatric Nosology, Social, Genetic and developmental Psychiatry Research Centre, Institute of Psychiatry, London

Carl Gray Medical Director, Consultant in Histopathology and Forensic Pathology, Harrogate and District NHS Foundation Trust, Harrogate District Hospital, Harrogate

Richard Gray   Senior Lecturer and Head of the Section of Mental Health Nursing, Institute of Psychiatry, King's College London

Peter Hill   Professor and Consultant in Child and Adolescent Psychiatry, Wimpole Street and Great Ormond Street Hospital for Children, London

Frank Holloway   Consultant Psychiatrist and Clinical Director, Croydon Integrated Adult Mental Health Service, and Honorary Senior Lecturer, Health Services Research Department, Institute of Psychiatry, King's College London

Gareth Holsgrove   Medical Education Advisor, Royal College of Psychiatrists, London; Section of Mental Health and Ageing, Health Services and Population Research Department, David Goldberg Centre, Institute of Psychiatry, King's College London

Kalyani Katz   Consultant Psychiatrist and Honorary Senior Lecturer, Park Royal Centre for Mental Health, London

Sheila A. Mann   Formerly Consultant in the Psychiatry of Old Age, North Essex Mental Health Partnership NHS Trust; correspondence c/o The Royal College of Psychiatrists, London

Jane Marshall   Consultant Psychiatrist and Senior Lecturer in the Addictions, National Addiction Centre, Institute of Psychiatry, King's College London

Hilary McCallion   Director of Nursing and Education, South London and Maudsley NHS Foundation Trust, London

Povl Munk-Jørgensen   Research Director, Chief Consultant, Professor, Unit for Psychiatric Research, Aalborg Psychiatric Hospital, Aarhus University Hospital, Aalborg, Denmark

Ross Overshott   Specialist Registrar in General Adult, Old Age and Liaison Psychiatry, Northwest Deanery

Femi Oyebode   Professor of Psychiatry, University of Birmingham, Birmingham

Pramod Prabhakaran   Consultant Psychiatrist, Northwick Park Hospital, Watford, Harrow

Rosalind Ramsay   Consultant Adult Psychiatrist, South London and Maudsley NHS Foundation Trust, London

Nick Rose   Formerly Consultant Psychiatrist and Honorary Senior Lecturer, University of Oxford; Regional Advisor for Psychiatry, Oxford Deanery; Chair, Royal College of Psychiatrists' Overseas Doctors Training Committee, Littlemore Mental Health Unit, Littlemore, Oxford

Alan Rushton   Programme Leader, MSc in Mental Health Social Work, Reader in Adoption Studies, Section of Social Work and Social Care, Health Services Research Department, Institute of Psychiatry, King's College London

Shekhar Saxena   Coordinator, Mental Health: Evidence and Research, World Health Organization, Geneva, Switzerland

Padmal de Silva Visiting Senior Lecturer, Department of Psychology, Institute of Psychiatry, King's College London

Mark Sutherland Presiding Chaplain, South London and Maudsley NHS Foundation Trust

Michael J. Travis Honorary Senior Lecturer, Section of Clinical Neuropharmacology, Institute of Psychiatry, London, and Associate Professor, Director of Residency Training, Western Psychiatric Institute and Clinic, University of Pittsburgh Medical Center, Pittsburgh, PA, USA

Peter Tyrer Professor of Community Psychiatry, Department of Psychological Medicine, Imperial College London

Stephen Tyrer Professor of Psychiatry, Royal Victoria Infirmary, Newcastle upon Tyne

Koravangattu Valsraj Specialist Registrar, South London and Maudsley NHS Foundation Trust, London; Consultant Psychiatrist, East London and The City University NHS Trust

Cleo Van Velsen Consultant Psychiatrist in Forensic Psychotherapy, The John Howard Centre, Hackney Hospital, London

Cecilia Wells Director, Astar Management Consultants Ltd, Non-Executive Board Member of the Office of the Parliamentary and Health Service Ombudsman and of the Office of the Independent Adjudicator for Higher Education, Chair of the Race Equality (Community) Network for Guy's and St Thomas' NHS Foundation Trust

Hilary Williams Lead Occupational Therapist – Research and Development, South London and Maudsley NHS Foundation Trust, Maudsley Hospital, London

CHAPTER 1

Psychiatric training: the next steps

Dinesh Bhugra

Psychiatry is one of the key medical specialties, and has close relationships with non-medical mental health disciplines, with biology and with primary care medicine. Psychiatry has to demonstrate its effectiveness in dealing with mental illness and distress, and the role of the psychiatrist has to include educating the public, other physicians and legislators as well as employers. Psychiatry has to rise above the 'psychobabble' of pop psychology. The role of psychiatrists has changed dramatically in the past 50 years or so as the services have evolved and changed.

In the 1950s psychological therapies, biological pharmacological innovations and social psychiatry influenced the way psychiatry was practised. In the 1960s, specific neurotransmitter hypotheses led to an expansion in biomedical clinical investigation in psychiatry. In the 1970s and 1980s, although newer forms of psychotherapy emerged, the challenges to service development led to closure of mental hospitals and a shift towards community-based services, with community mental health teams as the focus for service delivery. In the 1990s the introduction of sub-specialisation based upon employer-/government-led initiatives, such as home treatment, continuing care and crisis resolution, held sway.

Various aspects of being a good psychiatrist include psychological mindedness (understanding the patient's and the trainee's subjective responses; objective approach to behaviour; ability to make contact with psychiatric patients; understanding of signs, symptoms and syndromes; ability to conduct and organise investigations and treatment methods using physical, psychological and social approaches; and an understanding of the self; Walton, 1986). These characteristics remain important for the psychiatrist after more than two decades.

Good Psychiatric Practice (Royal College of Psychiatrists, 2004) lists attributes of a good psychiatrist in the areas shown in Box 1.1. The core attributes of a good psychiatrist listed in *Good Psychiatric Practice* are given in Box 1.2. It is clear that there is a tremendous area of overlap in qualities of an individual psychiatrist as well as the characteristics of a service that will be acceptable to the patients and their carers.

Box 1.1 *Good Psychiatric Practice* lists attributes of a good psychiatrist in these areas (Royal College of Psychiatrists, 2004)

- Trusting relationship
- Good clinical care
- Consent to treatment
- Note-keeping and inter-agency/inter-professional communication
- Confidentiality
- Availability and emergency care
- Working as a member of a team
- Referring patients
- Clinical governance
- Teaching and training
- Research
- Being a good employee and employer

The consultant of the future will have to have a range of competencies in clinical care, management, teaching, and research. The essential roles and key competencies are given in Box 1.3 and the attributes of a good consultant psychiatrist are shown in Box 1.4 .

Therefore, the training of psychiatrists will have to take on board a number of factors, including peer group-based learning, learning across disciplines and teams, and continuing professional development (CPD).

Certain driving forces within the profession have challenged our assumptions of training. These include continuing rapid expansion in our

Box 1.2 Core attributes of a good psychiatrist (Royal College of Psychiatrists, 2004)

- Clinical competence
- Being a good communicator and listener
- Being sensitive to gender, ethnicity and culture
- Commitment to equality and working with diversity
- Having a basic understanding of group dynamics
- Being able to facilitate a team
- Ability to be decisive
- Ability to appraise staff
- Basic understanding of operational management
- Understanding and acknowledging the role and status of vulnerable patients
- Bringing empathy, encouragement and hope to patients and carers
- Critical self-awareness of emotional responses to clinical situations
- Being aware of potentially destructive influence in power relationship
- Acknowledging situations where there is potential for bullying

Box 1.3 Essential roles and key competencies of a psychiatrist

Medical expert
- Demonstrate diagnostic and therapeutic skills for ethical and effective patient care: precise clinical history-taking, physical examination, investigation
- Apply relevant information and therapeutic options to clinical practice
- Demonstrate medical expertise in situations other than direct patient care
- Recognise personal limits of experience
- Demonstrate effective consultation skills with respect to patient care, education and legal opinions: present well-documented patient assessment

Communicator
- Establish therapeutic relationships with patients and their families
- Elicit and synthesise relevant information from patients, their families and communities: be aware of beliefs, age, gender, culture
- Listen effectively, foster understanding
- Discuss appropriate information with patients, their families and communities and other healthcare professionals

Team player
- Consult and liaise with other health professionals
- Recognise limits of personal competence
- Contribute effectively to multidisciplinary team activities (training, etc.)
- Aware of roles and expertise of other disciplines
- Integrate opinions of patients in decision-making

Manager
- Managing resources and time effectively to balance patient care, learning needs, outside activities and personal life
- Allocate finite healthcare and education resources effectively and work efficiently
- Utilise IT effectively to aid patient care

Health advocate
- Help promote health and prevent disability
- Identify social/cultural factors affecting health
- Recognise and respond to settings related to advocacy: populations at risk, policy awareness, development of policy

Scholar/educator
- Personal CPD strategy and learning needs and methods
- Be a critical appraiser of sources of medical information
- Educator: help others to define learning needs and development, provide feedback, adult learning

Professional
- Deliver highest quality care with integrity, honesty and compassion
- Appropriate personal and interpersonal behaviours: self-awareness
- Ethically acceptable/responsible: local laws

knowledge base and technology leading to changes in service delivery. Growth of sub-specialties and super-specialisation, changes in undergraduate education, arrival of increasing numbers of international medical graduates,

Box 1.4 Attributes of a good consultant psychiatrist

Medical knowledge
- Up-to-date knowledge needed to evaluate and manage patients

Clinical skills
- Demonstrate proficiency in history-taking
- Effective physical examination
- Organise and evaluate investigations
- Lead and manage diagnostic studies
- Propose interventions based on individual formulation
- Demonstrate practice skills
- Show proficiency in technical skills

Clinical judgement
- Demonstrate clinical reasoning
- Make sound diagnostic and therapeutic decisions
- Understand the limits of knowledge
- Incorporate cost-awareness and risk–benefit analysis

Interpersonal skills
- Communicate and work effectively with patients, families, other members of the team and agencies

Professional attitudes and behaviour
- Accountability
- Accept responsibility
- Maintain comprehensive, timely and legible medical records
- Be available for consultation
- Seek improvement in quality of care provided
- Facilitating learning of patients, communities, students and other disciplines
- Lifelong learning
- Evaluate critically new medical and scientific information
- Self-awareness
- Humanistic qualities
- Demonstrate integrity and honesty
- Demonstrate compassion and empathy
- Respect for privacy and dignity
- Ethical practice

Managerial skills
- Effective and efficient working
- Utilise IT

Health advocacy
- Health promotion and prevention
- Advocacy for patients, families and communities

and structural changes within the National Health Service (NHS) and medical profession all indicate that training and delivery of training need to change.

Training is becoming outcome-based. For psychiatry it is crucial to determine what is good clinical care and what the working life of consultants will look like in 10 years' time. The potential impact of documents such as *The Ten Essential Shared Capabilities* (Hope, 2004) cannot be overestimated. These shared capabilities are as follows.

- Working in partnership: developing and maintaining constructive working relationships with service users, carers, families, colleagues, lay people and wider community; working positively with any revisions created by conflicts of interest or aspiration that may arise between the partners in care.
- Respecting diversity: working in partnership with service users, carers, families and colleagues to provide care and interventions that not only make a positive difference but also do so in ways that respect and value diversity, including age, gender, race, culture, disability, spirituality and sexuality.
- Practising ethically: recognising the rights and aspirations of service users and their families, acknowledging power differentials and mini-mising them whenever possible; providing treatment and care that is accountable to service users and carers within the boundaries prescribed by national (professional), legal and local codes of ethical practice.
- Challenging inequality: addressing the causes and consequences of stigma, discrimination, social inequality and exclusion on service users, carers and mental health services; creating, developing or maintaining valued social roles for people in the communities they come from.
- Promoting recovery: working in partnership to provide care and treatment that enables service users and carers to tackle mental health problems with hope and optimism and to work towards a valued lifestyle within and beyond the limits of any mental health problems.
- Identifying people's needs and strengths: working in partnership to gather information to agree health and social care needs in the context of the preferred lifestyle and aspirations of service users, their families, carers and friends.
- Providing service user-centred care: negotiating achievable and meaningful goals, primarily from the perspective of the service users and their families, influencing and seeking the means to achieve these goals and clarifying the responsibilities of the people who will provide any help that is needed, including systematically evaluating outcomes and achievements.
- Making a difference: facilitating access to and delivering the best quality, evidence-based, values-based health and social care interventions to meet the needs and aspirations of service users and their families and carers.
- Promoting safety and positive risk-taking: empowering the person to decide the level of risk they are prepared to take with their health and safety. This includes working with the tension between promoting safety and positive risk-taking, including assessing and dealing with possible risks for service users, their families and the wider public.

- Personal development and learning: keeping up to date with changes in practice and participating in lifelong learning, personal and professional development for one's self and colleagues through supervision, appraisal and reflective practice.

Developments in medical education

Contemporary developments in medical education have led to a situation where we have both the understanding and the opportunity to make significant improvements, especially at postgraduate level. This opportunity has largely developed from the reforms in undergraduate medical education outlined in *Tomorrow's Doctors* (General Medical Council, 1993). These were astonishingly slow in coming about. For example, a minute of the General Medical Council as long ago as 1869 warned about the dangers of an excessively burdensome curriculum, and Thomas Huxley, in an address in 1876, said that

'the burden we place on the medical student is far too heavy .... a system of medical education that is actually calculated to obstruct the acquisition of sound knowledge and to heavily favour the crammer and the grinder is a disgrace'.

Progress since the first of the modern *Tomorrow's Doctors* curricula came into operation in 1990 has been much more brisk. Today, every UK medical school has a modern undergraduate curriculum and the spotlight has now turned to postgraduate medical education.

Developments in postgraduate medical education have been initiated and shaped by various initiatives such as the recommendations for senior house officer training from the Conference of Postgraduate Medical Deans (Conference of Postgraduate Medical Deans, 1995), the Academy of Medical Royal Colleges (Academy of Medical Royal Colleges, 1996), the General Medical Council (General Medical Council, 1998), and the Department of Health (2002, 2003, 2004) with *Unfinished Business* and *Modernising Medical Careers*.

Postgraduate Medical Education and Training Board

In 2003 the Postgraduate Medical Education and Training Board (PMETB) was established as the UK statutory body for standards in postgraduate medical education. Once established, PMETB became independent of government and set its own agenda and direction. Following the publication of *The NHS Plan* in 2000 (Department of Health, 2000), the stated aims for setting up PMETB included: cultural change (to 'modernise' the institutions of medicine and professional regulation of all the healthcare professions); resetting the constitutional checks and balances (an emphasis on professionally led regulation with public involvement); better connections between the institutions of postgraduate medical education and the needs of the NHS; more involvement of patients and the wider public;

bringing consistency and integration to the diverse collection of historical arrangements; and, perhaps most importantly, for one organisation to take on collective responsibility for postgraduate medical education and be accountable for ensuring that standards are met.

As PMETB itself acknowledges, its establishment was also influenced by negative impressions and experiences of the past which, although addressed by the relevant institutions, did not fully meet the ideals. Two additional factors were the perception that the Specialist Training Authority was a weak organisation, and that quality assurance of postgraduate medical education was not rigorous enough. Thus, the aim to bring about transparency and consistency to quality assurance functions led to the establishment of PMETB. Changes in the medical workforce, service provisions and patients' expectations were further triggers for the change. Modernising Medical Careers (MMC, see below) has set both short-term and long-term challenges for PMETB. Other factors that influenced the establishment of PMETB include international recruitment, a wish for a closer fit between the status and job titles of doctors and the work they do for the NHS, discrepancy in different regions of the UK, reforms in medical education and standard setting.

PMETB principles and guidance are set to shape a wide range of improvements under a new legislative framework. The key functions of PMETB are to deliver its stated and statutory functions, and to meet the needs of patients, doctors and the service through curriculum design, delivery, assessment and quality assurance in relation to the evidence base. The stated criteria for the success of PMETB are given in Box 1.5.

The PMETB came into force on 30 September 2005. The following priorities were set for its first year of operation:

- develop funding streams
- complete preparation to take on its role as the competent authority
- establish financial and contractual arrangements
- operate the first year of its certification processes efficiently and without delays
- deal with expected front load of applications under article 14
- operate first year of quality assurance arrangements
- play its full part in the quality assurance of the first foundation programmes
- further develop its standards for postgraduate medical education and communicate them effectively.

The PMETB is responsible for approving the curricula for each specialty. It defines curriculum as a statement of the intended aims and objectives, content, experiences, outcomes and processes of an educational programme, including:

- a description of the training structure (entry requirements, length and organisation of the programme, including its flexibility and assessment system)

Box 1.5 Stated criteria for the success of PMETB

- Evidence that standards for medical education are informed by the needs of patients
- Quality assurance arrangements that:
  - are consistent
  - involve structured evidence-based decisions
  - are proportionate and harmonised with other quality assurance arrangements
  - are transparent
  - are perceived as relevant to the needs of the service
  - involve the wider public
  - make a difference and are seen to do so
  - command the confidence of the NHS and other UK institutions
  - are highly regarded internationally
- Certification arrangements that:
  - are consistent and fair
  - involve structured evidence-based decisions
  - have a credible and sound approach towards doctors trained overseas
  - command the confidence of the NHS and other UK institutions
- Governance arrangements that match best practice and Board activity that is open to public and professional scrutiny
- An organisation fit for purpose, well run and recognisable as a learning organisation
- Efficient and financially sound, with genuine involvement of the wider public, trainee doctors and the NHS
- Real and perceived independence from the government
- International repute

- a description of expected methods of learning, teaching, feedback and supervision.

The curriculum should cover both generic professional and specialty-specific areas. The syllabic content of the curriculum should be stated in terms of what knowledge, skills, attitudes and expertise the learner will achieve. The standards for the curriculum are available from PMETB.

Modernising Medical Careers

Modernising Medical Careers (Department of Health, 2004) built upon the educational aims set out in the document *Unfinished Business* (Department of Health, 2002, 2003). The former's underlying educational principles are:

- outcome-based educational process
- defined competence
- assessment of competence
- lifelong professional development.

After graduating from medical school doctors now undertake an integrated 2-year foundation programme followed by specialist training with a unified training grade and a 6-year rotation within which the current training plan will broadly remain in place.

Foundation programme

The aims of the foundation programme are to develop generic skills, competencies and attitudes to ensure professional conduct that will reflect good medical practice. The experience of working in psychiatry in either the first or second year of the foundation programme will allow trainees to 'sample' the specialty and will improve and encourage recruitment. This will be an induction to what is currently basic specialist training (but may well change into specialist unified training). The foundation programme aims to help trainees develop competencies that will enable them to progress further in their chosen fields. Modernising Medical Careers recommends clear entry criteria for foundation programme training. The application procedure is under review (see http://www.mmc.nhs.uk/pages/home for latest details).

In foundation year 2 (FY2) the trainee will be expected to do at least three placements of 4 months each. Psychiatry offers unique training opportunities for working with multidisciplinary teams, culturally appropriate and ethical services. Essential elements of the programme as indicated in *Good Medical Practice* (General Medical Council, 2001) are professional competence, good relationships with patients and colleagues, and ethical clinical practice. The principles of multidisciplinary working and knowledge of the roles of individual team members and the basic provisions within mental health legislation are all essential components of the curriculum agreed across different specialties, as are a number of competencies, such as communication skills. Patient-based learning encourages trainees to gain experience in multiple settings and gain an understanding of the impact of biological, social, psychological (as well as broader spiritual and anthropological) factors on the genesis and perpetuation of mental illness. By following the patients' journeys throughout their contact with psychiatric services from the presentation of acute illness, through investigations – physical, psychological or social – to reach a diagnosis and obtain a basic understanding of the management plan, the trainees can start to synthesise the information and develop skills and competencies. Personal attention, with supervision at both educational and clinical levels will encourage trainees further to develop their competencies.

Educational supervisors will provide continuity of supervision over the 1-year period irrespective of the clinical job the trainee is doing. The responsibilities of educational supervisors will include assessment, appraisal, mentoring, career guidance and evaluation of educational and training programmes. Supervision is a formal process that allows the trainee to grasp an academic perspective on questions arising from direct patient care.

Assessment of trainees in FY2 includes monitoring how the trainee manages to: examine a patient's mental state; work within a multidisciplinary team; arrange investigations; collate third-party information; and understand how management plans are reached and acted upon. The aims, objectives and outcomes of the psychiatry programme are given in Box 1.6.

Key features of the foundation programme are set out below.

- Doctors in the programme will take responsibility for their own learning and take advantage of all the learning opportunities presented within the day-to-day work of each attachment.
- Competence and performance will be objectively assessed throughout the programme.
- The programme will instil in doctors the need for continuous professional development and lifelong learning.
- Successful completion of the first year of the foundation programme will fulfil the criteria for full registration with the GMC.
- Successful completion of the second year of the foundation programme will indicate that the doctor is professionally accountable for patient safety and ready to start a programme of further specialist training.

The foundation programme will enable medical graduates to:

- consolidate and develop their clinical skills, particularly with respect to acute medicine, enabling them to reliably identify and manage patients in whatever setting they present
- embed modern professional attitudes and behaviours in every aspect of clinical practice

---

Box 1.6 Aims, objectives and outcomes of the foundation programme in psychiatry

Aims
- To produce doctors with the knowledge and competency to treat common psychiatric conditions

Objectives
- To identify mechanisms underlying an exemplar condition, e.g. depression
- To develop skills in history-taking and mental state examination for an exemplar condition, e.g. depression

Intended learning outcomes
- To attain and utilise knowledge and skills required to treat common psychiatric conditions
- To identify and summarise mechanisms underlying an exemplar condition, e.g. depression
- To acquire and demonstrate skills in history-taking and mental state examination for an exemplar condition, e.g. depression

- demonstrate the acquisition of competence in these areas through a reliable and robust system of assessment
- explore a range of career opportunities in different settings and areas of medicine.

The curriculum puts quality of care and patient safety at the centre of clinical practice. The learning environment for the foundation programme will be:

- trainee-centred
- competency-assessed
- service-based
- quality-assured
- flexible
- coached
- structured and streamlined.

All foundation training will be delivered within a foundation training programme led by a foundation training programme director/tutor. There will be three types of appointments into foundation training programmes:

- 2-year appointment to encompass F1 and F2 training
- 1-year appointment to F1 (first year of foundation training)
- 1-year appointment to F2 (second year of foundation training).

Postgraduate deaneries

The postgraduate deaneries have operational responsibility and accountability for ensuring that the foundation programme is delivered to the national standards set by the GMC and the PMETB. The deaneries will need to ensure that there is an effective educational infrastructure to support the development of the foundation training programme by establishing foundation schools, which are responsible for the operational aspects of delivering the programme (see Fig. 1.1). This won't apply to all, as several deaneries have established Schools of Psychiatry and appointed Heads of these Schools in conjunction with the Royal College of Psychiatrists.

Foundation schools operate under the auspices of the postgraduate deans who will develop, in conjunction with the university and medical school/s in the deanery, the educational framework. In addition, close working with provider organisations will be essential to develop and maintain such supportive environments. Overall accountability for the quality of training delivered through the school will rest with the university and the postgraduate dean, with particular responsibility for the F1 year falling to the university.

Quality assurance for foundation training will be through a joint approach to be established by the GMC and the PMETB, which will quality assure the foundation training programme overseen by the deaneries. The deaneries will quality control the delivery of foundation training through the monitoring of educational contracts with NHS employers.

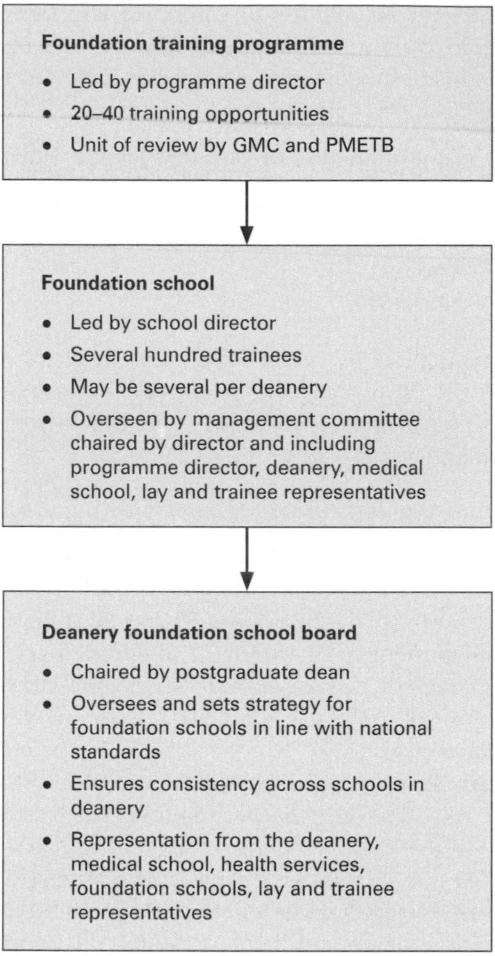

Fig. 1.1 Proposed delivery of the foundation training programme. GMC, General Medical Council; PMETB, Postgraduate Medical Education and Training Board.

Foundation schools will support no more than 20–40 combined F1 and F2 training opportunities (posts) providing foundation training, and normally one programme director/tutor will look after 20-40 posts and the trainees in them.

Deaneries may establish a foundation school management committee or school board, comprising the postgraduate deans, the directors of postgraduate general practice education, the dean of each medical school linked to a foundation school, the directors of each of the foundation schools, an NHS chief executive from each school, a lay representative, a trainee representative from each school, and others as deemed necessary locally. At each level sufficient administrative and infrastructure support must be available to allow training and education to progress smoothly.

Trainees will follow an individual foundation programme. It is possible for deaneries and training programme directors to look at the number of SHO posts and covert some into FY2 posts. As the unified training grade implies a columnar approach (with 5–10% attrition) rather than the current pyramid, it should be possible to 'shave off' some of the SHO numbers to convert them into FY2 posts; 33% of SHO posts in Scotland have been successfully converted to FY2 posts.

Specialist training

A unified training grade has been recommended as the way forward. The trainees for specialist training are being appointed for a 6-year rotation within which the current training plan will broadly remain in place (Fig. 1.2). The current three basic specialist training years will remain the same and the assessments for MRCPsych examinations will remain roughly at the same times.

The MRCPsych part I examination will be taken after at least 1 year of training and part II after 20 or 36 months. As PMETB is approving training schemes, the eligibility criteria for the examinations will have to change. The Royal College of Psychiatrists is exploring the possibility of offering MRCPsych examinations overseas. Further information is available from the College website (http://www.rcpsych.ac.uk/training.aspx).

The unified training grade will be called specialist training (StR) and the years of specialist training will be ST1–ST6. The first year of specialist training will have 6 months of general adult psychiatry and 6 months of old age psychiatry or rehabilitation psychiatry. In the first 3 years, 6 months of developmental psychiatry will be mandatory. From day one, specialist trainees will take on patients for 'long-term' psychotherapy and over the 6-year period they will be expected to treat at least two patients using 'long-term' psychotherapy, others using cognitive–behavioural therapy and two using behaviour therapy. They will be expected to be 'selected' into sub-specialty training at the end of 3 years. The entry criteria for specialty selection need to be confirmed but will be influenced by the criteria established by PMETB.

European Working Time Directive

The European Working Time Directive (EWTD) is the health and safety legislation adopted by the European Commission in May 2000. From August 2004 the NHS has been required to ensure that their employment of junior doctors adheres to EWTD legislation. The key points of the directive are that workers must have an 11-hour rest in every 24 hours – or a minimum 20 min break when their shift exceeds 6 hours – a minimum 24-hour rest in every 7 days, a minimum 48-hour rest in every 14 days, a minimum of 4 weeks' annual leave and a maximum of 8 hours work in every 24 hours for night workers.

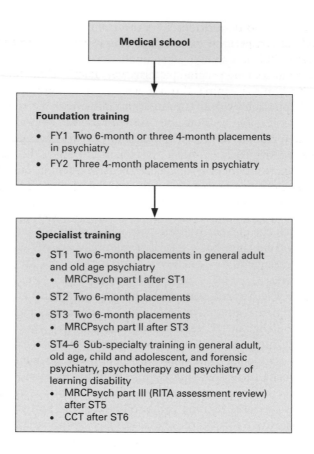

Fig. 1.2 Proposed training for psychiatrists after leaving medical school. RITA, record of in-training assessment; CCT, certificate of completion of training.

In some deaneries, trainees are being offered 4-month placements although Tooke (2007) in his interim report recommends 6-month placements.

Changes in service delivery will influence education and training. In addition, continuity of care and experience of long-term care may become difficult to achieve. Other problems that may emerge as a result of implementation of the EWTD include difficulties with regular educational supervision, with the likelihood of it changing its format. In addition to the EWTD, the subdivision of adult community psychiatry into home treatment, assertive outreach, crisis resolution and other teams will make delivery of educational supervision much more difficult and irregular. Sessions devoted to sub-specialty training will also have to undergo a change. The EWTD is also likely to affect acting up or acting down, in that emergency or routine cover may need to be provided by a team of doctors with varying grades and levels of competence, rather than doctors simply performing a set of preordained duties.

The introduction of new shift patterns will radically alter the opportunities for teaching and learning through face-to-face contact. The focus in training has to shift to self-directed learning where the trainees take on the responsibility for their training and optimisation of the limited contact between trainers and trainees. The trainee logbook will become an important component of overall assessment. The teaching will have three components: patient-based (ward rounds, topic-based bedside teaching, outpatient-based, case conferences, psychotherapy, audit and clinical governance); classroom-based (web-based learning, didactic teaching, journal clubs); and learner-based (educational supervision directly or indirectly using web-based methods, formal and informal study).

Patient-based learning activity will be systematic with emphasis on patient problem-based learning. The learning will not necessarily be apprenticeship, and formal documentation such as a logbook or portfolio of competencies achieved will be the core of future assessments. Individual patient encounters, on wards or in out-patient departments, will be assessed using direct observation and video links with reflective analysis as well as problem-based learning.

Classroom-based activities of the kind currently used in MRCPsych courses will change. The EWTD means trainees will miss many classroom-based teaching sessions because of rest or work requirements. Although an arbitrary figure of 75–80% attendance has been used by many courses to date, this is likely to decrease under the EWTD. The trainees will have to build upon their experience and record it individually or in a group. They will complete their logbook against their agreed learning plan and the logbook will be assessed and monitored at trainee appraisals and by educational supervisors. The Royal College of Psychiatrists may choose to randomly audit these logbooks.

Learner-based training will be self-directed and the trainees will keep their logbooks along with web-based learning. They may choose to record details of supervision, papers read, journals and book reports, distance learning, etc.

Educational supervision may need to follow the foundation year 2 (FY2) structure where one educational supervisor is responsible for a number of trainees and a distinction is made between clinical and educational supervisors. In addition, the educational supervisors will have dedicated programmed activity in their job plan agreed by the employing trust. It is expected that each educational supervisor will have between 8 and 10 trainees. The educational supervisor will not necessarily supervise all of them at the same time but will facilitate and provide supervision for a longer period. The clinical supervisor will continue to provide supervision in clinical settings. Educational supervision may occur through electronic means using email, web cam, video conferencing, etc.

Clinical experiences in sub-specialty training such as psychotherapy will have to be planned well in advance, and the trainees have to demonstrate in workplace-based assessment that they have acquired competencies as required and at the right stage during their training.

Workplace-based assessments

Many of the anticipated improvements in psychiatric training will be in the area of assessment, and the positive influence of PMETB on the curriculum in general and assessment in particular are already becoming evident. For example, all assessment systems must satisfy PMETB's *Principles for an Assessment System for Postgraduate Medical Training* (PMETB, 2004). Furthermore, the future design of assessment systems should ensure that the assessments are fit for purpose, and part of a coherent assessment strategy that also fulfils the requirements of *Good Medical Practice* (General Medical Council, 2001), the NHS appraisal for doctors in training framework (http://www.dh.gov.uk) and revalidation. An important aspect of 'fit for purpose' is to avoid unnecessary assessments – those that either duplicate other assessments or that are made too frequently to be of value.

The PMETB proposes an overarching assessment strategy consisting of workplace-based assessment and examinations of knowledge and clinical skills. It is recommended that this assessment strategy relates to the entire training period and that this is mapped to a blueprint. The balance between workplace-based assessment and formal examinations, and the methods used in each, is likely to vary from specialty to specialty and to alter over time.

A recent trend in medical education is to soften the distinction between formative and summative assessment. Formative assessment is typically undertaken to provide feedback to the doctor in training and their educational supervisor about progress and potential difficulties, but without contributing in any way to pass/fail decisions. Summative assessment, on the other hand, is traditionally concerned only with formal testing of attainment and forms the very basis of pass/fail decisions. Keeping the two quite separate has been useful in the past to both curriculum and test developers. The distinction still exists today, but is much softer and should always be in the trainee's favour. This is because the emphasis is moving rapidly away from gaining a certain number of marks in high-stakes examinations and far more towards gathering evidence of clinical competence and appropriate professional behaviour and attitudes. Much of this evidence cannot be captured in the kind of formal examinations that have traditionally been the primary focus in postgraduate training. It is demonstrated, day in, day out, in the workplace and is seen by educational supervisors, other team members, fellow healthcare workers, patients and their relatives and carers. Since it is both demonstrated and observed in the workplace, then it stands to reason that the workplace is where the evidence can be gathered. This is why workplace-based assessment will become increasingly important over the next few years.

From an educational perspective, there is good sense in developing workplace-based assessments given the contemporary view that assessment should be an integral part of educational planning in which teaching, learning and assessment are closely integrated. Furthermore, workplace-based assessment has the advantage of offering high validity, because of the authenticity of assessing performance in the workplace rather than by simulation or in the examination hall. For example, Jolly *et al* (1997: p. 232) noted that

'to achieve valid assessments of clinical competence it is plain that more use will have to be made of "real life" events and practice'.

We have long known that assessment is a potent driver for learning (Entwhistle, 1981; Newble & Jaeger, 1983; Stillman & Swanson, 1987; van der Vleuten *et al*, 1997). Indeed, 'assessment of attainment can prove to be the most powerful factor in the entire curriculum' (Holsgrove, 1997*a*: p. 181) and it commands a place of its own in consequential validity (e.g. Holsgrove, 1997*b*: p. 185), which is the aspect of validity that is concerned with the effect that assessment has on what and how students learn. It is therefore imperative that assessment focuses on what is considered important rather than what appears to be easiest to assess. Not only will this support appropriate learning but it is also essential given the increasing requirement for public reassurance that doctors are safe and competent. Therefore, in order to seek assurance that doctors are performing well, or to identify under-performing doctors, the focus of their professional development and its assessment must be based upon what they actually do in the workplace.

The assessments in the foundation programme will include multi-source feedback (including the Mini-Peer Assessment Tool), the Mini-Clinical Evaluation Exercise (mini-CEX), direct observation of procedural skills (DOPS) and case-based discussion. Trainees will keep a foundation learning portfolio, which will include personal development plans, self-appraisal tools, records of structured meetings and review forms. The reviews will occur at the mid-point and end of placement. An educational agreement will be signed between the trainee and the educational supervisor. The trainees will monitor their own reflective practice by evaluating learning experiences and untoward incidents. The trainees will also be required to provide information on their probity and health within the context of portfolio assessments.

Workplace-based assessments provide an excellent opportunity to ensure that teaching, learning and assessment are fully integrated and appropriate to the needs of the learner. They should ensure learning and professional development are monitored and supported by the systematic collection of evidence, with the assessment activity occurring mainly in the workplace. Procedures for triangulation of evidence and moderation of the summative judgments made, along with other means for quality assurance, must be properly planned, robust, explicit and publicly available. The requirements of PMETB will inevitably lead to significant developments in practice, both in the workplace and in the College examinations.

Postscript

Since this chapter was originally written in 2006, further developments have occurred. The selection process using the Medical Training Application Service (MTAS) had major problems that left nearly a quarter of applicants feeling suicidal (Lydall & Bhugra, 2007). Following this fiasco, an inquiry into MTAS was carried out and the government also established an independent inquiry chaired by Sir John Tooke, whose interim report *Aspiring to Excellence* has recently been published (Tooke, 2007). Among a total of 45 interim recommendations are the following: the decoupling of FY2 from FY1 and including it with families of specialties in core specialist training; the merger of PMETB into the GMC; an increase in the period of GP training to 5 years; a careful assessment of the role of the doctor; the linking of deaneries with local medical schools; harmonisation of FY1 with Year 5 in medical schools; making medical directors responsible for delivery of training; and establishing a Director of Training at the Department of Health. We wait for the government to announce which, if any, of these recommendations will be accepted and what the timescale will be for implementing them.

References

Academy of Medical Royal Colleges (1996) recommendations for Training Senior House Officers. Academy of Medical Royal Colleges.

Conference of Postgraduate Medical Deans (1995) *SHO Training: Tackling the Issues, Raising the Standards*. Conference of Postgraduate Medical Deans.

Department of Health (2000) *The NHS Plan: A Plan for Investment, A Plan for Reform*. Department of Health.

Department of Health (2002) *Unfinished Business: Proposals for Reform of the Senior House Officer Grade – A Paper for Consultation*. Department of Health.

Department of Health (2003) *Unfinished Business: Proposals for Reform of the Senior House Officer Grade: Consultation Outcome*. Department of Health.

Department of Health (2004) *Modernising Medical Careers*. Department of Health.

Entwistle, N. (1981) *Styles of Learning and Teaching*. John Wiley & Sons.

General Medical Council (1993) *Tomorrow's Doctors*. GMC.

General Medical Council (1998) *The Early Years – Recommendations for Senior House Officer Training*. GMC.

General Medical Council (2001) *Good Medical Practice*. GMC.

Holsgrove, G. (1997a) The purpose of assessing medical students. In *Teaching Medicine in the Community: A Guide for Undergraduate Education* (eds C. Whitehouse, M. Roland & P. Campion). Oxford University Press.

Holsgrove, G. (1997b) Principles of assessment. In *Teaching Medicine in the Community: A Guide for Undergraduate Education* (eds C. Whitehouse, M. Roland & P. Campion). Oxford University Press.

Hope, R. (2004) *The Ten Essential Shared Capabilities – A Framework for the Whole of the Mental Health Workforce*. Department of Health.

Jolly, B., Wakeford, R. & Newble, D. (1997) Requirements for action and research certification and recertification. In *Certification and Recertification of Doctors: Issues in the Assessment of Clinical Competence* (eds D. Newble, B. Jolly & R. Wakeford). Cambridge University Press.

Lydall, G. J. & Bhugra, D. (2007) MTAS – 'mental health of applicants seems to be deteriorating'. *BMJ*, **334**, 1335.

Newble, D. & Jaeger, K. (1983) The effect of assessment and examinations on the learning of medical students. *Medical Education*, **17**, 165–171.

Postgraduate Medical Education and Training Board (2004) *Principles for an Assessment System for Postgraduate Medical Training*. PMETB.

Royal College of Psychiatrists (2004) *Good Psychiatric Practice* (2nd edn) (College Report CR125). Royal College of Psychiatrists.

Stillman, P. & Swanson, D. (1987) Ensuring the clinical competence of medical school graduates through standardized patients. *Archives of Internal Medicine*, **147**, 1049–1052.

Tooke, J. (2007) *Aspiring to Excellence: Findings and Recommendations of the Independent Inquiry into Modernising Medical Careers*. MMC Inquiry.

van der Vleuten, C. P. M., Newble, D., Case, S., *et al* (1997) Methods of assessment in certification. In *Certification and Recertification of Doctors: Issues in the Assessment of Clinical Competence* (eds D. Newble, B. Jolly & R. Wakeford). Cambridge University Press.

Walton, H. J. (1986) *Education and Training in Psychiatry*. King Edward's Hospital Fund.

Part 1

CHAPTER 2

Global healthcare systems

Dinesh Bhugra and Shekhar Saxena

Healthcare systems in societies are influenced by a number of factors. Cultures in themselves are complex sets of shared mores, beliefs and norms among which individuals are born and brought up. The gaining of cultural values is incipient and individuals pick up cultural traits subconsciously. These are also communicated across generations and are acquired from institutions such as schools and universities, from peers and colleagues, and also from the media. Individuals acquire characteristics of culture without conscious learning, and it is the culture which allows individuals to develop methods of dealing with stress and distress. Cultures also empower individuals to cope with stressors, whereas the cultural values dictate what is normal and what is deviance. This also means that the culture and the society decide which condition should be treated and where it should be treated. As a result, cultures dictate what resources are made available, who gets these resources and how these are utilised. In addition, cultures determine what pathways individuals follow for their help-seeking and at what step of the pathways alternative therapies are chosen and utilised.

Healthcare systems

In many cultures more than one healthcare system coexists. Patients and their carers often choose a certain healthcare system because of their previous experience with that particular system, because someone with the same condition recommends it, or becasue other systems have failed to alleviate their distress. The patients bring to their clinicians a series of complaints which are their formulations in their own words and 'experiences of dissolved changes in states of being and in social function' (Eisenberg, 1977). These social functions are worth bearing in mind because they include the patients' ability to deal with social obligations. Help-seeking might reflect a need for social support or might have secondary gain reflected in the release (however temporary) from social obligations and other social processes which may or may not be directly related to the illness or symptom (Mechanic, 1975). Therefore, presentation to the doctor with physical symptoms (which may reflect underlying psychological distress) starts to make sense.

There is no doubt that different cultures see the role of the doctor in different ways. Patients may seek help from structured statutory healthcare if they believe that to be the right source or they may choose to take treatment in the personal or folk sector. Between 70 and 90% of all illness episodes in the USA are said to be managed within the popular sector (individual–family–social axis) according to Kleinman (1980). An additional factor highlighted by Kleinman (1980) based on Eisenberg's (1977) definitions is the distinction between disease and illness. Disease refers to a malfunctioning of the biological and/or psychological processes, whereas illness is the psychosocial experience and the perceived meaning of disease to the individual. Carers of course play a role in this. Kleinman (1980) points out that illness is a secondary, personal and social response to primary malfunctioning (disease) in the individual's physiological or psychological status (or both). Illness involves perception of and attention to symptoms, along with affective and cognitive responses directed at the disease and malfunctions resulting from it (Kleinman, 1980).

The disease affects individuals but illness affects others as well. Patients suffer from illnesses but doctors diagnose and treat diseases (Eisenberg, 1977). Thus illness can be construed as shaping of the disease into behaviour and experience. Helman (1990) argued that most cultures maintain a wide range of social norms which are considered appropriate according to age, gender, occupation, social rank and cultural minorities within the society. Thus every society has a spectrum extending between perceived normal and abnormal behaviour. It is important to bear this distinction in mind because epidemiological data which are based on disease for purposes of service development and provision will carry a different value. Moreover, cultural mores and values also have a role to play in terms of resources and models of healthcare delivery.

Global models

In various countries the model of healthcare delivery, including delivery of mental healthcare, depends upon existing healthcare policies, type of funding and political will. The World Health Organization (WHO) put forward a model for performance of national health systems in 2000 (World Health Organization, 2000). This identified three overall goals – good health, responsiveness to the expectations of populations and fairness of financial contribution. The model also identified four functions of health systems – service provision, resource generation, financing and stewardship. It should be noted that responsiveness to the expectations of populations, determined in part by their cultural belief systems, constitutes an important goal for a healthcare system that is performing well.

Box 2.1 Six domains considered to be essential components of a mental health system

- Policy and legislative framework
- Mental health services
- Mental health in primary healthcare
- Human resources
- Public education and links with other sectors
- Monitoring and research

Mental healthcare

The mental health system is defined as all the activities whose primary purpose is to promote, restore or maintain mental health. The mental health system includes all organisations and resources focused on improving mental health (World Health Organization, 2005a). The six domains considered to be essential components of a mental health system are given in Box 2.1.

A recent publication by the WHO (*Mental Health Atlas;* World Health Organization, 2005b) gives a detailed picture of the state of mental health in various nations around the world. Mental health policy, defined as a specific document written by the government or ministry of health detailing and prioritising the goals for improving national mental health and the main directions for attaining them, was available for between 48 and 72.7% of countries. More than half (53.5%) had initially formulated their mental health policy only in the last decade of the past century.

The components of mental health policy described in the *Mental Health Atlas* (p. 14) are shown in Box 2.2. These are advocacy, promotion, prevention, treatment and rehabilitation.

Box 2.2 Components of mental health policy according to the *Mental Health Atlas* (World Health Organization, 2005b)

- Advocacy: to raise awareness and gain political commitment, policy support, social acceptance and health support systems for mental health goals
- Promotion: enabling people to gain control over the determinants of their mental well-being and to improve it
- Prevention: organising activities in the community to prevent the occurrence of and progression of mental disorders
- Treatment: relevant clinical and non-clinical care aimed at reducing the impact of mental disorders and improving the quality of life of patients
- Rehabilitation: care given to people with mental illness to help them achieve their optimum level of social and psychological functioning

When one studies the details of existing mental health policies in different countries, it becomes clear that treatment issues take precedence over reduction of stigma, promotion of mental health and patient advocacy. However, the *Atlas* also noted (p. 15) that there was a significant association between the presence of mental health policy and a substance misuse policy, a national mental health programme, disability benefits, primary care training and community care facilities.

A national mental health programme is defined as a national plan of action that includes the broad and specific lines of action required in all sectors to give effect to this policy (*Mental Health Atlas*: p. 16). The programme describes and organises action aimed at the achievement of the objectives. It also indicates what is to be done, whose responsibility it is and the time frame and identified resources. Surprisingly, only 52.9% of countries in Europe have a national mental health programme compared with 90.9% of countries in the Eastern Mediterranean region. Again, more than half of countries formulated this plan only in the last decade of the past century. In community care, Europe is ahead of all other regions, with 79.2% of countries having a national mental health programme for community care; the lowest proportion (50%) was reported from South-East Asia. High-income countries had the highest proportion of community care facilities.

The lowest proportion of countries with mental health legislation in place (13.9%) was reported from the Western Pacific region and the highest (91.8%) from Europe. Again, most countries had developed their mental health legislation within the 1990s. Disability benefits were reported by all countries in Europe but only 45.5% in Africa. The availability of disability benefits was related to the income of the country. Most countries (83.9%) had a therapeutic drug policy or a list of essential drugs; this was developed in 61% of countries in the 1990s.

A specified budget for mental health (a proportion of a country's budget allocated for the achievement of mental health objectives) was reported to be available for 90% of the countries in South-East Asia but only 59.3% of countries in the Western Pacific.

Methods of financing mental healthcare are many and range from out-of-pocket payment, tax-based funding, social insurance, private insurance and external grants. Of the 180 countries in the *Mental Health Atlas* (p. 27) out-of-pocket payment was most common in Africa (38.6%) followed by South-East Asia (30%). In no country in Europe was this method the most common. Tax-based payments were reported from 54.5% of countries in Africa, 74.2% in the Americas, 68.4% in the Eastern Mediterranean, 55.1% in Europe and 70.4% in the Western Pacific. Out-of-pocket payment is the most important method for financing mental healthcare in 17.8% of countries worldwide (World Health Organization, 2005b). In 62.8% of countries the most important method is tax-based payment, in 14.4% of countries social insurance is the most important method, with private insurance in 1.7% of countries. There are variations across countries and interested readers should look for these in the *Atlas*.

Worldwide, 87.3% of countries provide basic preventive and curative mental healthcare often by the non specialist. High- and middle-income countries all have mental healthcare in primary care settings, but this is available in only 76.3% of low-income countries. Mental health training for primary care varies from a low of 27.3% in the Americas to 90% in South-East Asia. Rather intriguingly, only 55.9% of high- and middle-income countries offer training.

The median number of beds for mental illness per 10000 population varies from 0.33 in South-East Asia to 8.00 in Europe; the highest proportion in general hospital settings is 34.5% in the Western Pacific and the lowest 8.8% in the Eastern Mediterranean region. The median number of psychiatrists per 100000 population varies form 0.04 in Africa to 9.80 in Europe; the number worldwide is 1.20. Not surprisingly the lowest number of psychiatrists is 0.05 per 100000 in low-income countries and the highest 10.50 per 100000 in high-income countries. The median number of psychiatric nurses per 100000 population is roughly similar, with the lowest in Africa and the highest in Europe (0.16 in low-income countries and 32.95 in high-income countries). A similar picture emerges for psychologists and social workers working in the mental health field (with 0.05 in Africa and 3.10 in Europe for psychologists and 0.05 in Africa and 1.50 in Europe for social workers).

Compared with the earlier data from 2001 (World Health Organization, 2005*b*), there had been an increase in the number of mental health professionals worldwide, especially psychologists, although the number of psychiatric beds went down in some parts of the world. There had also been an increase in primary mental healthcare. However, the overall improvements in the availability of mental health resources worldwide have been very small. Regional imbalances have remained largely similar, especially across the high- and low-income countries.

Conclusions

This necessarily brief overview indicates that cultures and societies define, dictate and describe idioms of distress and indicate pathways people use. The allocation of resources for healthcare delivery and for training is also determined by the prevalent political, social and economic climate, as the figures from the *Mental Health Atlas* show. There is a need to enhance the resources earmarked for mental health and also to make their use more efficient and better suited to the expectations of the populations. It is important that mental health practitioners are aware of the system in which they are working so that appropriate use can be made of resources.

References

Eisenberg, L. (1977) Disease and illness: distinctions between professional and popular ideas of sickness. *Culture, Medicine and Psychiatry*, 1, 9–23.

Helman, C. (1990) *Culture, Health and Illness* (2nd edn). John Wright.

Kleinman, A. (1980) *Patients and Healers in the Context of Culture*. University of California Press.

Mechanic, D. (1975) Sociocultural and sociopsychological factors affecting personal response to psychological disorder. *Journal of Health and Social Behaviour*, 16, 393–404.

World Health Organization (2000) *World Health Report. Health Systems: Improving Performance.* WHO.

World Health Organization (2005a) *World Health Organization Assessment Instrument for Mental Health Systems*. WHO (http://www.who.int/mental_health/evidence/WHO-AIMS/en/index.html).

World Health Organization (2005b) *World Mental Health Atlas*. WHO (http://www.who.int/mental_health/evidence/atlas).

CHAPTER 3

History and structure of the National Health Service[†]

Ross Overshott, Alistair Burns and Dinesh Bhugra

It is perhaps important for everyone working in the National Health Service (NHS) to have some idea of the origins, development and current structure of what is one of the biggest and most complicated organisations in the world. A detailed analysis of the NHS and its history is beyond the scope of this chapter; suggestions for further reading are given at the end. The purpose of the chapter is instead to outline briefly how the NHS has evolved and to put into perspective the changes it was undergoing in 2006. For more recent developments the Department of Health's website (http://www. dh.gov.uk) should be consulted.

Healthcare before the NHS

Until the middle of the 19th century, the state had virtually no control over the medical profession. Doctors had developed their own organisational structure which satisfied the need for self-regulation. Members of the Royal College of Physicians mainly worked in the London teaching hospitals and treated those who could afford their fees. Members of the Royal College of Surgeons (which had been the Company of Barbers a century before) were more experienced in the practice of medicine and treated patients both in London (in competition with the physicians) and outside. The vast majority of people were treated by members of the Society of Apothecaries, who basically prescribed medication. For a considerable period of time churches provided forms of treatment to people with mental illnesses.

The state became more involved in the health of the population and regulation of the medical profession throughout the 19th and early 20th centuries. The 1834 Poor Law was an early acknowledgement that government had some responsibility for the care of the population. Among its effects were the statutory provision of a parish medical officer to care for

---

[†]This chapter has been previously published as Chapter 1 of Bhugra *et al* (2007).

the poor and the establishment of parish workhouses with sick wards where able-bodied inmates could be treated when they became ill (Levitt, 1976). Free services were offered by boards of guardians to those who could pass a means test.

The Public Health Act 1848 established statutory powers that enabled a local medical officer of health (an official of the local authority) to cater for the health of the local population. Following the Poor Law reforms, the medical officers' responsibilities were extended to some Poor Law hospitals, which were considered to be providing healthcare rather than welfare. By the 1930s, their responsibilities included control of environmental hazards, infectious diseases, the school medical service and district nursing/midwifery services.

Local acts (e.g. in London and Liverpool) had proved the benefit of providing care for people suffering from infectious diseases and for those with mental illness or intellectual disability. The establishment of the General Medical Council under the Medical Act 1858 granted the profession self-regulation by establishing a basic qualification for doctors and instituting a register of qualified medical practitioners.

In the first half of the 20th century there were some important changes in the mode of delivery of healthcare and in the organisation of the medical profession (Stacey, 1988). The profession had gained prestige and status but lacked tools; these became available with the development of microbiology, which led to the establishment of a scientific basis for medicine.

The National Insurance Act 1911 was passed to ensure that workers were afforded some protection in the event of sickness. It involved compulsory contributions from the employee, employer and the state. The 1911 Act concerned mainly general practitioners (GPs) and the working classes; the middle and upper classes could afford their own care and the Act, which covered the cost of GP care and medication, did not include the cost of hospital care, nor did it cover workers' families. A lack of space does not allow us to look at the effects of gender and class on the establishment and delivery of public healthcare (see Navarro, 1978; Stacey, 1988).

Before 1911, only a small proportion (5 million) of working-class people could afford GP care; where it was available, it was generally through membership of friendly societies or other agencies, which set up 'sick clubs' as a form of low-cost health insurance. These offered their members and sometimes their dependants treatment through the engagement of GPs, via a committee. Around this period GPs were perhaps the least contented of the medical professions and were also the most vociferous (Stacey, 1988). They were unable to choose their patients under this system, and to be controlled by a committee of working men was 'not a pleasant matter for an educated gentleman' (*British Medical Journal*, 1875, p. 484). The 1911 Act immediately covered 15 million people and by the mid-1940s covered about 24 million (half the population).

However, the scheme established by the 1911 Act was inefficient. Local insurance committees (the forerunners of family practitioner committees) and approved societies (private insurance companies, friendly societies and trade unions, all of which tended to be confined to a particular occupation or location) formed the administrative agencies. The approved societies brought the system into disrepute. As they were not allowed to be profit making, money was purposefully wasted, for example by increasing the number of staff. They paid sickness benefit and were able to pay for specialist care only if there was a surplus at the end of a defined period, which was rare, especially in those occupations where morbidity was high and which caused the greatest drain on resources of an individual society. Those earning over the income limit were excluded. Needless to say, this limit had to be changed regularly, always against the wishes of the doctors, because of inflation.

Whereas before the 19th century treatment for most conditions was almost always offered at home, by the 20th century treatment was gradually being shifted to hospitals, in the public domain. A major consequence of the increasing influence of hospitals was a greater differentiation between general practitioners and hospital consultants under the 1911 Act (Honigsbaum, 1979). Increasing specialisation among consultants and the development of a hierarchy were two major factors that were to affect the running of the NHS subsequently. Non-clinical advances (e.g. in social services) contributed to the development of special skills and interest in specialties such as psychiatry (Stevens, 1966).

By the time the NHS was formed, in 1948, there were about 2800 hospitals in England and Wales (just over 1000 were voluntary hospitals and the rest were municipal hospitals). The voluntary hospitals ranged from the London teaching hospitals, staffed by consultant specialists, to non-teaching hospitals with little money, staffed by local doctors who combined general with hospital practice. About one-third of the voluntary hospitals were larger institutions, where the beds were controlled by consultant specialists, who were unpaid and who therefore relied on private practice to generate income. An appointment to such a hospital was regarded as a stimulus to the recruitment of such patients. This part of the hospital system was affected by the rise of specialism in the 19th century, as only very large centres were able to support all specialties.

Voluntary hospitals were run from money gleaned from endowments, donations, public appeals and some schemes whereby care from the hospital was guaranteed by means of a regular weekly payment. The municipal hospitals provided about 80% of the total number of beds. They consisted of a number of Poor Law hospitals (the former workhouse infirmaries, handed over to the local authorities when the Poor Law was reformed, and run by the local medical officers of health) and local infectious disease hospitals. Mental asylums (also under local control) accounted for half the total number of beds. Although some of the Poor Law infirmaries were of a standard equivalent to that of the voluntary hospitals, they were mainly concerned with the care of the elderly and chronically sick.

The hospital component of the health service was therefore unsatisfactory. Many of the hospitals were old and ill equipped; scant provision was made for the ordinary worker and there was relatively little available between private medicine and the Poor Law. There was inequality in the distribution of services and a financial crisis developed in the London teaching hospitals towards the end of the 1930s.

The Emergency Medical Service (EMS) was an important development in the hospital system. It was established in 1939 by the Ministry of Health to coordinate the response to the expected number of war casualties and to arrange supporting services. The EMS took over financial control of the hospitals (but not ownership), divided England and Wales into 12 regions, and categorised each hospital by its particular function. Many of the voluntary hospitals became second-line hospitals (outside the main centres of population) and specialists worked in them on a salaried basis.

It is interesting to note that by the time the NHS was formed, many hospital specialists had been paid on a sessional basis for a decade. Thus, the payment system was never a political issue in the same way that it was for GPs, who maintained their freedom of practice despite the introduction of the first scheme of National Health Insurance in 1911. It was the threat to this independence that was at the root of the GPs' suspicion of the introduction of the NHS. The EMS proved that the central administration of the hospital system could work and it was the forerunner of the NHS.

The formation of the NHS

According to Jaques (1978), a description of the general features of the NHS which need to be taken into account must take as a starting point the objective of providing the following services:

- clinics, school services, education and other services for the prevention and detection of disease
- physical treatment (medical and surgical intervention for physical and psychological illnesses and impairment)
- psychological treatment (for psychological disturbances and related physical symptoms)
- educational procedures and provision of aids to enable patients to use their abilities as fully as possible.

These features are often ignored by politicians.

The NHS provides an administrative structure by which healthcare can be properly organised and financed. The essence of the NHS is that it provides, free at the point of service, healthcare to anyone who needs it, regardless of their ability to pay. The idea of the NHS originated as far back as 1911. The originator of the Insurance Bill (the then Chancellor of the Exchequer, David Lloyd George) had the idea that the Act would eventually be extended to cover dependants, specialist care and, eventually, hospital care.

With the creation of the Ministry of Health in 1919, an attempt to extend the Act was made, embodied within the Dawson report of 1920 (named after its author, Lord Dawson, a leading physician of the day). The report recommended that preventive and curative medicine be combined, that hospital inefficiency be corrected by elected regional authorities (each of which would have a principal medical officer in administrative charge) and, in an effort to increase standards, that all general hospitals be brought into line with teaching hospitals. No mention was made of the funding of these health services, but the report specifically warned of the dangers of a salaried service, suggesting that this would 'discourage initiative, diminish the sense of responsibility and encourage mediocrity'. However, the necessary political commitment to respond positively to the Dawson proposals was absent, and it took the threat of war and the consequent creation of the EMS in 1939 to resurrect these principles.

Other reports supported the notion of change. In 1929, the British Medical Association (BMA) produced *Proposals for a General Medical Service for the Nation*, which suggested that everyone should have a GP of their choice, through whom specialist services would be available. In addition it emphasised that prevention and promotion of health were as important as the treatment of disease, and that close coordination of medical services should be promoted. The service would basically have been funded by extending the National Health Insurance Scheme.

The independent research institute Political and Economic Planning published a report in 1937 that criticised existing services for being disorganised (Political and Economic Planning Group, 1937). It also reported regional differences in infant mortality in the UK, the tendency of GP's to work where a private practice income was guaranteed rather than where there was real need, and the association between environmental conditions and ill health.

Sir William Beveridge produced his report on *Social Insurance and Allied Services* in 1942. As part of an attack on the 'five giants' impeding social progress (want, disease, ignorance, squalor and idleness), he suggested that the burden of the cost of a health service should be borne by everyone, as such a service would make the nation healthier, thereby saving on social security payments and increasing national efficiency. However, he missed the point that better health, if it leads to longer life, inevitably leads during that longer life to a greater use of services (Godber, 1975).

The wartime coalition government accepted the principle of a national health service and set about finding a formula which would be acceptable to the medical profession, politicians, the voluntary hospitals and local authorities. The Minister of Health, Ernest Brown, proposed that the service would be administered by local authorities (with voluntary hospitals retaining their independence) and that GPs would be paid a salary. The doctors effectively rejected these proposals and they were dropped when Sir Henry Willink succeeded Brown in late 1943.

In February 1944, the government published a White Paper on the NHS. The plan was to make local authorities responsible for health, directly so in the case of the municipal hospitals (as they already were) and via contractual arrangements in the case of the voluntary hospitals. Hospital doctors would be salaried and GPs would have the choice of a salaried service or capitation fees. The BMA held a postal ballot and doctors (especially GPs) came out strongly against the proposals. They were opposed to the idea of local authority control and to a scheme that would be available to all, free at the time of use, as this would restrict the scope for private practice. In contrast, among the general public there was widespread endorsement of the proposals, in particular of the fact that the services would be free at the time of use.

Before a Bill could be drafted on the basis of the White Paper, a Labour government came to power with Aneurin Bevan as the Minister of Health. Bevan took a much harder line, claiming that Willink had merely cobbled together conciliatory proposals to keep everyone happy. He objected to the political erosion of the supremacy of Parliament and made the point that one should consult, but not negotiate with, outside bodies such as the medical profession. He felt that the Minister of Health should have total control of the service. His Bill was put forward in spring 1946 and was opposed by both the Conservative opposition and the BMA. The former argued that the nationalisation of the hospitals and the loss of independence of GPs would discourage initiative, and would deprive the profession and voluntary hospitals of their freedom. However, experience with the EMS had shown that central control of hospitals could be a success. The reasons why the medical profession objected were more complex – restriction of individual freedom was one, but it is possible that they were fuelled by resentment over the Labour government's supposed attack on the middle classes (through social reform for which the middle classes thought they were paying), from which the medical profession generally drew its members. The government criticism of doctors spanned the spectrum, on the one hand, of doctors being guardians of vested interests and, on the other hand, of doctors waging a war on the government on behalf of their class.

Both Bevan and the BMA (an incredibly complex negotiating machine where its leaders had very little room to manoeuvre) stood firm. The deadlock was broken when Bevan introduced an amendment saying that he could not introduce a fully salaried service for GPs without further legislation. Leaders of the BMA (helped by the Royal Colleges) saw the chance to save face and accepted the new service. The BMA ordered a plebiscite of all its members (instead of a further meeting of the representative body, whose opposition might have become entrenched had the dispute been allowed to continue) and it was apparent that, although opposition was still strong, sufficient numbers of doctors would be employed in the new service to make it workable. Thus, on 5 July 1948, the NHS was born.

The principle of universalism which characterised welfare and health legislation in the post-war period is perhaps manifested most dramatically in the NHS (Stacey, 1988): to provide good healthcare to the whole population without a financial barrier was its original aim.

The Health Service in Scotland

The Scottish Health Service was created in May 1947, on the same tripartite principles (of hospital care, and primary and local authority health services) as that in England and Wales. The hospital and specialist services were administered by five regional hospital boards, with 65 boards of management. The community and environmental health services were provided by 55 local health authorities and family practitioner services were administered by 25 executive councils. The Secretary of State for Scotland was responsible for the whole of the NHS in Scotland (Levitt, 1976).

Under the National Health Service (Scotland) Act 1972 health boards were created for each area of Scotland to act as the single authority for administering the three branches of the former tripartite structure. Two new bodies – the Scottish Health Service Planning Council and the Common Services Agency – were created.

Developments to 1974

The NHS developed a tripartite structure as much because of vested interests as from an overall view that this structure was the most efficient. What the founders of the NHS thought they were doing and what in fact emerged are two distinct matters, for there were undoubtedly a number of unintended consequences (Stacey, 1988). Out of the negotiations leading up to the brave new world of 1948, the consultants overall, but especially those in teaching hospitals, did better than the GPs. The nurses did less well and the ancillary workers were not considered at all. The role and function of the multidisciplinary teams need to be addressed in the light of this historical development.

The hospital system was nationalised and taken away from local authorities (mainly as a result of the profession's unwillingness to work under local authority control). The Minister of Health was responsible for hospitals through hospital management committees (336 in number) and non-elected regional hospital boards (of which there were 16). Teaching hospitals retained their independent status (not wishing to 'come down' to the level of all voluntary hospitals) and were responsible through 36 boards of governors to the Minister, independent of the regional hospital boards. The Public Health Laboratory Service and the specialist hospitals were directly responsible to the Minister, although the Blood Transfusion Service remained under regional control.

General practice was unaffected by the changes and retained its independent status. The National Insurance Act 1911 was extended to cover the whole population, and general practice was controlled by 134 executive councils (the successors of the local insurance committees). The rest of the service was left to the 174 local authorities' medical officers of health, essentially because no other influential medical interest wanted them. These residual services comprised the maternity and child welfare services, health visitors, health education and prevention, the ambulance service and vaccination/immunisation services.

It is of particular importance that the readers of this book appreciate the relationship between the NHS and doctors: it has been argued that doctors are the single most important profession within the service. Changes in the shape of the NHS are impossible without a change in the relationship of power within the NHS (Heller, 1978). This is the dictum that various governments have followed to reduce the power of various factions. At the inception of the NHS, GPs retained their independent status and consultants and specialists became salaried employees of the state (although, as has been noted, the EMS had been employers since 1938). Aneurin Bevan stated that he saw the function of the Ministry of Health as providing the profession with all it needed to be used fully and without control to the benefit of patients. Consultants and specialists thus considered themselves on a par with GPs as being able to do as they wished, unworried by considerations of cost and administration. The fact that medical practitioners were on regional boards and not the hospital management committees (in charge of the day-to-day running of the hospitals) strengthened this stance.

The problem of what doctors should be paid was apparent soon after the creation of the NHS. Sir Will Spens chaired three committees dealing with the pay of GPs, consultants and specialists, and dentists. The committee on consultant's pay recommended that the salary for a consultant aged about 40 should be £2500, compared with £1300 for a GP of equivalent age (both 1939 prices). Consultants' pay before the NHS had such a wide range (from a consultant in a non-teaching voluntary hospital to one in a London teaching hospital with income from private practice) that a salary scale incorporating both ends of the spectrum was impractical. The distinction award scheme was introduced as a solution to this problem, with the top grade doubling a consultant's salary. The committee that reviewed the pay of specialists in training recommended that this should be substantially increased, to allow doctors in these grades to devote a larger part of their time to professional training without the need to do alternative work (such as teaching) to supplement their income. Much discontent still existed following the Spens committees and it took a royal commission into doctors' and dentists' pay (the Pilkington Commission) to recommend the establishment of an independent review body to advise the Prime Minister directly.

The problem of the numbers of junior doctors soon emerged. By 1950 there were 3800 registrars and senior registrars, and only double that number of consultant posts. There also existed the grade of senior hospital medical officer (devised at the inception of the NHS to employ those practitioners in hospital practice who were not of consultant calibre), many of whom were still in competition for consultant posts. The Ministry of Health attempted to force hospitals to terminate contracts of time-expired senior registrars (after three years in higher professional training), but following an outcry from the profession it was decided that their contracts could be renewed annually. The suggestion was made that consultant numbers be expanded, but this was rejected by the Ministry on the grounds of cost, and by existing consultants for fear of added competition for private patients. The result was a review by Henry Willink (the ex-Minister of Health in the wartime coalition government) of the numbers of doctors required in the UK. The recommendation was a 10% reduction in intake to the medical schools. However, the review did not take into account the numbers of doctors emigrating and the increased numbers required because of advances in medical technology; this led to a shortage of junior doctors in the 1960s, with the attendant influx of foreign graduates to fill posts in unpopular specialties, of which psychiatry was one.

The need for change

Almost as soon as the NHS was established, there was recognition that reorganisation was necessary. It was noted as early as 1952, by Dr Ffrangcon Roberts in *The Cost of Health* – see Watkin (1978) – that Sir William Beveridge was wrong in assuming that the demand for healthcare was limited. The aphorism of the NHS, 'infinite demand, finite resources', was born. A committee was set up under the chairmanship of the Cambridge economist C. W. Gillebaud with the remit of reviewing the cost of the NHS and to make recommendations for changes in administration that would make the service more efficient. The committee's conclusion was that the service was not wasteful and that a major change in organisation was unnecessary (although Sir John Maude, a former parliamentary under-secretary in the Ministry of Health, appended a personal recommendation that the three arms of the NHS be unified). The Porritt Committee, set up by the Royal Colleges and the BMA (all the members of which were doctors), also reported (in 1962) that unification of the three arms of the service was highly desirable. Thus, there was general recognition for the need to unify the tripartite structure to ensure comprehensive planning of the service and better coordination of community, GP and hospital components.

Inequalities in the distribution of resources both geographically and within medical specialties highlighted deficiencies in the system; these caused embarrassment to successive Ministers of Health because of scandals concerning ill treatment in mental and geriatric institutions. It is not that the NHS in 1948 was perfect in any sense. Klein (1989) argues it was as much a product of messy compromises as of inspired visions, and the same remains true today.

In 1968, the government published a Green Paper on reorganisation, the basic proposals being integration of all services under 50 area boards (each to have 16 members) with responsibility for all hospital, general medical and community health services. Objections raised included the remoteness of the regional boards to local services, the problem of the continued independence of GPs and the mismatch of the 50 area boards with proposed local government reorganisation that would result in 90 local government units.

Following the merger of the Ministry of Health and National Insurance in 1968, a second Green Paper emerged, this one under Richard Crossman, the new Secretary of State of the combined departments, which recommended the following: 14 regional health councils advising the Secretary of State on planning; 90 area health authorities (the word 'authority' having replaced 'board' without explanation) to coincide with the 90 local government districts and to set up subcommittees to be responsible for services; and 200 district committees with at least half the members working in the district. The functions of the service were to be divided between health and local government, based on the skill of the provider rather than the need of the user (e.g. all social workers were to be employed by local government, all nurses by the health service).

Developments from 1974 to 1989

In 1971, the Conservative government published a further document, the thrust of which was embodied in the NHS (Reorganisation) Act 1973. The reorganisation came into being on 1 April 1974, which coincided with the reorganisation of local government. The reformed service was to have two characteristics: it was to be an integrated service and there was to be responsibility upwards to managerial authority.

The reorganisation led to the formation of regional health authorities, which for the first time had the responsibility to plan all services. The reforms led to a 30% increase in the number of administrators and the influence of managers increased, as well as to the creation of a managerial hierarchy.

The doctors insisted on retaining clinical autonomy, and this was noted:

'The distinguishing characteristic of the NHS is that, to do their work properly, consultants and general practitioners must have clinical autonomy, so that they can be fully responsible for the treatment they prescribe for the patients.' (Department of Health and Social Security, 1972)

This notion of a one-to-one doctor–patient relationship has been challenged by Stacey (1988). The clinical autonomy and security of tenure for the consultant were seen as advantageous (Beeson, 1980).

However, the final document differed from the second Green Paper in that regional health authorities were in line management with the area health authorities, and 90 family practitioner committees (replacing the executive councils) were co-terminous with the local government areas. Community health councils became essentially watchdogs of the Health Service. There were also 'district' management teams under the 1974 organisation. Some regions had 'single district areas', but more commonly each area had several such teams. It was this duplication that the 1982 reforms sought to abolish. Representatives of the professions and public were slightly different, with restriction of local authority appointees and the chairs of the regional health authority being chosen for personal qualities rather than as representatives of any particular interest. There was emphasis on professional management, with regional and area health authorities responsible for policy and teams of officers responsible for implementation. A detailed analysis of the political and practical ramifications of the relationship between central and local government and their representation on the authorities is given by Forsyth (1982).

In Scotland, the reorganisation of local government created new local authorities. The Scottish Health Service then constituted nine regional authorities divided into 56 districts and three island councils, and their boundaries were closely followed by the health board boundaries (Levitt, 1976). The 15 health boards were concerned with major policy matters and the broad allocation of resources; authority to manage the service was delegated to four senior officers of the board.

In 1982, in response to criticism of excessive administration of the NHS and the implementation of the Resource Allocation Working Party (RAWP) to ensure a more equitable distribution of resources between geographical areas and specialties, the area health authorities were abolished and replaced with 190 district health authorities.

Readers are recommended to read the account by Draper *et al* (1976) on the influence of the 1974 reorganisation on the NHS.

The Conservative government also introduced general management of hospitals following the Griffiths report in 1983. Sir Roy Griffiths, a supermarket executive, had been commissioned to review the management of hospitals. He concluded that the traditional NHS management by senior consultants and administrators had led to 'institutionalised stagnation'. The report's recommendations, including that hospitals should be managed by general managers, were accepted and in the middle of the 1980s they took over the role of managing hospitals. This change in emphasis brought about a large increase in general or senior managers in the NHS, from 1000 in 1986 to 26000 in 1995, with spending on administration rising dramatically over the same period (Webster, 2002). This also resulted in a number of managers begin 'classified' into their primary professions, for example nursing, also indicating that a number of people from professions were being brought into management. There was also a new business/commercial culture in the NHS, which led to the policy in the 1980s of 'contracting out' or 'outsourcing'. The clinical work of the NHS was retained in the public sector, but, to reduce costs, support services such as laundry, cleaning and catering were contracted out to private providers. The number of non-clinical NHS employees had nearly halved by the end of 1980s. To ensure they made a profit the private companies paid the support staff less, while the quality of service reduced; in fact, the cleanliness of hospitals is still a major issue for the NHS over 20 years later.

Four themes emerge from the history of the NHS since 1983 (Klein, 2001). First, there was a sharp turn towards centralisation. This led to the second theme – that of managerialism and bureaucratic rationalisation. Third, the expansion of private medicine continued apace, along with the privatisation of ancillary services within the NHS. Fourth, there was increasing consumerism within the health sector. The increase in demand for NHS funding was accompanied by the development of healthcare as a public-policy issue. A consumer-led service was being emphasised rather than a professional-led care system (Davies, 1987). Klein (2001) further argues that the 'politicisation' of the NHS between 1974 and 1989 was also related to the shifting of accountability from local to central authorities.

A crisis in the NHS developed in the second half of 1987. Since 1979, resources for the NHS had been increased by the Conservative government, from £7.7 billion in 1979/80 to £18.35 billion in 1988/89. Despite this, the Service was not doing well. Although resources were increasing, demand was outstripping this. The increasing elderly population, advances in medical technology and priority objectives (e.g. kidney transplants) meant that services had to be increased by 2% per annum just to keep up.

To reduce costs and stave off a crisis, some services provided by the NHS were effectively privatised in the late 1980s. Resources for dentistry in the NHS were reduced and as dentists were, like GPs, mostly 'independent contractors' they stopped taking on NHS patients and worked increasingly in the private sector, where they could earn more money. (By 2006 NHS dentists had become so scarce that all over the country there were large queues in the high street when spaces became available for NHS care.) In 1989, routine eye examinations became free only for children and the elderly. It was argued by the government that people could now afford to pay for tests, but the new policy led to a major reduction in examinations. Long-term care from the NHS was also eliminated, which stimulated the growth of private nursing and residential homes throughout the 1990s. These measures were implemented to reduce costs in an attempt to avert the financial melt-down of the NHS. However, they compromised one of the founding principles of the NHS – to provide a comprehensive service.

Following the June 1987 election, when Margaret Thatcher was returned for a third term, a financial crisis began facing the health authorities. Beds began to close, charities began to shore up NHS operations, cancer patients were being denied operations and both the Institute of Health Service Management and the King's Fund announced their own independent reviews of NHS funding. Despite this, the government continued to publicise statistics about how much more was being spent on the NHS. The poor showing of the Minister, John Moore, who unfortunately became ill during this time, compounded the issue.

In early December 1987, the lack of heart operations on children in Birmingham was publicised and nurses at St Thomas' Hospital picketed the Houses of Parliament in their uniforms. Probably the most significant event, and certainly a historical one, was when the Presidents of the Royal Colleges of Surgeons, Physicians, and Obstetricians and Gynaecologists issued a joint statement suggesting that the NHS was almost at breaking point (Hoffenberg et al, 1987). The BMA supported the Presidents and added to the media clamour for increased resources. The government responded on 16 December by announcing an extra £100 million for the NHS, but despite this the crisis continued and more nurses began to strike.

The Prime Minister reassured the public that the NHS was in safe hands and was not about to be abolished. She, however, was also still advocating tax cuts to encourage private health insurance. It was generally accepted that a government review of the NHS was inevitable. It was not until Thatcher announced it in a BBC television *Panorama* programme on 25 January 1988 that it gathered momentum (many cynics believe that she was tricked into saying this and that the Department of Health did not know of this review until she announced it).

Developments from 1989 to 1997

The results of the government's review were initially announced in the publication of the White Paper *Working for Patients* (Department of Health, 1989) on 31 January 1989. A year later the NHS and Community Care Act followed. These two policy papers instigated what was at the time the most radical reform the NHS had undergone since its inception in 1948. The policies were criticised for lacking strategic planning and many were unhappy that there had been no consultation inside the NHS. The following three measures were perhaps the principal changes made by the Act.

- *Self-governing hospitals.* Stand-alone hospital trusts were established; these were separate from the health authority and were accountable directly to central government. They were to be managed by a board of directors with a chair appointed by the Secretary of the State for Health. The hospital trusts were able to contract out services and buy and sell assets, borrow capital, employ staff on local terms and advertise their services. The government's idea was to move decision making as near to patients as possible.
- *Fund-holding GPs.* Fund-holding GPs were created. They were given their own budget, to buy hospital services directly from source. The scheme was voluntary for GPs but provided financial incentives to encourage them to sign up. Initially only larger practices (i.e. with lists of at least 11 000) could apply to be fund-holders and their budgets covered just elective surgery, out-patient and diagnostic services, prescribing and staff costs.

- *The internal market*. The 'internal market' was advocated by the US Defense Department economist Alan Enthoven, who was highly thought of by the UK government. To create an internal market, the NHS was split into 'purchasers' – health authorities and fund-holding GPs – and 'providers' – hospital and community trusts and non-fund-holding GPs. It was envisaged that providers would compete with each other (though all still within the NHS) to secure contracts with purchasers by offering higher-quality, more responsive and efficient services.

Most attention and scrutiny focused on those three reforms but there were other significant changes at this time.

- *Funding and contracts for hospital services*. A new formula on a capitation (population-weighted) basis for purchasing services for a given population replaced the RAWP. The amount to be spent was to be determined on the basis of population, with adjustments made for cross-boundary referrals and allocations to budget-holding GP practices. It was hoped this would promote resource equity between regions and allow services to be developed to meet local needs.
- *Drug budgets*. Each GP practice now has to monitor its prescriptions closely.
- *Capital charges*. The intention is to stimulate fair competition between public and private healthcare by limiting the amount of capital the government effectively provides free to the public health sector.
- *Medical audit*. This was defined in *Working for Patients* as 'systematic, critical analysis involved in clinical care' so that 'the best quality of service is being achieved within the resources available'.
- *NHS consultants*. Job descriptions were to be reviewed annually; managers were given the right to sit on appointments committees; distinction awards were to be reviewed every 5 years and were not to be awarded less than 3 years before retirement; and progression to the higher awards was not limited to those with a 'C' award.
- *Implications for family practitioner committees*. New chief executives were to be appointed and were to be responsible for organising cash-limiting budgets for GPs and monitoring the cost of GP prescribing.

The internal market did not lead to the benefits the government thought it would produce. Hospitals could not truly compete with each other as the government could not, for political reasons, allow less competitive hospital trusts to go out of business, as would happen in the real commercial world. GP fund-holding was also an unpopular policy. A two-tier system was therefore created. Fund-holders' contracts with healthcare providers gave their patients quicker access to hospital services than patients from non-fund-holding practices. There were distinct advantages for patients whose GP belonged to a fund-holding practice (the 'haves') over patients whose GP was part of a non-fund-holding practice (the 'have-nots'). The reforms of 1989 severely compromised the premise of equity that the NHS had been founded on.

The Conservatives under John Major won the 1992 general election and continued to develop the internal market in the NHS. Many still feared privatisation, as part of the 1989 reforms allowed hospital trusts to raise income from other sources, such as private beds. The collectivist model of the NHS was being threatened, although the 1992 White Paper *The Health of the Nation* (Department of Health, 1992) appeared to address the government's responsibilities for the health of the country. The document moved towards health promotion and set out 25 specific policy targets, including reducing the suicide rate by 15%, as well as reducing the proportion of the population who were obese, smokers and heavy-drinkers. The White Paper was criticised for setting targets that were easily achievable and for failing to address the effect poverty, inequality and unemployment have on health. Kearney (1992) concluded that the policy had no strategy at all and was merely 'window dressing'.

The Patient's Charter (Department of Health, 1991) reinforced the consumerist model the government had been encouraging. The document explicitly set out patients' rights, some of which reflected the original philosophy of the NHS (e.g. 'to receive health on the basis of clinical needs, regardless of ability to pay'). Other standards were promised for patients, such as waiting no more than 2 years once placed on a waiting list and to be seen within 30 minutes of a specific out-patient appointment time. A performance guide was published in 1994 (Department of Health, 1994) and hospital trusts were rated (using a five-star system) on whether they had achieved its standards. This system gave the public information on how their local NHS services were performing. Despite being 'well informed consumers', patients had no true power to choose between different NHS providers, only to opt out of the NHS and to choose private services, which they would have to pay for.

The reforms of the 1990s moved the power base of the NHS away from hospitals and towards primary care. The advent of GP fund-holders altered the relationship between hospitals and GPs. The hospitals were now in effect answerable to the GPs and therefore in essence the patients. Community service providers were also encouraged to establish themselves as separate trusts from acute hospital services, which promoted community services over hospitals.

The multitude of reforms did not lead to an improvement in services, however, although GP fund-holding was a moderate success, as a relaxation of entry requirements had allowed approximately 50% of GPs to become fund-holding by 1996. Many, however, had joined under duress, as they felt they would be left behind if they did not become fund-holders. The cost of reorganisation (e.g. the purchaser/provider split) had been covered by two short increases of funding to the NHS in 1992/93 and 1994/95. The extra money was quickly absorbed and no benefits were seen to services. The government remained prudent but its belief that the NHS would become more efficient and save money if there were strict financial pressures was misguided.

Further reorganisation was implemented and by 1996 the regional health authorities had been abolished and replaced by eight regional offices of the NHS Executive. There were 425 NHS trusts, which acted as 'providers' of services, and 8500 GP fund-holders, who were 'purchasers'. In addition to fund-holders, there were still non-fund-holding GPs, under the management of 100 health authorities. This fragmentation of the NHS into purchasers and providers made it difficult for the NHS to plan and distribute resources on the basis of the population's health needs. Many NHS trusts were failing financially and waiting lists remained static. The NHS had lurched from reform to reform, nearing a crisis many times, to the extent that come the eve of the 1997 general election the *Sun* newspaper (4 May) told its readers that they had '24 hours to save the NHS'.

Developments since 1997

The Labour Party's general election victory in 1997 brought new hope to the NHS, which in many people's eyes had been in a permanent state of crisis for over 20 years. The public were ready for change and returned Tony Blair's party with a majority of 179 following the largest two-party swing since Clement Attlee's victory in 1945. This was, however, a very different Labour Party to the one that had overseen the genesis of the NHS. Eighteen years in opposition had forced it to instigate major policy reform. Traditional party beliefs in nationalisation, central planning and state paternalism, which had underlain the creation of the NHS, were abandoned. The new government adopted what was to be known as the 'third way', mixing notions of equality and social justice with privatisation and free-market competition (Blaine, 1998). The 'third way' of running the NHS was based on partnership and driven by performance, and has led to the period of biggest reform in its history.

The newly elected government was committed to keeping to the overall expenditure plans of the previous Conservative government for the first 2 years of its term. An extra £1.2 billion was, however, invested immediately into the NHS, and was just the beginning of increased resources for the service. Following the Wanless report (Wanless, 2002), which recognised that the NHS was and had for many years been under-funded, UK taxes were increased to finance extra NHS expenditure, which for the next 5 years averaged an increase of 7.4% a year in real terms. This was to raise total health spending in the UK from 6.8% of gross domestic product (GDP) in 1997 to an estimated 9.4% in 2007/08, which would make the UK one of the higher spenders on health in Europe (Stevens, 2004).

Extra investment in the NHS coincided with a programme of major reforms, which focused on reorganising services and raising standards of health and care. In 1997 the UK's first Minister for Public Health was appointed. Subsequently, the policy document *Our Healthier Nation* (Department of Health, 1998*a*) was published to replace *The Health of the*

Nation. The new policy set a national target of saving 300000 lives over the next decade, specifically focusing on cancers, coronary heart disease, stroke and mental illness. *Our Healthier Nation* shifted the focus away from the policies of the 1990s, which implied that individuals were responsible for improving their own health, and recognised that there needed to be a framework to empower individuals, as well as strategies to reduce inequality and poverty.

The first significant health reforms by the new Labour government were set out in the White Paper *The New NHS. Modern, Dependable* (Department of Health, 1997). Although the reforms were extensive, they were by no means radical. The paper proposed the dismantling of the internal market, but many components of it were maintained. The purchase/provider split remained, but the emphasis was on cooperative relationships rather than competition. GP fund-holding was abolished and instead all general practices were obliged to join a primary care group (PCG). Primary care groups covered populations that ranged in size from 30000 to 250000 and functioned both as providers of primary care and as purchasers of secondary care. They were led by GPs, although their boards also contained representation from community groups and the health authority. The PCGs were allowed to retain any surplus from their budget, which could be spent on services or facilities of benefit to patients. Although competition was disapproved of by the Labour government, purchasers (i.e. the PCGs) were still able to switch to other providers if they were dissatisfied with the services they received.

The 1997 White Paper also began to address quality and standards in the NHS and was expanded upon by *A First Class Service: Quality in the New NHS* (Department of Health, 1998b) a year later. Clinical governance, which was at the time seen as a radical idea, was introduced to the NHS and a statutory responsibility for the quality of care was placed upon trust and health authority chief executives. Hospital trusts and PCGs developed systems and committees to meet the clinical governance requirements of quality assurance, audit and risk management. There has been criticism that the implementation of clinical governance in the NHS was impeded by lack of time and resources, that is, that there was too much change, implemented too quickly and with a lack of clear guidance (Roland *et al*, 2001).

The government also set up two new national bodies: the National Institute for Clinical Excellence (NICE), which was renamed in 2004 the National Institute for Health and Clinical Excellence (while retaining the acronym unaltered), and the Council for Health Improvement, which evolved into the Commission for Health Improvement (CHI), in 2000. In 2002 CHI was replaced by the Commission for Health Audit and Inspection (CHAI), which combined its work with that previously done by the Audit Commission. The CHAI also had responsibility for regulation in private healthcare (e.g. private nursing homes and hospitals). The work of the CHAI was in turn taken over by the Healthcare Commission in 2004. In simple terms NICE was expected to set standards while the Council for Health Improvement enforced them.

NICE's aim to address the lack of national standards and resultant wide variations in quality of healthcare was at first very popular. There had been growing public concern over 'postcode prescribing', where the availability of effective treatments depended on where in the country the patient lived. NICE's assessment of the effectiveness of drugs and other medical technologies led to it recommending their use in virtually all cases. A large part of NICE's remit was to attempt to limit the growth of the NHS drug bill, but even when its experts asserted that the anti-viral drug zanamivir had little therapeutic benefit, they back-tracked on their original judgement and still recommended its use. The work of NICE remains controversial. In 2005, it was criticised for the speed of its evaluation of the cancer drug trastuzumab (Herceptin) and its withdrawing of support for anti-dementia drugs on cost-effectiveness grounds rather than purely on the grounds of their clinical effectiveness.

National Service Frameworks (NSFs) set out new standards for service delivery, emphasising effectiveness and outcomes. The first wave of NSFs included protocols for the management of cancer, coronary heart disease and mental health. The Council for Health Improvement instigated a rolling programme of reviews of every NHS trust (acute and primary care) every 3–4 years. Its objective was to review the clinical governance of trusts as well as their implementation of the NSFs and other guidance from NICE. CHI inspections proved truly effective only when discovering gross incompetence and negligence, as they had few solutions to offer still under-resourced trusts which were not meeting the performance standards (Day & Klein, 2002).

Other innovations to modernise the NHS and change the ways it had previously worked included NHS Direct and the National Programme for Information Technology (NPfIT). NHS Direct is a nurse-led 24-hour telephone advice service. Five years after its inception in 1998 it was handling over half a million calls a day; it expanded into an equally busy online service in 2001. The NPfIT is an ambitious project which originally aimed for NHS trusts to have electronic patient records in place by 2005 (NHS Executive, 1998). It has, however, been riddled with logistical and technical difficulties, and now aims for electronic patient records to be implemented in all acute trusts by the end of 2007 (Hendy *et al*, 2005).

The NHS Plan

The New NHS. Modern, Dependable (1997) was only the beginning of the reforms the Labour government intended for the NHS. In July 2000, its full programme to modernise the NHS was announced in *The NHS Plan* (Department of Health, 2000*a*), which described the government's vision for the NHS for the next 10 years. The Plan was enterprising, impressive in scope and in places daring. It concentrated on the areas of capacity, standards, delivery and partnership, but the central aim was to create a patient-led health service. It proposed an NHS that responded to the needs and preferences of patients, rather than their choice being prohibited by 'the system' or health professionals. The implementation of the NHS Plan coincided with an increase in spending on the NHS by 6.3% in real terms. Significant improvements were, however, expected for this investment:

- *More health professionals.* Over the 5-year period the extra money was expected to provide 7500 more hospital consultants (a rise of 30%), 1000 more special registrars, 2000 extra GPs and 450 more trainees. There would also be 1000 more medical school places each year, on top of the 1000 places that had been announced before the NHS Plan.
- *More hospitals and beds.* Provision was made in the Plan for 100 new hospitals over a 10-year period and 7000 more hospital and intermediate care beds.
- *National standards for waiting times.* By 2005, the maximum waiting time for out-patients was expected to be 3 months and 6 months for in-patients. No one should be waiting more than 4 hours in accident and emergency departments by 2004. It was also promised that all patients would be able to see a GP within 48 hours by 2004. Waiting lists for hospital appointments and admissions would be abolished by the end of 2005 and replaced with a booking system designed to give patients a choice of a convenient time.
- *Performance monitoring.* The performance of hospital trusts and primary care groups would be rated using a traffic light system by the CHI. 'Green light' organisations, the 'best performers', would receive funds from the National Performance Fund and be given more autonomy. A 'red light' rating would lead to intervention from government agencies and if necessary the installation of new management. (The traffic light system was later replaced by the equally loathed star rating system, where trusts were evaluated against performance standards such as finances and waiting lists and awarded up to three stars.)
- *Development of partnerships.* All hospitals would have a new patient and advocacy service. There would also be increased involvement and scrutiny of the NHS by local authorities.
- *Expansion of nursing roles.* To make up the shortfall of doctors, the NHS Plan also proposed training for around 20000 nurses, who would be able to prescribe a limited range of medicines.

The NHS Plan also promised to deliver an expanded NHS Direct and further national standards for more clinical specialties.

To implement the NHS Plan, the government set up the National Modernisation Agency and local modernisation boards for each regional office of the NHS. The *Implementation Programme for the NHS Plan* (Department of Health, 2000b) was published at the end of 2000 and included provisional milestones and key targets for the early years of the Plan. More targets followed and many working in the NHS felt overwhelmed by the pace of change.

The reorganisation of the NHS

The NHS Plan promised greater power and authority for patients and the public. *Shifting the Balance of Power Within the NHS* (Department of Health, 2001) attempted to give that greater authority to patients as well as to decentralise decision-making. The NHS Executive was dismantled, and all English and Welsh health authorities were abolished. They were replaced with 28 new strategic health authorities, which have a strategic role in improving local health services and also in monitoring local health trusts' performance.

The PCGs evolved into new primary care trusts (PCTs), which inherited the health authorities' powers, responsibilities and resources. PCTs have become the new powerhouses of the NHS. They are responsible for health improvement, and developing and delivering primary care, but also for commissioning hospital services. PCTs hold approximately 75% of all NHS resources. While there were nearly 100 health authorities, there are now over 400 PCTs, each covering an average population of 175 000.

One of the most controversial reforms was the proposal to establish foundation trusts. Initially only top-performing trusts could apply for foundation trust status, but it is now envisaged that all NHS trusts and PCTs will eventually be eligible. Becoming a foundation trust offers more financial freedom, with organisations being allowed both to retain operating surpluses and to access a wider range of options for capital funding to invest in new services. They are also able to recruit and employ their own staff. Although they must still deliver on national targets and standards, they are not under the direction of the Department of Health and the regional strategic health authorities. There has been much resistance to foundation trusts, as many feel they indicate the break-up of the NHS, with individual hospitals having almost complete independence and determining their own priorities. Even their detractors in some hospital trusts and PCTs have realised that they are a reality, and feel obliged to prepare to apply for foundation trust status, as otherwise they, and their patients, will be left behind and disadvantaged. This is similar to the situation that GPs found themselves in over 10 years previously with regard to fund-holding.

The NHS and the private sector

For the NHS to reach the targets of the NHS Plan, it needed to increase its capacity, but extra resources to build new hospitals were unavailable. Previous governments had utilised the Private Finance Initiative (PFI), where private capital was used to build hospitals. Hospital trusts would then lease the buildings from the private companies, under contracts lasting 25 years or more. The NHS gained new buildings without raising taxes, as the public's payment was deferred, although in the long term it would be more expensive than if the buildings had been built using public money. The 2002 White Paper *Delivering the NHS Plan* announced that 55 major hospital schemes would be carried out, mostly through the PFI system (Department of Health, 2002). The PFI schemes have been renamed 'public–private partnerships' (PPPs). Some NHS services, such as psychotherapy, are contracted out to private companies. This has again been done in the hope of increasing capacity and meeting targets. Most contracts involve elective surgical procedures or diagnostic tests. The primary concern of private healthcare providers is profit and so they are prone to choose activities that will yield a profit and to leave less financially attractive services to the NHS. Because there were concerns about the quality of work provided by the private companies, contracts now specify expected performance levels. There have also been concerns that the NHS is slowly being privatised through PPPs, although at the time of writing the government is committed to a maximum of 15% of the NHS's output being provided by the private sector. For an in-depth discussion of the relationship between the NHS and the private sector, readers are recommended *NHS plc* (Pollock, 2005).

The results of the recent reforms, and the future

There has been massive investment in the NHS in the period 1997–2006: NHS spending increased from £46 billion a year to £94 billion a year. This investment has led to some modest improvements; for example, nearly 200 000 extra front-line staff have joined the NHS. Over half of the extra money has been spent on pay and pensions for staff, most significantly, in increased National Insurance contributions. General practitioners and hospital consultants received new contracts, which, while increasing the scrutiny and accountability of their work, considerably increased their pay. The average GP now earns more than £100 000 a year, making UK doctors some of the highest paid in the world outside the USA. Extra funding is due to cease in 2008.

There have been some successes. The number of patients on waiting lists, a favourite marker of success for politicians, is at an all-time low, but average out-patient waiting time has been reduced only to 6.6 weeks, compared with 7.7 weeks in 1997. In-patient waiting lists have fallen more substantially but on the whole it must be concluded that too much has been spent on delivering too little. NHS productivity has not increased enough and the Service has ended up costing more and delivering less value for money.

At the time of writing (summer 2006) the NHS in England has a net deficit of £512 million, equivalent to 0.8% of its turnover. Services in some areas are being cut, leading to staff redundancies as trusts try to balance their books. This is likely to continue as the current level of NHS spending cannot continue. From 2008, annual increases for the NHS are expected to decrease from the current 7% to 3–4%. Further reform in 2006 included plans set out in a new White Paper to expand care outside of the hospital, with 5% of resources to be shifted from hospitals to GPs over the next 10 years. The new emphasis is on community provision of healthcare. Services previously provided by hospitals will be offered by GPs or by privately run, but NHS-funded, clinics. This will place more financial pressure on hospitals, as they will competing with each other for work: since 2005 patients have been able to choose from at least four hospitals, including one in the private sector. Under the new payment by results scheme hospitals will be paid only for the work they do, rather than being given a budget at the start of the year. Each procedure, whether it be a surgical operation or an out-patient follow-up appointment, has an attached national tariff/price and the hospital receives this payment only if it completes the activity. This system will increase the competition between hospitals, and a hospital that fails to attract enough work will face considerable financial adversity, as many already have financial deficits and are tied into long, expensive PFI contracts.

Financial difficulties will inevitably lead to further reorganisation of the NHS, but it is difficult to assess how much appetite the already reform-weary NHS staff have for further change.

Changes in the NHS management structure since 1974 are summarised in Table 3.1.

Further sources and directions of change

The Postgraduate Medical Education and Training Board (PMETB) and Modernising Medical Careers (MMC) are two key factors that will change the face of training and assessment in psychiatry. The third prong of this change is the European Working Time Directive (EWTD).

Modernising Medical Careers introduces a 'foundation year 2', with the aim of exposing trainees to three further specialties before they have to make their selection. This is a generic foundation programme for the first two postgraduate years (F1 and F2), to be followed by a Unified Training Grade (UTG) with no midpoint reselection.

The EWTD restricts the working hours of trainee doctors to a maximum of 58 hours per week, and the trainee cannot work continuously for more than 13 hours without a minimum 11 hours off; also, trainees are considered to be working if they are required to be in the hospital, whether awake or asleep. As of 30 September 2005, the PMETB is the single competent authority for postgraduate medical education, training and assessment throughout the UK. The PMETB will be responsible for all postgraduate medical education and assessment of doctors completing final postgraduate training and will be in charge of establishing, maintaining and monitoring standards relating to medical training in the NHS and elsewhere. It will issue certificates of Completion of Training and statements of eligibility for specialist registration. It has three main committees – Quality Assurance, Training and Assessment. The PMETB has taken over the approved visits

Table 3.1 Some important changes in NHS management structures since 1974

Year	Initiative
1975	*Better Services for the Mentally Ill* published, a White Paper based on a report from the Audit Commission
1982	The Korner report, from the Department of Health and Social Security's Steering Group on Health Services Information, concerning the collection and use of information on hospital clinical activity
	Abolition of NHS area health boards
1983	Management budgeting experiment started
1983	Griffiths report on Health Service management
1986	Introduction of the 'resource management initiative'
1987	*Achieving a Balance* published, which recommends staffing levels for doctors
1988	NHS review announced
1989	*Working for Patients* and *Caring for People* published – White Papers leading to the 1990 Act
1990	The NHS and Community Care Act (reforms effective 1 April 1991) and introduction of the purchaser/provider split
1991	Postgraduate and continuing medical education introduced
	First wave of trust hospitals
1992	Second wave of trust hospitals
1993	Managing the new NHS – new proposals
1994	Fourth and last wave of trust hospitals
1997	*The NHS. Modern, Dependable* published. GP fund-holders abolished. Moves away from competition. PCGs established
1998	*A First Class Service* published and clinical governance introduced
2000	The NHS Plan: increased resources, performance monitoring (traffic light system)
2001	*Shifting the Balance of Power* launched. PCTs set up. NHS executive replaced by strategic health authorities
2002	Wanless report highlights under-funding of the NHS
2003	Health and Social Care Act presents concept of foundation hospitals and trusts

from the medical Royal Colleges and the assessments and training have to comply with PMETB standards and principles. The assessments will be largely workplace based and trainees will become increasingly responsible for their own learning and assessment; the assessments will focus on what doctors do rather than simply knowledge. These changes will have major effects on service delivery and training. Curricula for psychiatrists have been approved and the assessment matrix has been provisionally approved.

Conclusion

It is hoped that this brief precis of the history of the NHS will act as an introduction to the doctor interested in management and the complex organisational structure in which we work. Two things can be learned immediately from taking this historical overview: first, that history repeats itself and it is remarkable how current plans for the NHS are similar to old ideas; second, as an administrative machine the NHS is continually evolving, and that should be borne in mind by all of us who intend to plight their troth to it for the vast majority of our professional careers.

References and further reading

Allsop, J. (1986) *Health Policy in the National Health Service.* Longman.

Beeson, P. B. (1980) Some good features of the British National Health Service. In *Readings in Medical Sociology* (ed. D. Mechanic), pp. 328–334. Free Press.

Beveridge, W. (1942) *Social Insurance and Allied Services.* TSO (The Stationary Office).

Bhugra, D., Bell, S. & Burns, A. (eds) (2007) *Management for Psychiatrists.* RCPsych Publications.

Blaine, A. R. P. (1998) *The Third Way, New Politics for a New Century.* Fabian Society.

British Medical Association (1929) *Proposals for a General Medical Service for the Nation.* British Medical Association.

British Medical Association (1989) *Special Report on the Government's White Paper, 'Working for Patients'.* British Medical Association.

British Medical Journal (1875) Provident institutions and hospitals. II Outpatients reforms. *British Medical Journal*, 483–484.

Davies, C. (1987) Things to come: the NHS in the next decade. *Sociology of Health and Illness*, **9**, 302–317.

Day, P. & Klein, R. (2002) CHI. Who nose best? Commission for Health Improvement. *Health Service Journal*, **112**, 26–29.

Department of Health (1989) *Working for Patients.* TSO (The Stationery Office).

Department of Health (1990) *National Health Service and Community Care Act.* TSO (The Stationery Office).

Department of Health (1991) *The Patient's Charter.* TSO (The Stationery Office).

Department of Health (1992) *The Health of the Nation.* TSO (The Stationery Office).

Department of Health (1994) *Hospital and Ambulance Services: Comparative Performance Grade 1993–1994.* TSO (The Stationery Office).

Department of Health (1997) *The New NHS. Modern, Dependable.* TSO (The Stationery Office).

Department of Health (1998a) *Our Healthier Nation.* TSO (The Stationery Office).

Department of Health (1998b) *A First Class Service: Quality in the New NHS.* TSO (The Stationery Office).

Department of Health (2000a) *The NHS Plan: A Plan for Investment, a Plan for Reform.* TSO (The Stationery Office).

Department of Health (2000b) *Implementation Programme for the NHS Plan.* TSO (The Stationery Office).

Department of Health (2001) *Shifting the Balance of Power Within the NHS.* TSO (The Stationery Office).

Department of Health (2002) *Delivering the NHS Plan: Next Steps on Investment, Next Steps on Reform.* TSO (The Stationery Office).

Department of Health and Social Security (1972) *Management Arrangements for the Reorganised Health Service.* TSO (The Stationery Office).

Draper, P., Grenholm, G. & Best, G. (1976) The organization of health care: a critical view of the 1974 reorganization of the National Health Service. In *An Introduction to Medical Sociology* (ed. D. Tuckett). London: Tavistock.

Forsyth, G. (1982) Evolution of (the National Health Service). In *Management for Clinicians* (eds D. Allen & D. Grimes), pp. 18–35. Pitman.

Godber, G. (1975) *The Health Service: Past, Present and Future.* Athlone Press.

Godber, G. (1988) Forty years of the NHS. Origins and early development. *BMJ*, **297**, 37–43. (Subsequent articles in the same issue, pp. 44–58, are also of interest.)

Heller, T. (1978) *Restructuring the Health Service*. Croom Helm.

Hendy, J., Reeves, B. C., Fulop, N., *et al* (2005) Challenges to implementing the National Programme for Information Technology (NPfIT): a qualitative study. *BMJ*, **331**, 331–336.

Hoffenberg, R., Todd, I. P. & Pinker, G. (1987) Crisis in the National Health Service. *BMJ*, **295**, 1505.

Honigsbaum, F. (1979) *The Division in British Medicine: A History of the Separation of General Practice from Health Care 1911–1968*. Routledge & Kegan Paul.

Honigsbaum, F. (1989) *Health, Happiness and Security – The Creation of the National Health Service*. Routledge.

Jaques, E. (1978) *Health Services*. Heinemann.

Kearney, K. (1992) Strategy for improvement or window dressing? *The Guardian*, 9 July.

Klein, R. (1989) *The Politics of the National Health Service* (2nd edn). Longman.

Klein, R. (2001) *The New Politics of the National Health Service*. Pearson Education.

Levitt, R. (1976) *The Reorganised National Health Service*. Croom Helm.

Navarro, V. (1978) *Class Struggle, the State and Medicine: An Historical and Contemporary Analysis of the Medical Sector in Great Britain*. Martin Robertson.

NHS Executive (1998) *Information for Health. An Information Strategy for the Modern NHS 1998–2005*. NHS Executive.

Political and Economic Planning Group (1937) *The British Social Services. The British Health Services*. Political and Economic Planning.

Pollock, A. (2005) *NHS plc*. Verso.

Roland, M., Campell, S. & Wilkins, D. (2001) Clinical governance: a convincing strategy for quality improvement? *Journal of Management in Medicine*, **15**, 188–201.

Stacey, M. (1988) *The Sociology of Health and Healing*. Unwin Hyman.

Stevens, R. (1966) *Medical Practice in Modern England: The Impact of Specialization and State Medicine*. York University Press.

Stevens, S. (2004) Reform strategies for the English NHS. *Health Affairs*, **23**, 37–44.

Timmins, N. (1988) *Cash Crisis and Cure – The Independent Guide to the NHS Debate*. Newspaper Publishing PLC.

Wanless, D. (2002) *Securing Our Future Health: Taking a Long-Term View*. HM Treasury.

Watkin, B. (1978) *The National Health Service: The First Phase 1948–1974 and After*. George Allen and Unwin.

Webster, C. (2002) *The National Health Service: A Political History* (2nd edn). Oxford University Press.

CHAPTER 4

The College

Gareth Holsgrove, Vanessa Cameron and Dinesh Bhugra

The Royal College of Psychiatrists is the professional and educational body for psychiatrists in the UK and Ireland. The College also has international Divisions (Pan-American, Western Pacific, South Asian, Middle Eastern, European and African).

The College promotes mental health by:

- setting standards and promoting excellence in mental healthcare
- improving understanding through research and education
- leading, representing, training and supporting psychiatrists
- working with patients, carers and their organisations.

History

The Royal College of Psychiatrists has been in existence in some form since 1841, first as the Association of Medical Officers of Asylums and Hospitals for the Insane (later changed to the Medico Psychological Association), then, in 1926, receiving its Royal Charter to become the Royal Medico Psychological Association and finally, in 1971, receiving a Supplemental Charter to become the Royal College of Psychiatrists we know today.

Structures and function

Like any large organisation, the structures within the College have developed and evolved since its inception. The Chief Executive of the College has overall responsibility for the management of the College and is assisted by the Deputy Chief Executive. The Registrar is responsible for policy, public education and other related matters. The President is elected by the College membership for a 3-year term and the Registrar, Dean and Treasurer for 5-year terms. The Dean is the principal academic officer responsible for training and assessment.

There are several departments in the College. As part of its responsibility for public education, the College has an external affairs department, including a public affairs officer, a policy analyst and a campaign and communications administrator. The Library and Information Service supports both the profession and the public, with a small specialist library for members, access to electronic journals and a large range of public information materials, including excellent leaflets and books for patients, their families and carers, produced by the College.

The External Affairs and Information Services Department promotes the College's interests with the media, government and other organisations and works closely with the President and Registrar. The Department played a major role in the Partners in Care Campaign (January 2004 to October 2005), a very successful collaboration between the College and the Princess Royal Trust for Carers, which has led to the increasing involvement of patients and carers in psychiatric education. This involvement is now enshrined in the new curriculum for specialist training in psychiatry.

The Facilities Department is responsible for the smooth running of the building and related office services. The financial aspects of the College are the responsibility of the College Treasurer, who works closely with staff in the Financial Services Department.

The Postgraduate Educational Services Department is responsible for a wide range of tasks that support the College's educational remit. This includes supporting the many educational committees and working groups, scrutinising applications from psychiatrists who want to go onto the Specialist Register, representing the College at careers fairs and dealing with international issues. Some of the College meetings and conferences, such as the annual education and training conference, are organised by the Postgraduate Educational Services Department. It also supports the Dean and two of the Associate Deans who deal with training and with the equivalence of overseas qualifications.

The Examinations Services Department is responsible for the massive task of organising and running the College Membership examinations. This includes maintaining the question banks, receiving and processing applications from candidates, coordinating marking and informing candidates about their results. This department supports the Chief Examiner, the team of Examiners and the Examination Board. There are two Deputy Chief Examiners.

The College has a thriving Publications Department which publishes books under the imprint RCPsych Publications (formerly Gaskell). The department also publishes four journals (*The British Journal of Psychiatry, Psychiatric Bulletin, Advances in Psychiatric Treatment* and *International Psychiatry*) and jointly owns a fifth (*Evidence-Based Mental Health*). All of the journals are available online. The College also produces a series of online interactive learning modules for the continuing professional development of mental health professionals (http://www.psychiatrycpd.co.uk). The Publications Department also designs and maintains the College website (http://www.rcpsych.ac.uk).

The Deputy Chief Executive's Department has many functions, including support for Faculties, Sectors and Special Interest Groups. The Conference Unit is within this Department and provides support staff for the College annual conference and several other specialist conferences. The Department supports the divisional offices, which are located in Belfast, Birmingham, Bristol, Cardiff, Dublin, Edinburgh, Leeds and London. A recent development has been the establishment of the Psychiatrists' Support Service, which provides a confidential helpline to psychiatrists in distress.

College Research and Training Unit

The College Research and Training Unit (CRTU), based in Aldgate in east London, is made up of four centres: College Centre for Applied Research, College Education and Training Centre, National Collaborating Centre for Mental Health and College Centre for Quality Improvement. The Unit enjoys an international reputation and has been extremely successful in obtaining competitive grants for a number of projects dealing with health services research. The CRTU has a number of full-time researchers under the direction of Professor Paul Lelliott and is a major source of evidence on matters concerning mental health. Many influential research papers are based on work carried out in the College Centre for Applied Research.

The College Centre for Quality Improvement offers an inspection and approval service for electroconvulsive therapy (ECT) provision throughout the UK and accreditation of acute in-patient mental health services. Other quality improvement networks include those for child and adolescent and perinatal mental health services, among others.

The College Education and Training Centre was established in 2005. The Training Centre has the responsibility for developing and delivering specialist courses and educational conferences for psychiatrists and mental health professionals on a wide range of issues such as the Mental Health Act, sharing patient information, etc. It is envisaged the Centre will take on the role of training assessors and educational supervisors, and will offer training in workplace-based assessment and how to manage trainees who are in difficulty. The Centre has a Head of Training and has been developing web-based learning packages and the first training package should be available in early 2007.

Future directions

The next few years seem certain to see considerable changes to the activities of all of the medical Royal Colleges as a result of the many significant changes taking place in postgraduate medical education under Modernising Medical Careers (MMC) and the Postgraduate Medical Education and Training Board (PMETB; http://www.pmetb.org.uk). Some of the functions of PMETB were formerly undertaken by the Colleges and the Specialist Training Authority.

The PMETB is now responsible for approving the curriculum developed by the Royal College of Psychiatrists (http://www.rcpsych.ac.uk/training/curriculumpilotpack.aspx), awarding certificates of completion of training, and approving training schemes.

The Royal College of Psychiatrists is well to the fore in anticipating and preparing for these changes. A new, modular curriculum has been approved by PMETB. Unlike the present system of basic and higher specialist training, under MMC there will be a unified training grade, and the new curriculum is designed with this in mind. It is also hoped that mental health professionals other than psychiatrists will be able to access relevant parts of the curriculum. Over the next few years there will be a greater emphasis on workplace-based assessments and this is accounted for in the new curriculum. The Membership examinations will also need to be assessed and modified so that they meet PMETB principles and standards. In order to support trainers and trainees through these changes, the College has already started to organise seminars and workshops via the Education and Training Centre.

The College will still be committed to advancing the science and practice of psychiatry, furthering public education and promoting research. In some instances, departments will be relatively unaffected by the changes. However, those concerned with education, training and examinations are likely to undergo quite substantial change in order to meet new statutory requirements and ensure that the College's educational and professional mission remains of the highest standard.

CHAPTER 5

The General Medical Council

Sheila A. Mann

The objective of the General Medical Council (GMC) is to protect, promote and maintain the health and safety of the public by ensuring proper standards in the practice of medicine. To achieve this the GMC is responsible for:

- setting the standards of good medical practice that society and the profession expect of doctors throughout their working lives
- assuring the quality of undergraduate medical education in the UK and coordinating all stages of medical education
- administering the systems for the recognition and licensing of doctors to control their entry to, and continuation in, medical practice in the UK
- dealing with doctors whose fitness to practise is questioned.

History

The GMC was first established as the single statutory medical regulatory body of the UK by the Medical Act of 1858. Previously there had been a considerable number – over a dozen – of licensing bodies and many doctors were not licensed at all. The purpose therefore was to ensure that there was one body that held the names of qualified doctors whom the public could consult when necessary.

The Medical Act 1858 empowered the GMC to erase from the Medical Register any doctor found guilty of a criminal offence or 'infamous conduct in a professional respect'. For nearly a century this Act remained in force.

In 1950 a further Medical Act established a Disciplinary Committee to investigate and if necessary remove a doctor's name from the Register. This Act introduced a right of appeal to the Court, a requirement for a legal assessor to advise the committee and the power to restore a doctor following erasure if deemed appropriate.

In the late 1960s and 1970s a dispute arose between the Council and some members of the medical profession over funding. The GMC was unable to manage within its funding structure (a one-off registration fee) and sought to introduce an 'annual retention fee'. Such was the depth of feeling in the profession that many were prepared to take strike action and, seeking to avoid this, the government of the day set up the Merrison Committee which reported in 1975 (Merrison, 1975). It was given very wide terms of reference – effectively to consider all aspects of medical regulation, how it should be provided and constituted, and to make recommendations.

The main proposals of the Merrison Committee are shown in Box 5.1. The Committee proposed that the Council should have a professionally elected majority of members to ensure that it would be representative of those directly involved in patient care. It was recommended that the number of elected medical members should exceed the number of appointed medical and nominated lay members.

The Penal Cases Committee, which had been responsible for considering referrals, should be abolished and replaced by the Complaints Committee (later the Preliminary Proceedings Committee) and the Disciplinary Committee should be abolished (later to be replaced by the Professional Conduct Committee).

The Preliminary Proceedings Committee was given power to order temporary interim suspension or conditional registration where there was clear evidence to suggest that continued registration would be a serious danger to the public.

Of particular interest to psychiatrists, the Merrison Committee looked at problems arising from a doctor's ill health. Previously there had been no power to restrict the practice of a doctor with mental illness (unless they committed an offence, which might involve the Professional Conduct Committee) however much their illness compromised patient care.

The GMC had, however, been concerned about these doctors and had wished to set up local machinery to supervise them. The Merrison

---

Box 5.1 Main proposals of the Merrison Committee

- The GMC should have a professionally elected majority of members
- The Penal Cases Committee should be replaced by the Preliminary Proceedings Committee and the Disciplinary Committee by the Professional Conduct Committee
- The Preliminary Proceedings Committee should be given power to order temporary interim suspension or conditional registration
- A Health Committee should be established which could impose conditional registration, allowing a flexible means of supervising sick doctors or, if deemed necessary, suspending their registration
- An Education Committee should be established to take over the GMC's role in promoting and coordinating medical education
- The GMC should be given the power to give advice to doctors on standards of professional conduct and ethics.

Committee did not accept this and instead recommended the establishment of a Health Committee that could impose conditional registration, allowing a flexible means of supervising sick doctors or, if deemed necessary, suspending their registration.

The Committee emphasised that in its view the Fitness To Practise procedures should aim to protect the public not to punish the sick doctor. From the report, members clearly felt strongly about this and their opinion has been supported subsequently by judgments delivered by the Judicial Committee of the Privy Council. The considerable number of doctors with addictive disorders was remarked on from the beginning.

The Committee recommended that the legislation should be amended to impose a duty on the GMC to promote high standards. An Education Committee should be established to take over the GMC's role in promoting and coordinating all stages of medical education.

It was also recommended that the GMC should be given the power to give advice to doctors on standards of professional conduct and ethics. The Committee believed that it was necessary for the GMC to take a more active role in maintaining standards.

The Medical Act 1978 embodied the major part of the Merrison Committee proposals which government accepted. Guidance to the medical profession on standards was given in *Professional Conduct and Discipline: Fitness to Practise* (General Medical Council, 1993). The guidance aimed to cope with exceptional misconduct. Although some patient-orientated advice was given, for example that failure to organise treatment or to visit patients when appropriate could amount to serious professional misconduct, much advice related to professional matters (i.e. advertising, canvassing for business, entering into an improper relationship or issuing a false medical certificate).

However, during the 1980s increasing concern was felt within and outside the profession that (other than the health procedures) most guidance limited itself largely to these matters. There was an increasing belief that the Council ought to be equally if not more concerned with questions of competence and clinical performance.

From 1995 guidance was no longer issued in what was previously called colloquially the 'Blue Book' but in a document *Good Medical Practice*. This set out systematically the principles of good practice that would be expected of all doctors and has been revised every few years. A summary will be found in the next section.

In addition the GMC has prepared, and when necessary updated, a considerable number of booklets dealing with specific aspects of practice, such as confidentiality, consent, etc. (Box 5.2).

With rising concern over the need for a system that could deal with persistently poor or deficient performance, the GMC began to work with the medical Royal Colleges and others to create a framework that could be used to identify impaired performance (i.e. not conduct or health).

Box 5.2   GMC booklets for doctors in training

The Duties of a Doctor Series
- *Good Medical Practice*
- *Seeking Patients' Consent*
- *Confidentiality: Protecting and Providing Information – FAQs*
- *Confidentiality: Questions*
- *Management for Doctors*
- *Research – The Role and Responsibilities of Doctors*
- *Duties Folders*
- *Withholding and Withdrawing Life-Prolonging Treatments*
- *0–18 Children: Guidance for Doctors*

Education Series
- *Principles of Good Medical Education and Training*
- *The New Doctor*
- *Tomorrow's Doctor*
- *Continuing Professional Development*
- *Medical Students: Professional Behaviour and Fitness to Practise*

Referral Series
- *Guide for Doctors referred to the GMC*
- *How to Complain about a Doctor – Patients*
- *How to Complain about a Doctor (for Health Professionals)*

Referral Series
- *2007 Annual Review*
- *2007 Business Plan*

The Royal College of Psychiatrists participated, as did other Royal Colleges and professional associations, in looking at ways of assessing performance in the specialty. The recommended performance procedures were approved and introduced in 1997. As with the health procedures, experienced specialists from psychiatric practice contributed greatly to the assessment and advice given to poorly performing doctors.

It will be appreciated that over the past 60 years or so the GMC has been constantly scrutinising procedures and publications. As readers will be aware, there have been major concerns and criticism from the public and from the profession at times that the GMC is too 'secretive', supports doctors even if they may be at fault or does not support doctors when they or the profession as a whole are criticised.

Further reforms

Further reforms were proposed in 2001 (Box 5.3) and began to be implemented in 2003. It should in future be possible to introduce reforms, like these, rather

---

Box 5.3   Further reforms of the GMC

- Reduction in size and constitution
- Reforms to registration
- Reforms to fitness to practise procedures
  - Separation between those investigating and those adjudicating
  - More integrated approach
  - Responding to serious concerns not requiring action on registration
  - Streamlining and speeding up processes
  - New procedures must be linked to other organisations protecting patients
  - Implementing the planned process of revalidation

---

more quickly since the Health Act 1999 confers in section 60 the power to speed up changes in the law. The Medical Act 1983 (which was made 'to consolidate the Medical Acts 1956–1978 and certain related provisions ...'), as amended by subsequent legislation, is still the statutory basis for the regulation of the medical profession today. Before the section 60 Order, changes in the law took a considerable time to be agreed and passed by Parliament. It is now possible for the Medical Act 1983 to be amended through a statutory instrument, which is generally very much quicker than previous proceedings. This has been used, for example, to give the Council more flexible powers to impose interim restrictions on a doctor's practice, to obtain and disclose information needed for fitness to practise investigations and to amend procedures governing restoration to the Register following erasure by the Professional Conduct Committee or Fitness to Practise Panel.

Following a number of high-profile inquiries in recent years, including the Ayling, Kerr/Haslam, Neale and Shipman inquiries, the government announced a review of clinical performance and medical regulation. In 2006, the Chief Medical Officer Sir Liam Donaldson published a report setting out proposals to strengthen the system to assure and improve the performance of doctors and protect the safety of patients (Department of Health, 2006). This was followed, in 2007, by a government White Paper on the regulation of health professionals (Department of Health, 2007).

Reduction in size and constitution

The further reforms include reduction in the size and constitution of the GMC. Previously there were 104 members, which made it unwieldy, for example, to make rapid decisions. The Council now comprises:

- 19 elected members
- 2 appointed members (1 by the Academy of Medical Royal Colleges and 1 by the Council of Heads of Medical Schools)

- 14 lay members (appointed by the Appointments Commission as before but through a more open and transparent selection process).

In the smaller Council there is a substantial increase in the proportion of lay members from 25% to 40%.

Further changes are expected to the size and constitution in 2008. It is proposed that:

- Council should be smaller
- all council members should be appointed by the Appointments Commission, against competencies
- the GMC should put in place 'better systems for patient and public involvement panels within the regulatory bodies, with terms of reference to ensure that wider societal interests and concerns are taken into account in the conduct of councils' business and the shaping of their policies
- there should be proactive programmes to engage more widely with public, patient and parliamentary opinion on issues where there are obvious tensions between patient and professional interests
- governance should be more open and transparent, with papers published and meetings open to the public
- the GMC should be under a statutory duty to ensure that the interests of all stakeholders are considered
- Council should assume statutory responsibility for the overseeing of medical education, because of the interlocking nature of the GMC's functions.

Reforms to registration

Reforms to registration involved creation of a simpler means of dealing with doctors' registration which is fair, objective, transparent and non-discriminatory. This involved the creation of registration panels and will be discussed further below.

Reforms to fitness to practise procedures

Separation between those investigating and those adjudicating

This was a major change which was seen by those within and outside the GMC as being important. It proposed that Council members (who previously sat as constituted medical members of panels) not be eligible to sit on panels. Instead appointed GMC panellists selected against clear and transparent criteria would adjudicate.

More integrated approach to fitness to practise

Instead of there being three concepts (serious professional misconduct, serious health impairment and seriously deficient performance), the aim of the revised procedure was to consider whether the doctor's fitness to practise was 'impaired to a degree justifying action on registration'.

Responding to concerns which, although serious, do not require action on registration

A system has been developed whereby a warning can be issued to a doctor where there has been a significant departure from good medical practice or cause for concern about performance as a whole, although any individual shortcomings are not serious enough to justify restriction of registration.

Streamlining the fitness to practise processes

It is hoped that the new structure will abolish the serious delays that led to potential further risk to patients in some instances and to considerable stress for the doctor awaiting the result.

New procedures must be linked to other organisations protecting patients

Recognition that new procedures must be linked to other organisations protecting patients has meant making arrangements for sharing information in a responsible and appropriate way with employers, the NHS and other regulatory bodies.

Implementing the planned process of revalidation

The Merrison report (Merrison, 1975) considered two possibilities for changing the GMC's role in regulating fitness to practise. One was 'exception reporting' as had been the case in the past and is largely still today. The alternative, which was considered but not recommended, was relicensing.

In 1999 the GMC became increasingly concerned about high-profile cases where medical incompetence had not been reported although the deficiencies had been known for a considerable time.

In 2000 the GMC conceived a form of 'revalidation' that would be based on a 'revalidation folder' containing information about practice. It was expected that this would contain a broad range of information, including evidence that continuing professional development had been satisfactory, patient satisfaction surveys, complaints, compliments, audits and comments from clinical governance visits.

The plan was that these folders would be reviewed at the annual appraisal, and that every 5 years every doctor would go before a revalidation panel which would be made up of doctors, including a colleague in a similar field, and a lay person. If the panel was not satisfied that the doctor was performing satisfactorily, then the doctor would be referred to the GMC to undergo consideration as to whether it was necessary to invoke fitness to practise procedures, to issue a licence with conditions, or indeed to suspend the doctor.

Even with this proposed elaborate mechanism it was accepted that incompetent doctors might not be picked up at a very early stage. It became obvious that this system of revalidation, although seemingly thorough, would be expensive in terms of both time and money, particularly with regard to the revalidation panels, which might be expected to contain members from other areas than the doctor's own locality in order to provide impartiality. This would involve much extra work and travel for doctors involved in this process.

The GMC therefore proposed a different system in 2003 based on the appraisals that had been introduced on an annual basis. Arrangements were in place for revalidation to start when concern arose that this system was not in fact sufficiently robust to pick up poor practice. Overall concern was expressed that this was again going to lead to doctors being regarded as competent unless there was evidence that they were not, rather than having to prove that they are competent.

The GMC is preparing to introduce licences to practise with periodic renewal ('revalidation'), based on positive evidence that a doctor remains up to date and fit to practise. The government's White Paper (Department of Health, 2007) proposed that revalidation will consist of two core components: relicensing for all doctors and recertification for specialists. Relicensing and recertification will depend on an objective assessment of a doctor's fitness to practise against clear standards. *Good Medical Practice* (General Medical Council, 2006) will form the basis for those standards.

The GMC, in consultation with key interest groups, is working to translate *Good Medical Practice* into a framework that will support annual appraisal of individual doctors (by the NHS and other employing or contracting bodies) and provide a sound basis for GMC decisions about their relicensing.

The Academy of Medical Royal Colleges will lead work to develop the standards for specialist recertification, working closely with the GMC to ensure that these standards are consistent across specialties and that the process will provide sound evidence to support the GMC's decision on revalidation.

Trainees will almost certainly be in a different situation since they are appraised regularly by their educational supervisors, but it is worth noting that it seems likely that a very high standard of recording clinical and education matters will be required.

Trainee contact with the GMC

Trainees will inevitably have contact with the GMC. There follows a brief description of the major aspects of the GMC that are likely to be of concern to trainees.

Education

The GMC oversees the education of medical students in the UK in order that it is appropriate for the current practice of medicine. If medical education is completed successfully, medical schools will render the student trained sufficiently to enter postgraduate training.

Until recently, as well as graduates of UK medical schools and those obtaining the qualification of the United Examining Board, candidates qualifying from Australia, New Zealand, Hong Kong, Singapore, South Africa and the West Indies were entitled to practise medicine in the UK and to obtain a preregistration house officer post. This has now been discontinued and new arrangements, as outlined below, put in place.

The GMC sets outcomes and standards for undergraduate medical education in *Tomorrow's Doctors* (General Medical Council, 2007a). A system called quality assurance of basic medical education (QABME) reviews medical schools against those outcomes and standards. With the Medical Schools Council, the GMC has also published guidance for medical students on professional behaviour and fitness to practise (General Medical Council & Medical Schools Council, 2006).

From August 2008, new graduates will enter the foundation programme, provided that they have obtained provisional registration with the GMC.

During the first year they are provisionally registered with the GMC. If they successfully demonstrate the outcomes required by the GMC in *The New Doctor 2007* (General Medical Council, 2007b), they obtain full registration and enter the second year of the programme. Each year is made up of a number of posts (usually three 4-month posts) in differing specialties, including general practice and laboratory medicine. The GMC and Postgraduate Medical Education and Training Board (PMETB) jointly set standards and ensure that these are met through the Quality Assurance of the Foundation Programme (QAFP). After completing the foundation programme doctors may enter specialist or general practice training.

Registration

The process of gaining registration generally depends on the country where the doctor obtained their primary medical qualification and on their nationality. There are three main types of registration (provisional, full and specialist), with a different application for each type. All doctors wishing to practise medicine in the UK must be registered with the GMC and satisfy the GMC of their fitness to practise before registration will be granted. The GMC's website (http://www.gmc-uk.org) contains general information about the different types of registration and a number of factsheets to help doctors identify the type that applies to them and the evidence requirements. Application forms can be downloaded from the website, and online application should be possible from 2008. Registration issues vary according to the country of origin and of medical training. This is a complex arrangement and while the more common situations are given here, any trainee who is at all uncertain should contact the GMC as soon as possible moment to ascertain what is required.

Provisional registration

This allows a newly qualified doctor to undertake the general clinical training needed for full registration. This usually follows the award of a medical degree and lasts for 12 months, during which the newly qualified doctor is under supervision. After successfully completing the year, the doctor will be eligible to apply for full registration.

Full registration

This allows unsupervised medical practice within the UK. This is granted following successful completion of suitable training, usually from provisional or limited registration (see below). This has typically been granted following successful completion of a preregistration house officer post (now called a foundation year one post).

Following recent changes, instead of being able to undertake whatever medical work the individual wishes following the satisfactory completion of foundation year one, all graduates from the UK will be expected to do a second year of training: this usually means that they will complete six posts, each of 4 months duration. Assuming that they have satisfied requirements in the first year's posts, they will be granted full registration for the second (foundation year two) posts.

For the first 12 months of full registration, UK and international medical graduates are required to work within an approved practice setting (APS). This is a setting that has systems for the effective management of doctors, systems for identifying and acting on concerns about doctors' fitness to practise, systems to support the provision of relevant training or continuing professional development and systems for providing regulatory assurance.

Approved practice settings were introduced to ensure that all medical graduates, especially those unfamiliar with current UK medical practice, work in an environment where supportive and quality assured systems are in operation and aiming to improve standards.

Following successful completion of the second foundation year, trainees may enter specialty training or their chosen field of medicine.

Limited registration

Limited registration was introduced in 1979 for international medical graduates. It was abolished in October 2007. Those who held limited registration at that time were transferred to either full or provisional registration. Those who had held limited registration in the past but did not hold it in October 2007 were required to apply for either provisional or full registration.

International medical graduates now have the same opportunity as UK graduates and EEC counterparts in applying for provisional or full registration.

Specialist registration

Doctors must hold specialist registration in order to take up a substantive or honorary consultant post within the NHS or to become a principal in general practice.

The Registrar and GMC registration decisions panels

Under the GMC's decision-making structure, the Registrar makes registration decisions within a framework set by the Council. Council guidance specifies the considerations that the Registrar should take into account when making a decision. Where cases fall outside the guidelines, the Registrar may seek advice from a registration decisions panel. The vast majority of all registration applications are granted by the GMC's members of staff who operate many of the day-to-day functions of the Registrar under delegate authority in accordance with criteria set down by the Council.

The purpose of the registration decisions panels is to advise the Registrar on any matter arising in the course of his or her consideration of an application for registration. The panels do not have the power to make decisions on registration, except in cases of fraudulently procured registration or incorrect entries to the register. The procedures allow for a matter referred by the Registrar to a registration decisions panel to be considered at a meeting or before a hearing of a panel. Meetings of a panel are held in the absence of the parties. Hearings of a registration decisions panel are generally held in public, but either party may request for a hearing to be held in private. At a hearing the GMC is represented either by a solicitor or by counsel. Similarly the doctor may be represented either by a solicitor, or by counsel, or by a representative from any professional organisation of which the doctor is a member. At the discretion of the panel, a member of the doctor's family or another person may represent the doctor.

Under the new GMC procedures it is the Registrar who decides the appropriate registration. In case of doubt or disagreement, the Registrar can refer to a registration decisions panel for advice. Registration decisions panel meetings are held in the absence of the doctor and his representative.

Where the Registrar is aware of a dispute about the facts of the case or where he is considering making a direction of erasure of limited registration, the matter may be heard by a registration decisions hearing. At the hearing the doctor may be present and may be represented, although they can choose to present their case in person.

Doctors have a right to appeal certain registration decisions made by the Registrar. Schedule 3A to the Medical Act sets out the appealable and non-appealable decisions. A doctor wishing to appeal a decision of the Registrar can do so by giving notice of appeal to the Registrar. Any such notice of appeal must be given before the end of the period of 28 days beginning with the date on which the Registrar gave notice of his or her decision. A hearing of a registration appeal panel is usually held in private – the panel will deliberate in the absence of the parties – unless the doctor requests the panel to sit in public. Where a hearing of a panel takes place in public, the panel may decide to exclude the public for any part of the proceedings provided that it is satisfied that a decision to exclude the public causes no prejudice to the doctor, and is made after hearing representations from the parties.

If the doctor wishes to appeal the decision of a registration decisions panel, then the case will go to a registration appeal hearing. Panels do not normally hear oral evidence but the doctor is able to put their case to the panel and to give reasons for the appeal. Witnesses may be involved. The doctor can again be represented if they wish. It is the duty of the appeal panel to arrive at a decision but also to agree the reasons for the decision whatever the outcome. Costs may be awarded in an appeal, including costs against the appellant or the GMC, and this is explained to the parties before the appeal is heard. Further appeal against a decision of an appeals panel can be made to the Higher Court.

Fitness to practise

Hopefully, few trainees will experience referral to fitness to practise procedures. In the past there were three divisions – conduct procedures involving the Professional Conduct Committee, health procedures which might be 'voluntary' or dealt with by the Health Committee, and since 1997 the performance procedures. Since the reforms in 2004, this has changed. There is now one service for all complaints involving fitness to practise.

On receipt of a complaint or notification of other matters that might be of concern regarding a doctor's fitness to practise (e.g. referral from employers or evidence of conviction) the GMC undertakes checks, for example making sure that the complaint is about a doctor on the GMC register (many are not), whether the complaint seems appropriate for the GMC to deal with, and if both of these are fulfilled the GMC carries out a preliminary investigation and then, if appropriate (and if there is sufficient information to make a decision), the case is passed to the case examiners for a decision as to what, if anything, should be done.

If the complaint does not raise concerns that will require action on registration, then the GMC may refer the matter to local authorities and ask the employer to report back on the outcome of their enquiries. Once preliminary enquiries have been completed, including seeking the doctor's observations, these cases will be considered by both a medical and lay case examiner. These are individuals appointed after public advertisement. Both lay and medical case examiners are employed by the GMC. (Previously those dealing with fitness to practise issues were Council members of the GMC but not employed by it.) The case examiner has to decide whether there is any substance to the complaint and whether it should go forward. Two case examiners (one medical, one lay) are required to make the decision and to agree.

A new addition to the GMC's range of options is to issue a formal warning. Warnings have been issued by other committees, notably the Preliminary Proceedings Committee in the past, but these have not been made public and did not appear on the doctor's registration. Formal warnings from the case examiners do.

If the doctor disagrees with the warning they have the right to request an oral hearing before the Investigation Committee. The Committee will then make a new decision as to whether the warning should stand or not.

If the case examiners decide there could be substance in the complaint and that a warning is insufficient, the case will be passed to a fitness to practise panel. Such panels are comprised of individuals who have been carefully selected and have undergone an extensive assessment and training programme. Fitness to practise panels hear cases involving conduct, health and performance issues. The hearings are held in public, unless the matter is concerned with the health of the doctor, in which case they are held in private. This change separates the two aspects of the procedures – a long-standing criticism has been that the GMC acted as 'judge and jury'.

Acknowledgements

The content of this chapter is the responsibility of the author and does not necessarily represent the views of the Royal College of Psychiatrists or the GMC. I would like to thank my secretary, Pauline Gardner, and particularly colleagues at the GMC for their assistance.

References

Department of Health (2006) *Good Doctors, Safer Patients: Proposals to Strengthen the System to Assure and Improve the Performance of Doctors and to Protect the Safety of Patients.* TSO (The Stationery Office).

Department of Health (2007) *Trust, Assurance and Safety: The Regulation of Health Professionals.* TSO (The Stationery Office).

General Medical Council (1993) *Professional Conduct and Discipline: Fitness to Practise.* GMC. http://www.gmc-uk.org/guidance/archive/prof_cond_dis_fitness_to_practice_dec_1993.pdf

General Medical Council (2006) *Good Medical Practice.* GMC. http://gmc-uk.org/guidance/good_medical_practice/index.asp

General Medical Council (2007a) *Tomorrow's Doctors.* GMC.

General Medical Council (2007b) *The New Doctor 2007: Outcomes for the First Year of the Foundation Programme.* GMC. http://www.gmc-uk.org/education/documents/Outcomes_for_F1_270307.pdf

General Medical Council & Medical Schools Council (2006). Medical students: professional behaviour and fitness to practise. GMC & MSC.

Merrison, A. W. (1975) Report of the Merrison Committee. *Proceedings of the Royal Society of Medicine,* **68**, 763.

CHAPTER 6

Ethical reasoning in psychiatry

Gwen Adshead

Ethics is the discourse of 'ought' and 'should' in clinical practice. During clinical training we learn what is clinically possible: what we 'can' do. Ethical reasoning is the process of thought and reflection that we engage in when we ask ourselves 'What ought I to do in this situation? What should the good psychiatrist do now?'

Medical ethics has been part of ordinary clinical practice for hundreds of years. In general medicine, ethical dilemmas often arise in unusual or life-threatening situations, or when there is a clash of values between the patient and the doctor. Many of the medical ethical cases that came before the courts in the 1960s involved a clash of values between patients wishing to exercise autonomy of choice in healthcare and the medical profession wishing to fulfil their duty of beneficence. Respect for autonomy and a duty of beneficence are two of four ethical principles that underpin ethical reasoning in medicine; the other two principles are non-maleficence and respect for justice (Box 6.1).

However, in psychiatry, ethical dilemmas are part of everyday clinical practice for a number of reasons. First, psychiatry is an evolving discipline empirically, so it is possible for clinical facts to be interpreted in different ways. For example, one act of self-harm may indicate a high level of suicidality in one patient and not in another, but the current evidence base may make it difficult to tell which is which. Good-quality facts are essential to ethical reasoning, but good clinicians may interpret facts differently, so they will also see the ethical dilemmas differently.

Box 6.1 Four ethical principles in bioethics (Beauchamp & Childress, 2001)

- Respect for autonomy
- A duty of beneficence
- A duty of non-maleficence
- Respect for justice

Second, there are often many different people involved in ethical dilemmas in psychiatry, all of whom will have a different ethical perspective. For example, an elderly male in-patient with a mild degree of Alzheimer's disease wishes to go home. His carers may take one view, his doctors another, his social worker and key nurse yet another. Each person's perspective on the problem may make sense in terms of the ethical principles and attention to the consequences, yet they may be in conflict. Ethical reasoning involves reflection on, and respect for, different sets of values, especially when there appears to be no way to resolve the difference (Woodbridge & Fulford, 2004). Such irremediable clashes of values are an inescapable part of human life in social communities (Berlin, 1991).

Finally, psychiatrists have to engage daily with ethical dilemmas about how best to fulfil their duty to respect patient autonomy and dignity, and the scope of that duty. The autonomy of psychiatric patients is compromised by their mental disorders, to varying degrees over varying timescales, so that they need others to take decisions for them. Some psychiatric patients will be in long-term dependency relationships with both their psychiatrists and their carers: so their autonomy is both relational and complex (Agich, 1993; Adshead, 2002). However, mental disorders do not always compromise autonomy, so it may be hard to know if a patient's choices reflect their true will or if they are actually a product of an abnormal mental state. This is particularly so in relation to choices that involve outcomes that others disapprove of (such as refusal of treatment) or antisocial/criminal behaviour. Finally, psychiatrists are the only doctors who can compel patients to have treatment against their will and in the face of a flat refusal. This means that there is an imbalance of power in most therapeutic relationships that is not found to the same degree elsewhere in medicine.

Ethical advice can found in the General Medical Council's guide to ethics entitled *Good Medical Practice* (General Medical Council, 2006). The Royal College of Psychiatrists (like the other Royal Colleges) has its own version, entitled *Good Psychiatric Practice* (Royal College of Psychiatrists, 2004). There are also other College documents on ethical issues in psychiatry which can (and should) be accessed when needed (Royal College of Psychiatrists, 2002, 2006). The purpose of this chapter is to outline some of the most common ethical dilemmas in psychiatric practice and to offer some ways to initiate an ethical reasoning process. Both the MRCPsych curriculum and the proposed competency frameworks require psychiatrists to have gained some capacity for ethical reasoning during their training.

Common ethical dilemmas in psychiatry

Capacity to consent and refuse treatment

Mental disorders may impair the capacity to make decisions of any kind. For example, advanced dementia may result in the loss of capacity to make legal decisions, such as making a will. Psychiatrists will often be asked to assess an individual's capacity to make a decision, especially in relation to medical treatment. Under English law it is not possible for doctors to make people have treatment for physical disorders against their will, so if patients refuse life-saving treatment there is often concern that they lack capacity to make a legally competent decision.

The ethical dilemma centres around the question of whether the person really has a mental disorder that is affecting their thinking, or whether they are just thinking in ways that other people don't like. For example, a woman with a borderline personality disorder was refusing to eat. Her team wanted to force-feed her with a nasogastric tube. She took them to court, saying that although she had a severe personality disorder, she was still capable of making a legally valid refusal of treatment, which must be respected, even if the consequences were dire for her. The court agreed.

There have been many other similar cases, most of which centre on whether people have a right to make rational decisions and, crucially, whether mentally ill people have a similar right. At present, psychiatric patients are the only patients who do not have a right to refuse treatment for their disorder. They can refuse medical treatment for physical disorders, if they are deemed to have capacity to refuse; but even if they have capacity, they cannot refuse treatment for mental disorders.

There are now several studies of how different mental disorders affect capacity to make decisions (e.g. Grisso & Appelbaum, 1995; Tan *et al*, 2003; Palmer *et al*, 2004). The evidence seems to suggest that diagnosis means very little in terms of capacity; it cannot be assumed that everyone with a diagnostic label of 'schizophrenia' is incapable of making decisions for themselves. Rather, each case must be assessed on its own merits. It is also worth noting that the social trend (at least in legal terms) is respect for the dignity of personal choice over possible harmful consequences.

Forced treatment and detention

One aspect of many mental disorders is that the patient does not accept that they are ill. Other patients accept they are ill but do not wish to have treatment. Some disorders may result in the patient neglecting or endangering themselves; rarely, some disorders (mainly paranoid states) mean that patients present a risk to others. What should psychiatrists do when faced with a patient who is clearly mentally ill but refusing treatment?

This ethical dilemma is one of the most common in mental healthcare. Nearly all countries have developed mental health legislation to address this. Most legislations give powers to mental health professionals to detain people against their will for treatment of their mental condition. Some legislations (including the UK) allow for enforceable involuntary treatment.

The ethically competent psychiatrist will be knowledgeable about mental health law and what can be done using legal powers. There will still be the question of whether the psychiatrist should use those powers. In most

73

cases, the psychiatrist will need to be thoughtful about their duty to help the patient, their duty to do no harm and their duty to act justly. Even if the patient is too ill to consent to treatment, they can (and must) still be treated with respect; dissenting voices (such as those of family or other professionals) also need to be heard. Patients who are forced into treatment against their will may feel distressed and angry; it is part of the psychiatrist's therapeutic duty of beneficence to attend to those feelings, as well as to treating the patient's disorder. Psychiatrists will also have to come to terms with the fact that current legislation means that it is possible to detain people who are perfectly capable of making decisions for themselves and who may resent a psychiatrist's intrusion into their lives. Psychiatrists may also find themselves detaining patients solely for the benefit of other people (usually for the prevention of some anticipated harm). Since one can never know if the harm would have happened if one had not detained the patient, this usually is experienced by the patient as a public safety measure and not a therapeutic one. How many of us would like to be detained in hospital on the basis of a possible harm that we might do in the future?

It might be argued that if we were very sure that the harm was going to happen, then the benefit in preventing harm would outweigh the injury to the patient's sense of dignity and the insult to their claim to liberty and free choice. This brings us to the question of risk assessment (a common practice in psychiatry) and the problems of variations in interpreting facts. Risk is assessed using facts, which may not be interpreted the same by each person. Risk assessments may be both inconsistent and unreliable, but they may be used to justify detention. Would you be happy to be detained on the basis of the risk assessment tools used in your hospital? There is another ethical question about risk assessment: if it is a therapeutic intervention which is part of an overall care plan, then should the good psychiatrist get consent from the patient before carrying out a risk assessment?

Consent to disclosure: truth telling and when to breach confidentiality

The ethical principle of respecting patient confidentiality is an ancient one in medicine. It is taken as a given principle by doctors and patients alike. However, it is common in psychiatry for doctors to want to share information about patients with other people, usually on the grounds that it will be of benefit to the patient, or that it may avert some sort of harm to others. It is ironic that few practitioners worry about confidentiality until they want to breach it!

Any analysis of this dilemma begins with consent. If the patient consents to their material or data being disclosed to another person, then there is no dilemma. It is both courteous and respectful to discuss the issue with the patient and tell them what you intend to tell the other person. It is current NHS policy for patients to receive copies of clinic letters about themselves, and many psychiatric practitioners already make it their practice to discuss with patients the contents of reports and letters to third parties, such as general practitioners (GPs). The main ethical issue here is that it is no longer ethically justifiable to withhold information from patients in case it upsets them, even if they are mentally vulnerable. Rather, all doctors have a duty to deal honestly with patients and to acquire the necessary communication skills to deal with patients' emotional reactions. The current legal position is that patients own their personal information and have right of access to it at all times, the only exception to this being if access to personal information would put others at serious risk of harm.

The much more common situation is when the psychiatrist wants to breach confidentiality but does not want to tell the patient, either because they suspect that the patient would refuse consent to disclosure and/or they think that telling the patient would be risky in some way. Most often these situations arise when the psychiatrist thinks that the patient poses a risk to someone (themselves or others) and that by disclosing information about the patient harm can be averted. For instance, the psychiatrist may wish to warn a potential victim that a patient has made threats against them, or may wish to tell the police that a patient is missing, or may wish to inform the GP that further detention is planned, and in each case may not wish to discuss consent to disclosure with the patient.

These are uncomfortable situations for psychiatrists, because they involve not only a breach of confidentiality without consent but deception of the patient (in the sense of withholding information). If and when patients find out about these disclosures, what they often most object to is the deceit and the sense of being treated like a child. The justification for the ethical insult to autonomy (and injury to feelings) is the benefit obtained by the prevention of serious harm to others. Some would argue that it is beneficial to patients not to be allowed to harm others, although this is not an argument that is routinely used for ordinary citizens (Adshead & Sarkar, 2004). The General Medical Council (GMC) and the courts have taken the view that it is justifiable for doctors to breach patient confidentiality in order to prevent harm to others, especially when those others are actually identifiable and there is good evidence that the breach really will reduce the risk. There are practitioners who regularly advise patients on first meeting that it is their policy to breach confidentiality in situations of possible harm to others, but also that they will discuss those breaches with the patient if at all possible.

Professional boundary violations

It is perhaps not commonly known that, internationally, psychiatrists are over-represented at professional misconduct and unfitness to practise hearings. This suggests that there is something about the practice of psychiatry that makes boundary violations more common. Sexual boundary violations with patients most often come to public attention (probably because they have the potential to cause most harm), but there are other more common types of professional boundary violation that do not, such as financial impropriety, dilemmas to do with receiving gifts and inappropriate self-disclosure, such as sharing personal details about oneself with the patient.

It is worth thinking briefly here about the purpose of professional boundaries. They delineate the therapeutic space between the patient and the professional and demarcate between the doctor's personal identity (and needs and wishes) and their professional identity (and needs and wishes). Boundary violations occur when: (a) aspects of the personal identity creep into the professional space; and (b) there is exploitation of the power differential between the patient and the doctor.

Boundary violations may be more common in psychiatric practice because patients are especially vulnerable in relation to their psychiatrists. Not only do psychiatrists have power in terms of knowledge, they also have actual legal powers to deem someone mentally ill, incompetent to make choices and to detain them involuntarily. Patients have increased vulnerability in terms of their mental conditions and their ordinary distress. In addition, many psychiatric patients have experienced abuse or neglect from care-givers in their childhood and may be especially vulnerable to exploitation by authority figures.

There is a complex issue about the use of personal identity in professional spaces that also may explain why boundary violations are common in psychiatry. Mental healthcare professionals need to be able to use aspects of their personal identity to be effective therapeutic agents. Patients value genuine warmth, humanity and empathy in their psychiatrists, and these personal characteristics enhance therapeutic outcomes. However, if these aspects of personal identity are not carefully reflected on, then they may act as possible triggers for boundary violations. For example, empathy involves reflecting on a patient's emotional experience from their point of view ('I think I can see how that must have seemed to you'). Sympathy involves the sharing of experience ('I felt something similar when that happened to me'). Sympathy involves a sharing of personal information that could potentially lead to a (minor) boundary violation. This is not to say that sympathy is always inappropriate, rather that it is an interpersonal strategy that carries more risk, if only because most major boundary violations begin with minor ones (Sarkar, 2004).

Personal information sharing may be more likely when the psychiatrist is feeling vulnerable. Psychiatrists are a particularly vulnerable professional group in terms of their mental health. They are more likely than other doctors to develop mental health problems, especially depression, anxiety and substance misuse problems. They are at increased risk of suicide compared with most other specialties. These vulnerabilities may explain why psychiatrists can come to rely on their patients to make them feel better, and in that moment bring their personal identity strongly into the professional space.

Although sexual boundary violations have been prohibited by medical ethical codes since Hippocrates, it is remarkable how they persist as a form of misconduct. It is worth repeating that it is ethically unjustifiable to have sexual relationships with patients at any time, even if the patient seems willing. Such misconduct will nearly always result in erasure from the medical register, as well as possible negligence proceedings. Relationships with ex-patients are at least unwise, if not ethically questionable.

Research into boundary violations suggests that all psychiatrists are at potential risk of becoming involved in such behaviours. Seniority, training and experience do not necessarily reduce the risk. The best advice is to pay attention to any sense of anxiety that one has about relationships with certain patients, and to talk about it as early as possible with a trusted colleague. If a minor boundary violation occurs, much better to talk about it with a colleague than let it develop into something more major.

Ethical reasoning in practice

There are many other ethical dilemmas that junior psychiatrists will meet in training, apart from those listed above. Given that we will have to come up with solutions to ethical dilemmas in psychiatric practice, we have an overarching moral duty to make the best-quality decisions we can, so we can be the best psychiatrists we can be. We are not likely to achieve this straight away in our working lives, rather the capacity for ethical reasoning is one that we all engage with and will hopefully continue to develop throughout our working lives.

When faced with an ethical dilemma it is worth reflecting on the following issues.

- What are the facts of the case? Does everyone agree about the facts? Where are the areas of uncertainty? Can these be improved?
- What is the 'should' question? Is there more than one? For example, the casualty officer wants you to admit a patient. You can, in clinical terms: but should you? Are there other values at stake here apart from clinical ones?
- Discussion with other people aids the reflective process. What other ethical perspectives need to be taken into account? Have you considered the ethical point of view of carers or staff? Is there anyone who seems to have a lone dissenting voice in the discussion? (Ignoring dissent in group discussions often leads to bad decisions; Surowiecki, 2005).
- What feelings are involved here? All evaluative reflective processes also involve reflection on feelings. Many ethical positions may be fuelled by anxiety that on reflection is not justified.
- Ethical reflection needs equal consideration of ethical principles involved as well as the consequences of any decision. Medical technical reasoning tends to favour only paying attention to the avoidance of bad consequences and the promotion of good. The problem with this type of reasoning is: (a) that it is not clear whose view of the consequences should count; and (b) it tends to bias discussion in favour of the person who can imagine the worst consequences.

- It is worth documenting the discussions, especially when none of the outcomes is without cost to someone. It may be reassuring to others to let them know how much thought and consideration went into a difficult ethical decision; that the decision was made 'in good faith'.
- The ethical reflective process may lead you to the conclusion that your own position, no matter how heartfelt, may not be the most compelling!

Conclusions

The purpose of medical ethical education is said to be twofold: to create virtuous doctors and to provide a way for doctors to think about ethical dilemmas in practice (Eckles *et al*, 2005). This chapter is intended to offer some ways of improving thinking about common ethical dilemmas in psychiatry. To become a virtuous psychiatrist involves reflection on our own stories of why we became psychiatrists: the narrative of our personal and professional identities. But that, as they say, is another story.

References

Adshead, G. (2002) A different voice in psychiatric ethics. In *Health Care Ethics and Human Values* (eds K. W. M. Fulford, D. Dickenson & T. Murray), pp. 56–62. Blackwell.

Adshead, G. & Sarkar, S. (2004) Ethical issues in forensic psychiatry. *Psychiatry*, **3**, 5–16.

Agich, G. (1993) *Autonomy in Long Term Care*. Oxford University Press.

Beauchamp, T. & Childress, J. (2001) Principles of Biomedical Ethics (5th edn). Oxford University Press.

Berlin, I. (1991) *The Crooked Timber of Humanity*. Fontana.

Eckles, R. E., Meslin, E. M., Gaffney, M., *et al* (2005) Medical ethics education: where are we? Where should we be going? A review. *Academic Medicine*, **80**, 1143–1152.

General Medical Council (2006) *Good Medical Practice 2006*. GMC.

Grisso, T. & Appelbaum, P. (1995) The MacArthur Treatment Competence Study III: abilities of patients to consent to psychiatric and medical treatment. *Law and Human Behaviour*, **19**, 149–174.

Palmer, B. W., Dunn, l. B., Appelbaum, P., *et al* (2004) Correlates of treatment-related decision making capacity among middle aged and older patients with schizophrenia. *Articles of general Psychiatry*, **61**, 230–236.

Royal College of Psychiatrists (2002) *Vulnerable Patients, Vulnerable Doctors: Good Practice in our Clinical Relationships* (College Report CR101). Royal College of Psychiatrists.

Royal College of Psychiatrists (2004) *Good Psychiatric Practice* (2nd edn) (College Report CR125). Royal College of Psychiatrists.

Royal College of Psychiatrists (2006) *Good Psychiatric Practice: Confidentiality and Information Sharing* (College Report CR133). Royal College of Psychiatrists.

Sarkar, S. P. (2004) Sexual boundary violations in psychiatry and psychotherapy: a review. *Advances in Psychiatric Treatment*, **10**, 312–320.

Surowiecki, J. (2005) *The Wisdom of Crowds*. Abacus.

Tan, J., Hope, A. & Stewart, A. (2003) Competence to refuse treatment in anorexia nervosa. *International Journal of Law and Psychiatry*, **26**, 697–707.

Woodbridge, K. & Fulford, K. W. M. (2004) *Whose Values?* Sainsbury Centre for Mental Health.

CHAPTER 7

Compulsory treatment, capacity and consent

Jonathan Bindman

This chapter provides an overview of the legal basis for compulsory psychiatric treatment, considering broad principles used in a range of jurisdictions but also considering the Mental Health Act 1983 in England and Wales as a specific example of mental health legislation. Legal compulsion forms part of a spectrum of coercive pressures exerted upon patients to take treatment against their will, and the role of the law is placed in the context of coercion more generally.

The ethical justifications for compulsory treatment are then considered. These are not always explicitly considered in legislation. The Mental Health Act 1983, for example, allows wide scope for paternalistic clinical judgements about the necessity for treatment against the patient's will. However, other ethical approaches to such judgements may be of value to the clinician when faced with difficult clinical decisions. Indeed, even in England and Wales it may be essential. For example, although proposals to introduce a clear ethical framework, based on assessment of mental capacity, into a new mental health act for England and Wales have not been accepted, the Mental Capacity Act 2005 does require doctors to apply a test of decision-making capacity in a range of circumstances, as does recent legislation in Scotland (the Mental Health (Care and Treatment) (Scotland) Act 2003). Accordingly, an ethical framework for compulsion based on the consideration of capacity is outlined. When an explicitly ethical approach is taken to compulsion, various forms of advance decision-making, such as advance directives, become important in those mental disorders which result in fluctuating capacity, and these are therefore described.

General principles of compulsory treatment

The use of the law to compel treatment is only one aspect of a more general issue, coercion. It has been suggested that coercion can helpfully be understood as forming part of a spectrum of 'treatment pressures'. For example, Szmukler & Applebaum (2001) conceptualise a hierarchy

---

Box 7.1 Hierarchy of treatment pressures (Szmukler & Applebaum, 2001)

- Persuasion
- Leverage
- Inducements
- Threats
- Compulsion (including the use of physical force)

---

of 'treatment pressures' (Box 7.1) which may assist in understanding and making decisions to treat involuntarily.

Persuasion, leverage and inducement

These may be described as 'positive pressures' to take treatment – the 'carrots' rather than the 'sticks'. The lowest level of treatment pressure is persuasion, in which the professional sets out the benefits for the client of a particular course of action and attempts to counter objections. The patient is free to reject advice. The next level of pressure, leverage, assumes an interpersonal relationship between the client and professional which has an element of emotional dependence. This gives the professional power to pressure the client by demonstrating approval of one course of action or disapproval of another. Greater pressure may be exerted by inducement, in which acceptance of treatment is linked to material help, such as support in accessing charitable or welfare funds over and above any basic entitlement.

Threats and compulsion

These 'negative pressures' are overtly coercive. A threat could be made to withdraw services on which the client normally relies (which is more coercive than simply failing to offer inducements over and above normal services) or to detain in hospital. Finally, legally sanctioned compulsory treatment is at the highest level of the hierarchy of pressure, carrying with it the power to use physical force to overcome resistance to treatment.

The use of coercion as a routine part of care fundamentally distinguishes psychiatry from other areas of medicine, in which the autonomy of the competent patient to refuse treatment is more usually assumed. The association of physical restraint with mental healthcare has historic roots, preceding the English law of 1714 which permitted Justices of the Peace to secure the arrest of any person 'furiously mad and dangerous' and to lock them up securely for as long as 'such lunacy and madness shall continue'.

Historically, compulsory treatment has usually involved detention in a hospital, although this has also long been associated with restrictions which could be applied after discharge to the community, using the threat of readmission (conditional discharge). As community care has developed in many countries during the past 40 years, it has been increasingly argued that as the locus of treatment moves from hospital to community, so should the powers of compulsion. Compulsory treatment in the community (known as involuntary out-patient commitment in the USA and by a range of local terms such as community treatment orders elsewhere) has spread through a number of jurisdictions in recent decades, but this has also resulted in controversy and calls for restrictions on its use. The extent to which the need for it is supported by evidence is contested and is considered further below.

Compulsory treatment in different jurisdictions

The legal structures that govern the use of involuntary commitment vary in their detailed application between jurisdictions. However, some common themes can be identified.

- High-income countries all have specific laws that regulate the commitment of those with mental illness. They are therefore assumed from a legal point of view to be distinguishable from other people who may require control by the police, or from those who are in need of medical treatment but are unable to consent to it owing to temporary or permanent mental incapacity (such as those with dementia or learning disability). However, as definitions of mental disorder tend not to be universally accepted, lawmakers must decide to what extent to leave the judgement of who is mentally ill to professionals and to what extent to set legal limits upon it. In England and Wales the law relies upon clinicians to diagnose a degree of 'mental disorder' justifying compulsory treatment, but also states that substance misuse problems or unusual sexual behaviours are insufficient in themselves to justify the diagnosis.
- The law must state the criteria for compulsion. The criteria usually included are considered further below. A distinction is usually also made between the stringency of the criteria to be applied in an emergency or to detain for a short period of assessment, and those applied for longer term treatments, and additional safeguards may be required for treatments that are controversial or irreversible such as electroconvulsive therapy (ECT) and psychosurgery.
- The law must describe the way in which compulsion will be exercised, the roles assigned to police, doctors, other professionals such as social workers or nurses, and the role of the courts. The courts may have the primary role in authorising detention (as they did in the UK prior to 1959) or this may be left to mental health professionals who can use varying degrees of police powers to enforce treatment. However, even in systems where mental health professionals are given a wide

discretion to manage compulsion, they are likely to rely on the police to support them in physically removing patients to hospital.

- The law will include rights of appeal whereby a patient subject to compulsion, or an authorised representative, can challenge professional decisions. Relatives or carers may also have specified rights either to seek compulsory treatment or to oppose it.
- A distinction is usually made between the application of mental health legislation to people who have committed criminal offences and have mental disorder, compulsory psychiatric treatment being one of the 'disposal' options available to the courts, and those who have not committed offences and are therefore subject to civil measures.

Criteria for compulsion

Criteria for compulsion, although varying in different jurisdictions, also have common themes. It is usual for them to include the presence of mental illness, a consequent risk to the patient or to others and the likelihood of treatment having a positive effect. The 'least restrictive principle', that treatment should be given with the least restriction of liberty possible, may be stated.

A useful version of these criteria is that prepared by the WHO (World Health Organization, 2005) in their *Resource Book on Mental Health, Human Rights and Legislation*, which recommends minimum standards to be applied in all jurisdictions (see Box 7.2).

Although these are desirable criteria, and most appear in some form in jurisdictions in which mental health legislation is well developed, there is

---

Box 7.2 Criteria for involuntary commitment (World Health Organization, 2005: p. 47)

- A person may be admitted involuntarily to a mental health facility ... if ... a qualified mental health practitioner authorised by law determines ... that the person has a mental illness and considers:
  - that because of that mental illness, there is a serious likelihood of immediate or imminent harm to that person or other persons; or
  - that in the case of a person whose mental illness is severe and whose judgement is impaired, failure to admit ... is likely to lead to serious deterioration ... or will prevent the giving of appropriate treatment that can only be given by admission ...
- In the latter case a second such mental health practitioner, independent of the first, should be consulted where possible ...
- A mental health facility may receive involuntarily admitted patients only if the facility has been designated to do so by a competent authority prescribed by domestic law.

room for debate. For example, the WHO criteria include both the concept of mental illness, as judged by an expert practitioner, and the concept of impaired judgement (also known as impaired capacity to make decisions). It can be argued that if impaired capacity (assessed by a doctor or by another legal process) is present, then the criterion of diagnosed mental illness is redundant. By this argument, people with mental illness but without impaired capacity should be allowed to determine their own treatment, whereas people with impaired capacity may be treated involuntarily, in their own best interests, regardless of diagnosis.

The criteria allow wide latitude for clinical judgement, not only about the presence of mental illness but also about the seriousness or imminence of risk (notoriously hard to assess accurately), the likelihood of deterioration without treatment, or what treatment is appropriate. Legal criteria provide a framework for clinical decisions but do not determine them.

Ethical basis of compulsory psychiatric treatment

The usual justifications for pressurising patients to accept treatment involve risks to the health or safety of the patient or the safety of others, although these risks are often rather poorly defined and rarely quantifiable. Deciding what level of pressure is commensurate with the risk is not straightforward, but it may be helpful to try to apply an ethical framework commonly used to assist decision-making in general medicine. This requires consideration of the person's capacity to take treatment decisions in their best interests. Decision-making capacity (subsequently referred to just as 'capacity') is usually defined as the ability to understand and retain information about the proposed treatment and to weigh in the balance the consequences of alternative decisions. People with capacity can determine what treatment is in their own best interests, even where their views do not accord with those of clinicians, and minimal pressure, perhaps limited to persuasion, is all that can be justified. If capacity is lacking, the treatment that is in the person's best interest may need to be determined by clinicians, although taking account if possible of the past and present wishes of the patient and the views of significant others. The minimal level of pressure necessary to achieve the objectives of this treatment can then be exerted.

Although the application of this framework is helpful in clarifying the decision to be taken, community teams are often faced with situations where a simple judgement of capacity is not easy to make. A client may, apparently through choice, live in squalor or even on the streets. Does such an apparently irrational choice necessarily imply a lack of capacity or must delusional reasoning be established? Even if capacity seems to be absent, what minimum standard of living is in the best interests of a patient who expresses no desire for material comforts?

The use of alcohol or drugs may complicate the issue further. Again, if a patient uses substances that are clearly detrimental to health and well-being, does this in itself imply impaired capacity or is it necessary (or possible) to distinguish between 'normal' self-harming behaviours (which are of course very common in most societies), chosen with full capacity, and those that arise from 'mental disorder'? The Mental Health Act 1983 in England and Wales specifically excludes a substance use disorder as providing evidence for mental disorder of the kind justifying compulsion, but clinicians may still be faced with difficulties where substance misuse coexists in a complex relationship with altered mood or psychosis.

Faced with such complex issues, it is tempting to resort to the traditional medical approach of assuming that best interests are best determined by a beneficent doctor. However, attempting to apply a capacity-based approach makes it clear that it is the client's reasoning about their own situation that is the starting point for the decision, and makes it less likely that the values, anxieties, or prejudices of others will prevail over the client's expressed views. Sharing difficult decisions with multidisciplinary teams, carers and advocates similarly reduces the risk of poor or hasty judgements.

Although the Mental Health Act 1983 in England and Wales allows compulsion on the grounds of risk to others, and mental health services are exposed to strong societal expectations that they should prevent violence by their patients, attempting to take an ethical approach to treatment pressure on these grounds presents considerable difficulties. There are very few circumstances in which citizens without mental disorder can be detained preventatively on the grounds of risk, and it is hard to justify taking a different approach to clients of mental health services with capacity. The challenge for community mental health services is to avoid being pressured into applying an ethical double standard, in which behaviour that would not justify significant sanction in the absence of mental disorder is used to justify loss of liberty, or levels of treatment pressure that are not commensurate with the actual level of risk.

Advance statements, decisions and directives

An advance statement is a declaration made by a service user about preferences for treatment should future episodes of psychosis impair capacity to make their own decisions. The statement is intended to influence the practice of professionals towards practice more acceptable to the service user. It provides a way in which clinicians can be helped to determine what is in a service users 'best interests' when attempting to apply ethical reasoning to complex decisions about compulsion.

However, the criteria used in mental health legislation may not specifically require that the clinician consider the client's 'best interests' in its legal sense, in which case it will be possible to override an advance statement. A study in Bradford (Thomas & Cahill, 2004) sought to encourage service users to develop advance statements, but the principal finding was that only a very small proportion of service users made statements and the project generally 'failed to enthuse them'. It was suggested that although intended to empower service users, the advance statements were not in fact perceived as doing so, possibly because they can be overridden. This leaves open the question of whether, if clinicians were bound by such statements, they might be perceived as empowering by service users and be more widely taken up.

Joint crisis plans

These are also a form of advance statement but differ from a simple statement of treatment preferences in two crucial aspects. First, they are formulated together with the care team (hence 'joint' plans) and resolution of any conflicts between service user preferences and the care team is sought when drawing up the plan rather than being left to cause difficulties when a crisis arises. Second, a neutral facilitator works with the service user and care team to draw up the plan. The resource requirements, both in terms of time and for the facilitator, are therefore greater than simply asking the service user to prepare a statement. A randomised controlled trial in the UK (Henderson *et al*, 2004) has reported that joint crisis plans can reduce the use of detention under the Mental Health Act 1983. Of the 80 service users who had joint crisis plans, 10 (13%) were detained over a 15-month follow-up period compared with 21 of 80 (27%) in the control group ($P = 0.03$). Admissions were slightly reduced but not to a statistically significant extent, the risk of admission in the intervention group being 0.69 of that in the control group ($P = 0.07$) and the mean number of bed days only being reduced from 36 to 32 ($P = 0.15$).

However, only 36% of service users who could have taken part actually agreed to do so, and hence as with the Bradford study (Thomas & Cahill, 2004) there are clearly obstacles to take up. The authors suggest that these include the belief that the plans would not make any difference, reluctance to consider the possibility of becoming ill again and that existing plans were felt to be adequate.

Crisis cards

These were developed by service user movement 20 years ago as an early version of advance statements. They are designed to be carried by service users to provide immediate information on preferences in crisis situations. A crisis card was used in a pilot study in Croydon (Sutherby *et al*, 1999) which preceded the trial of joint crisis plans, and this and various other versions have been adopted by some local services. Crisis cards differ from joint crisis plans in that there is no specific process by which differences between the service user's and professional views of treatment in crisis are identified and resolved.

Crisis plans

The term 'crisis plan' is often used in services; it is a list of actions to be taken in a future crisis which may form part of care programme approach

(CPA) documentation. Crisis plans tend to be drawn up by clinicians, possibly with no service user involvement. However, if carried out as part of a CPA review at which the service user's preferences for future treatment in crisis are recorded, they would have the characteristics of an advance statement.

Conclusions

Legal compulsion is commonly used by psychiatric services and although laws differ between jurisdictions there are common themes concerning the nature of legislation and the criteria for deciding who should be subject to it. Coercive treatment is even more commonly used and legal compulsion is at the extreme end of a spectrum of treatment pressures. The law usually allows for psychiatric patients to be compelled to accept treatment in a way that is distinct from other forms of medical treatment, despite the difficulty of making any absolute distinction between the ability of people with mental disorder and the ability of anyone else to make decisions about their treatment. Even where the law does not require clinicians to do so, it may be valuable to attempt to apply general principles of medical ethics to coercive treatment in psychiatry. This does not provide a simple guide to action but may contribute to treatment decisions that are more acceptable to patients and carers, and also to doctors.

References

Henderson, C., Flood, C., Leese, M., *et al* (2004) Effect of joint crisis plans on use of compulsory treatment in psychiatry: single blind randomised controlled trial. *BMJ*, **329**, 136.

Sutherby, K., Szmukler, G., Halpern, A., *et al* (1999) A study of crisis cards in a community psychiatric service. *Acta Psychiatrica Scandinavica*, **100**, 56–61.

Szmukler, G. & Appelbaum, P. (2001) Treatment pressures, coercion and compulsion. In *Textbook of Community Psychiatry* (eds G. Thornicroft & G. Szmukler), pp. 529–544. Oxford University Press.

Thomas, P. & Cahill, A. (2004) Compulsion and psychiatry – the role of advance statements. *BMJ*, **329**, 122–123.

World Health Organization (2005) *WHO Resource Book on Mental Health, Human Rights and Legislation*. WHO. http://www.who.int/entity/mental_health/policy/who_rb_mnh_hr_leg_FINAL_11_07_05.pdf

Part 2

CHAPTER 8

Bio-psychosocial models of aetiology and management

Peter Tyrer

There have been dramatic changes in the way in which psychiatry has perceived its task over the past two millennia but the most rapid changes have been in the past 200 years. At the beginning of the twentieth century the predominant view of most psychiatric disorders was that they are degenerative conditions that can only be prevented by advances in neuroscience or control of infections such as syphilis. This remained the prevailing view well into the latter part of the twentieth century. In this model the patient was a passive recipient of treatment that was designed to counteract neurological and pathophysiological abnormalities. This model was promoted and reinforced by the apparently successful introduction of prefrontal leucotomy, electroconvulsive therapy and insulin coma therapy, and the psychopharmacological revolution which began with the introduction of chlorpromazine in 1950.

Nevertheless, psychologists and social psychiatrists began to express their dissatisfaction in the 1930s and the attack on what became 'the medical model' increased in ferocity in the last quarter of the century. The introduction of successful psychological treatments and the demonstration that psychological problems could be created, or at least triggered, by life events also changed attitudes. The notion gradually developed that there was much more to psychiatric disorders, and indeed most physical disorders, than simple pathogens or constitutional defects, and both the psychological and social manifestations of illness assumed much greater prominence.

The important turning point came with an article by George Engel in *Science* in 1977. Engel was based at the University of Rochester and, with the help of the first Chair of Psychiatry at the university, Professor John Romano, he developed a curriculum based on the bio-psychosocial model for all undergraduates at the university covering all disciplines. Engel's article in *Science* used both schizophrenia and diabetes as exemplars and emphasised that the bio-psychosocial model applied to all illnesses. Engel was not a psychiatrist but the bio-psychosocial model has perhaps been embraced most readily by those working in the field of mental illness.

It is now generally accepted that the bio-psychosocial model is the most appropriate single model for use in medical practice. However, one has to be careful not to be use Engel's model in a holistic way at all times. This is because it is impossible to accommodate all aspects of the model when treating an individual patient, particularly in an emergency. We (Tyrer & Steinberg, 2005) have argued that there are four models operating at different times within psychiatric practice (and indeed in other areas of medicine) and that these need to be harnessed appropriately at different times. The four models are the disease, psychodynamic, cognitive–behavioural and social models.

Disease model

The disease model implicitly assumes that every aspect of mental pathology is accompanied by physical pathology. It also assumes that the classification of this pathology allows mental illness to be ordered in exactly the same way as physical medicine, in which all illnesses have characteristic common features. As with physical illness it also assumes that mental illness is disabling and is disadvantageous to the individual, and that the cause of mental illness is directly explicable by its physical consequences.

The procedure used to identify the mental disease is the same as in general medicine but uses somewhat different processes. So the identification of physical signs is replaced by the investigation of mental signs (phenomenology), and the taking of the history includes much more than may often be necessary with a physical disease. The process of providing a systematic mental examination of behaviour, speech, thought and cognition is analogous to the systematic examination of each organ system in medicine, and the special terminology (often inappropriately called jargon) to describe the abnormal features of the mental state (e.g. command hallucinations) is the equivalent of clinical abnormalities such as 'hepatomegaly' in medicine. The 'diagnostic formulation' that is completed at the end of this assessment is similar to the provisional diagnosis of a medical problem.

The second stage of the medical model is to identify the pathology associated with the abnormal clinical features identified in the first stage. This is clearly missing for many mental illnesses but in the longer term would probably become essential. Thus the widespread use of computed tomography (CT) and magnetic resonance imaging (MRI) scans of the brain are helping to unravel many of the abnormal signs that are found in different mental illnesses. This is clearly true of many organic psychoses, particularly the dementias, but is now also becoming relevant in schizophrenia and other psychoses. Clearly for most of the common mental disorders tests of pathology are really only introduced to exclude other causes, but it is to be expected in the future that specific biological tests will identify the abnormalities associated with each specific disorder, and this is the intent of the authors of the fifth edition of the *Diagnostic and Statistical Manual of Mental Disorders* (DSM–V) (Kupfer *et al*, 2002).

Psychodynamic model

Although many regard the psychodynamic model as a stage in the development of psychiatry, it still constitutes an important element of psychiatric thinking. The central process in the psychodynamic model is the analysis of patterns of feeling. These are often difficult to access and we rationalise a large proportion of them. However, they are shown in various ways, often disguised, and this requires further and often subtle analysis. Much of this revolves around the notion that a large part of our thinking goes on at an unconscious level and our conscious assumptions about how our thoughts and feelings have developed may often be quite wrong.

An associated principle is that those feelings that are kept unconscious are often deliberately kept under wraps because they are considered dangerous or uncomfortable to expose openly. 'Unblocking' these pathways is an important part of the psychodynamic process and may be associated with considerable resistance. Following from this, the difficulties we have in our relationships with others, which are largely a product of our underlying feelings, tend to repeat themselves across settings and across time. It is therefore reasonable to assume that difficulties in one setting and with one person may therefore spread to others, and that the same patterns of difficulty may re-emerge on each occasion. Many of these abnormal patterns seem to be established during childhood.

It is also assumed in psychoanalytical theory, but not necessarily in all psychodynamic understanding, that the therapist ought to be fully aware of the nature of the interactions and feelings (transference and countertransference) and therefore should have special training (if not a personal analysis) in order to understand these difficulties. This will help the therapist to understand mental mechanisms such as projection and denial, which might not be recognised fully.

It is also important in psychotherapy for the therapist to be non-judgemental and neutral in all areas. It is also wise to assume that there are deficiencies in everybody that are to varying extents hidden, and that there is no innate superiority in any one individual. The variation introduced by different schools of psychotherapy is relatively unimportant in the model itself. Much of psychodynamic therapy could be regarded as 'guided exploration' in which untrained people can quickly get lost.

Cognitive–behavioural model

The cognitive–behavioural model is now very well known but it is important to recognise that it was preceded by a simple behavioural model, best illustrated by early studies of phobias (e.g. Watson & Raynor, 1920), and

91

has only more recently added the cognitive component. The basic tenet of the model is that peoples' thinking determines their view of the world, that this cognition influences symptoms, behaviour and attitudes, and thereby the features of mental illness. Persistence of mental illness is often the consequence of continuing errors in both thinking and maladaptive behaviour. Changes both for the better or worse in mental disorder are always associated with significant change in cognition and behaviour. In most circumstances the cognitive–behavioural model tests current thinking and attitudes but it can extend to long-standing beliefs or schemas (for example in the treatment of personality disorder; Tyrer & Davidson, 2000). The model is a collaborative one and the patient must be closely engaged in its development. Hence the therapist does not know exactly where it is going at the beginning of treatment, but has a set of rules that are more explicit than those in psychotherapy that allow the therapist to decide when the process is approaching its end. Virtually every mental illness has been subjected to the cognitive–behavioural model with a degree of success.

The model has essentially developed through the efforts of one man, Aaron Tim Beck (1976), a psychoanalyst who became unhappy with the conventional methods of psychoanalysis and concentrated instead on changing the patterns of thinking of his patients. The cognitive–behavioural model is very much an empirical model that takes evidence from individual patients, integrates it with a general approach to treatment and then provides specific rational interventions that change the patients' patterns of thinking so that they are more adaptive and positive. The preceding behavioural model was much more limiting and was motivated as much by a reaction to the psychodynamic model as to the need for a separate structure for behaviourism. When Hans Eysenck attacked psychoanalysis he argued that learning theory does not postulate any unconscious causes and regarded neurotic symptoms as simply learned habits: there is no neurosis underlying the symptom but merely the symptom itself. 'Get rid of the symptom and you have eliminated the neurosis' (Eysenck & Rachman, 1965). He was highlighting the frustration caused by psychoanalysis being preoccupied with past events and feelings but forgetting the present, and the fact that there were no reliable methods of getting rid of the symptoms except in a few specific cases, notably the phobias. The cognitive–behavioural model, however, has much greater adaptability and covers a whole field of psychiatric distress, from the simple effects of distress to the disintegrating effects of schizophrenia. Although there must be limits to the advance of cognitive–behavioural approaches, they do not appear to have been reached yet.

Social model

The social model in its most extreme form attempts to 'de-medicalise' all mental illness. It regards psychiatric disorder as a direct consequence of societal forces and events that create problems for the individual which are subsequently labelled as 'illness'. This is immediately understandable for conditions that are clearly related to external stress (for example those that have a 'Z' code in the *ICD-10 Classification of Mental and Behavioural Disorders*; World Health Organization, 1992). It is much less clear for many chronic and more serious mental illnesses. The best example is the famous theory of Ronald Laing and others which postulated that schizophrenia was a consequence of individuals being exposed to sets of conflicting messages from which the only escape was into a different form of reality: a psychotic reality that was not a true representation of the world but at least made more logical sense.

The social model is relevant at all stages of psychiatric illness. It is particularly apposite at the beginning of end of contact with services. Thus the initial access to services and the willingness for people to take advantage of their availability is governed strongly by social factors. Even in a sophisticated country such as the United States, where mental illness is discussed openly in all sections of society, at any one time 20–28% of people with psychiatric illness are not in contact with any services (Regier *et al*, 1993). Of course, those not in contact with services might have minor conditions that can be dealt with without any specialist input, which would indicate that the threshold for diagnosis is perhaps too low, but it could indicate that many of those who could be helped are not seeking assistance because of prejudice and stigma, and because of the social implications of attending mental health services.

After the acute phase of a psychiatric illness, the social model is also very much to the fore. After discharge from a psychiatric hospital there are major problems in adjusting to life outside and the individual is faced with all sorts of changes that have taken place as a consequence of their psychiatric care. These are often major changes and appropriate adjustments can be difficult. This is illustrated by the high rate of suicide in the initial 4 weeks after discharge from psychiatric hospital, a rate which is 400 times that expected in equivalent populations (Goldacre *et al*, 1993).

The natural consequence of adopting a social model is that a broader societal view has to be taken of mental illness and its management. This not only involves examining the impact of illness on the patient and changes that are necessary to return to equilibrium, but also examining the individual in the context of society, beginning with family and friends and extending to the community as a whole. This is particularly relevant when dealing with conditions that may be associated with violent or antisocial behaviour (for example schizophrenia and antisocial personality disorder) and explains why such conditions have attained such prominence in this context.

Integrating the four models

Although many practitioners insist glibly that they follow the bio-psychosocial model, in practice they frequently do not. Only recently the then President of the American Psychiatric Association, Steven Sharfstein, commented 'the bio-psychosocial model is increasingly being converted into the bio-bio-bio model by the influence of the pharmaceutical industry' (Sharfstein, 2005). It is also not easy to adopt all facets of the model simultaneously. Many practitioners insist they are doing so when they adopt what is often called a 'holistic approach', and this is particularly popular with those who practice complementary or alternative therapies. In practice, this just means being pleasant, accommodating and enquiring about peoples personal circumstances, wishes and needs, and then applying a specific therapy which is applied anyway in such a case and is not a direct consequence of the information obtained.

We have suggested that the best way of integrating the four models described above is to adopt a hierarchical approach (Fig. 1; Tyrer & Steinberg, 2005). In the hierarchical model it is first important to decide at which level each patient is in the hierarchy. At the very top level the patient is extremely ill, often psychotic, and frequently lacks capacity. The model illustrated in Fig. 1 bears some resemblance to a hierarchical model proposed by Foulds over 40 years ago (Foulds, 1965). The highest level of the latter model was 'disintegrating psychoses'. However, in addition to such psychoses, of which the most common examples are schizophrenia and the psychotic phases of bipolar disorder, we also place organic conditions such as Alzheimer's disease and other related dementias, psychoses associated with substance misuse (Korsakoff's syndrome) and psychotic depression in this highest level. At this level it is necessary to employ the disease model to produce effective intervention. Thus, for the patient who presents in a catatonic stupor and is not eating or drinking it is quite inappropriate to expect that any model based on conversational interaction with the patient is going to produce a dramatic effect. The important thing is for the patient

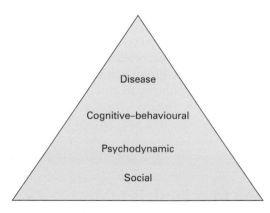

Fig. 8.1 Hierarchical relationship between the four models used in psychiatry. Note that in a true hierarchy all higher levels include those below in the hierarchy.

to eat and drink and have their basic bodily needs attended to before they can be engaged in other forms of treatment. In extreme instances it is therefore appropriate to give life-saving treatment such as electroconvulsive therapy without consent, as long as proper procedures are followed, including seeking one or more second opinions.

At the second level, the cognitive–behavioural level, the patient is able to engage in discussion and debate, and is able to formulate responses to questions and engage in quite complex interactive processes. This is the time that cognitive–behavioural approaches can be used, both in schizophrenia when the acute phase and its management has been completed, and in less serious conditions such as anxiety, depression and phobic disorders in which there is considerable distress but no impairment of reality constructs. Debate will take place over whether intervention is necessary with drugs or psychological treatments, or if a combination in what proportion, and the patient's views will be taken into account when making these decisions.

The third stage, the psychodynamic stage, is necessary when a level of improvement has been obtained and choices in how to move forward have to be made. Having an understanding of hidden motivation and past conflicts may be of particular value here and is particularly relevant when choosing long-term plans to promote good mental health. Issues of transference and countertransference are also relevant here; if the patient is irritating there may be a strong tendency to prescribe and so close the interview.

The social model is at the lowest level of the hierarchy, but this does not mean that it is the least important. The final integration of a person back into society in a form that is satisfactory for both the individual and for societal components is very important, and in many instances will determine whether that individual relapses in the future.

At this level the usage of treatments, particularly drug treatment, is very difficult to justify. This is a current area of concern because the need for pharmaceutical companies to increase market penetration often leads to symptoms that represent normal variation being treated with drugs, with a great increase in prescriptions but no improvement in symptoms or function. An example is the use of antidepressants in Iceland (Helgason et al, 2004), a study in which it was found that sales of antidepressants increased eightfold over 25 years but had no effect on suicide or disability due to depression.

Summary

The bio-psychosocial model is alive and well but needs to be structured before it can be fully implemented. Aquilina & Warner (2004) have summarised the model well across the areas of aetiology and management.

- Predisposing: what made this problem likely?
- Precipitating: why did it start then and not before?
- Perpetuating: why is it still going on?

Using their three 'Ps', predisposing, precipitating and perpetuating factors, it is easy to identify relevant elements from each of the four models above as well as the three elements in the bio-psychosocial model. This also helps enormously in the functioning of the multidisciplinary team, where the different models are held in varying esteem by its members, and recognition of these differences is the first step towards resolution of these difficulties.

References

Aquilina, C. & Warner, J. (2004) *A Guide to Psychiatric Examination*. PasTest.

Beck, A. T. (1976) *Cognitive Theory and the Emotional Disorders*. International Universities Press.

Engel, G. L. (1977) The need for a new medical model; a challenge for medicine. *Science*, **196**, 129–136.

Eysenck, H. & Rachman, S. (1965) *The Causes and Cures of Neurosis*. Routledge & Kegan Paul.

Foulds, G. (1965) *Personality and Personal Illness*. Tavistock Press.

Goldacre, M., Seagroatt, V. & Hawton, K. (1993) Suicide after discharge from psychiatric inpatient care. *Lancet*, **342**, 283–286.

Helgason, T., Tómasson, H. & Zoega, T. (2004) Antidepressants and public health in Iceland: time series analysis of national data. *British Journal of Psychiatry*, **184**, 157–162.

Kupfer, D. J., First, M. B. & Regier, D. E. (2002) Introduction. In *A Research Agenda for DSM–V*, p. xix. American Psychiatric Association.

Regier, D. A., Narrow, W. E., Rae, D. S., *et al* (1993) The de facto US mental and addictive disorders service system: epidemiologic catchment area prospective 1-year prevalence rates of disorders and services. *Archives of General Psychiatry*, **50**, 85–94.

Sharfstein, S. S. (2005) Big Pharma and American psychiatry: the good, the bad, and the ugly. *Psychiatric News*, 19 (August 19), 3.

Tyrer, P. & Davidson, K. (2000) Cognitive therapy in personality disorders. In *Review of Psychiatry: Personality Disorders* (eds G. O. Gabbard & J. Gunderson), pp. 33–64. American Psychiatric Press.

Tyrer, P. & Steinberg, D. (2005) *Models for Mental Disorder: Conceptual Models in Psychiatry* (4th edn). Wiley.

Watson, J. B. & Raynor, R. (1920) Conditional emotional reactions. *American Journal of Psychology*, **55**, 313–317.

World Health Organization (1992) *ICD–10 Classification of Mental and Behavioural Disorders*. WHO.

CHAPTER 9

Clinical psychology

Padmal de Silva

Clinical psychology is a well-established discipline in healthcare, although its formal beginnings in the UK date from after the Second World War. Clinical psychologists are essentially healthcare professionals, working primarily in the field of mental health. It is important to recognise, however, that there has been rapid expansion of the scope of clinical psychology into areas other than mental health in the past two decades. For example, clinical psychologists now work directly with general practitioners (GPs), in settings of general medicine and surgery, in the care of the elderly and the dying, in HIV/AIDS services and in social service settings. Despite these developments, clinical psychology is still as a profession most closely connected with mental healthcare.

Clinical psychologists are both practitioners and scientists, and the profession has repeatedly stressed this dual role. Clinical psychologists apply the principles and methods of psychology, which may be defined as the science of behaviour and experience, to the investigation, assessment and treatment of psychological disorders, and other aspects of behaviour. In practice, in mental health settings this consists of:

- the assessment of patients and their problems, both with established psychological tests and instruments, and through intensive individual investigation
- the treatment of various disorders and specific behavioural problems using psychological techniques
- the evaluation of the effects of psychological and other interventions
- research into aspects of mental disorder.

Trained clinical psychologists engage in these various activities with different emphases and time allocations, depending on the setting and the job requirements. Many also engage in a certain amount of formal and informal teaching, both of trainees and/or junior psychologists and of members of other professions. In their research activities, many psychologists engage in collaborative research, with medical and other colleagues.

Training

The special skills and knowledge that the clinical psychologist brings to the multidisciplinary team derive from two formal stages of training. The first is undergraduate training in the science of experimental psychology, which includes skills in observation, experimentation and evaluation, and knowledge of the large and growing literature on normal human behaviour, including the principles of learning, basic psychological processes such as perception and cognition, and social and other influences on behaviour. It also includes familiarity with literature on animal behaviour, which has contributed significantly to the development of the theories of learning.

The more obviously 'clinical' skills and knowledge are acquired during postgraduate training, which is required for entering the profession of clinical psychology. This training in the UK usually consists of a 3-year university course. Until relatively recently, many universities ran 2-year courses, but the expansion of the scope of the subject has led to courses being extended to 3 years. These courses usually lead to a practitioner doctorate (e.g. DClinPsy). The training includes academic teaching on abnormal psychology; relevant areas of other subjects, including psychiatry, neurology and pharmacology; training in clinical skills, including assessment and treatment techniques; supervised hands-on clinical experience; and supervised empirical research into a selected topic in the clinical field. Service-oriented research and single case studies are also part of the requirements for qualification in clinical psychology.

Clinical psychology training is monitored by the British Psychological Society, which accredits courses on a regular basis. This ensures comparable course content and standards across the various training programmes. In recent years, the Society has emphasised the need to encourage trainees to develop a reflective attitude in their work, in addition to working within the well-established scientist–practitioner model.

After qualification, the psychologist is entitled to enrol as a chartered clinical psychologist. Each year a clinical psychologist has to obtain a practising certificate from the British Psychological Society. Clinical psychologists are expected to acquire further training and skills as part of continuing professional development. Many acquire additional skills in specialist areas through formal or informal courses. The profession places much value on continuing professional development and the annual practising certificate now depends on this.

Contribution in psychiatric settings

In mental health settings, clinical psychologists contribute to both in-patient and out-patient services. Many patients are treated by psychologists on an out-patient basis: those with phobias, obsessive–compulsive disorder, or sexual problems are obvious examples of groups who can be treated in this way. Of course, patients with severe problems may need to be treated in hospital. When patients are admitted to hospital with, for example, severe depression or acute psychosis, psychologists may contribute to their care by devising observation programmes, carrying out assessments and – where relevant – using psychological techniques for the treatment of specific aspects of the disorder (e.g. hallucinations, negativism). Clinical psychologists will also contribute, when needed, to the rehabilitation of the patient. Group treatment may also be undertaken in both in-patient and out-patient settings. Conditions for which group treatment is commonly used include social skills deficits and substance misuse.

Specialist assessment skills include intelligence testing, personality assessment, and neuropsychological testing of patients suspected, for example, of brain damage or dementia. Assessment of scholastic attainment is also undertaken, this being almost routine in the case of children and adolescents. Assessment of vocational interests and aptitude is also part of the remit of clinical psychologists, although the need to use these is less frequent.

The theoretical orientation of a practising clinical psychologist will reflect their own interests and training. Most, however, have the basic cognitive–behavioural orientation as their main approach. Clinical psychology training courses provide a firm grounding in this for trainees. They also provide exposure to other models such as the systemic and the psychodynamic models, but specialist skills and expertise in these alternative approaches are usually mastered by those who have an interest after the basic clinical training.

The key role of the cognitive–behavioural approach has been particularly emphasised in recent years as a result of the trend towards evidence-based practice in medicine, including psychiatry. The guidelines provided by the National Institute for Health and Clinical Excellence, after close scrutiny of the available evidence, underpin the efficacy of the cognitive–behavioural approach for many disorders.

The multidisciplinary team

In a well-established and harmonious multidisciplinary team, psychologists will contribute in some or all of the ways noted above with regard to individual patients. They will contribute more generally by being active team members, particularly in discussing and making management decisions about all patients seen by the team, by helping the nursing staff to set up and carry out observation regimes and behavioural programmes where necessary, by participating in the teaching of all professional groups, including supervision of the treatment of patients, and by carrying out or contributing to relevant research programmes. Although this is the ideal situation, in practice psychologists may operate on a referral basis because of a lack of time allocated for psychologist input into each clinical team.

Patients will be referred to the psychologist with a specific request for assessment and/or treatment. This latter arrangement, although common, is much less satisfactory both for the clinical psychologist and the team, than the active team participation outlined above.

For a mental health team with an in-patient unit of about 12 beds, which also runs a parallel out-patient facility, the service of a full-time clinical psychologist should be provided. More limited provision will lead to the psychologist's service becoming primarily referral based.

Professional hierarchy

There are four grades of clinical psychologists:

- assistant psychologist – a graduate working as a helper or technician
- trainee clinical psychologist – a psychologist officially in clinical training
- A grade clinical psychologist – a qualified clinical psychologist
- B grade clinical psychologist – a qualified clinical psychologist at a higher level of the profession.

B grade psychologists hold more responsible positions, usually as heads of specialties within a district. The designations of individual psychologists who are qualified (i.e. A and B grades) are not uniformly specified, and it is up to each district or employing authority to give a designation (e.g. district psychologist or unit psychologist) as needed. Increasingly, many B grade psychologists in senior positions are given the designation 'consultant clinical psychologist'.

Recent developments

Recent changes introduced by the government's Agenda for Change place psychologists on an amalgamated pay structure with other healthcare professionals except medical staff. In this structure, there are nine bands, with sub-bands. Upon qualification a clinical psychologist enters band 7, and the B grade psychologists are placed in the top sub-bands of band 8 at entry. The Agenda for Change also stresses the need for clear job descriptions indicating levels of responsibility. The assimilation into the new structure has led to the formulation of new job descriptions for most psychologists in the health service.

The profession has for several years been actively considering its position and the contribution it can make to mental healthcare in the current, fluid circumstances. This has been done through seminars, study days, working papers, and committees. The Clinical Division of the British Psychological Society and other specialist groups have been taking an active part in this. The need to provide and expand services to the community has been fully recognised. The need to increase the output of trained psychologists has been stressed and representations have been made to government. The shortage of trained clinical psychologists in the UK at present is significant, and the current training schemes cannot meet this demand. The British Psychological Society runs a scheme for psychologists not trained in clinical psychology in the UK to obtain a Certificate of Equivalence on the basis of meeting all the training criteria. Some specialist courses are now available for the candidates to top-up their training so that they can obtain this certificate. The scheme is also open to British-trained psychologists whose background is not in clinical psychology but in another area, such as counselling psychology or health psychology.

The psychologist's role in relation to the Mental Health Act of 1983 needs to be noted. There are a number of clinical psychologists who function as mental health commissioners. Under sections 57 and 58 of the Act, where the involvement of a team member other than a doctor or a nurse is needed, clinical psychologists often fulfil this role. They are also increasingly involved in the statutory planning of after-care.

Some clinical psychologists have also gone into management within the National Health Service (NHS), especially as unit managers for mental health services. However, the number of psychologists in general administrative positions within the NHS is still relatively low. In the overall NHS management structure, the management of clinical psychologists is through a section head (e.g. head of adult services) who is accountable to the head of the psychology service, for example a district psychologist, who is in turn responsible to the overall manager or the chief executive of the service.

The future

Several trends are emerging. Because of the shortage of trained clinical psychologists, more and more are likely to have to work in consultative and training/supervisory capacities. Training policy and strategy continue to be under review for the same reason. Some of the work traditionally covered by clinical psychologists has also become the province of less highly trained groups, such as healthcare psychologists, counsellors and technicians. There is a significant movement towards the private sector and – as the demand appears to be increasing – this is likely to continue and possibly accelerate. Within the NHS, the expansion into areas other than mental health is likely to continue, particularly into health psychology/behavioural medicine. Despite these developments, the main contribution of clinical psychologists is likely to continue to be in the field of mental health. The relationship with psychiatry, which has had its vicissitudes in the past, is likely to remain strong and to grow, with increased collaborative work in both hospital and community settings.

CHAPTER 10

Occupational therapy

Hilary Williams

'It is neither wealth nor splendor, but tranquility and occupation which give happiness' (Thomas Jefferson, 3rd President of USA, 1743–1826)

The use of occupation therapeutically has been documented throughout the ages. However, occupational therapy as a concept is relatively recent. The American psychiatrist Meyer noted the importance of a 'balance of activities', of giving opportunities to work, to do, to plan and create, and he is generally regarded as one of the founders of occupational therapy in the USA (Mayers, 2000). The term 'occupational therapy' was introduced in the early 20th century by Barton, who benefited from directed occupation in his own recovery from illness. He later established an institution in the USA where people with chronic ill health used occupation to retrain or to adjust to gainful living. Shortly after this time, Henderson, a prominent Scottish psychiatrist, and then Casson, one of the first women doctors in the UK, introduced and influenced the development of occupational therapy in the UK (Paterson, 2001).

Occupational therapy in mental health practice in the UK is best understood in the wider context of the social and medical history of psychiatry. The treatment of mental illness in Britain moved from large county asylums to district general hospitals with the development of the National Health Service (NHS), with the emphasis in the past two decades on community care (Community Care Act 1990), social inclusion (Office of the Deputy Prime Minister, 2004) and recovery (Ralph & Corrigan, 2004). Occupational therapy interventions have evolved with these changes (see Chapter 3).

The aim of this chapter is to describe occupational therapy in mental health practice in the UK today by detailing its underlying philosophy, the value of occupationally focused practice in a multidisciplinary team and the future direction of occupational therapy practice in this field.

Occupational therapy today

Occupational therapists focus on the nature, balance, pattern and context of occupations and activities in the lives of individuals, family groups and communities. They are concerned with the meaning and purpose people place upon occupations and activities, as well as the impact that illness, disability and social or economic deprivation have on their ability to carry out these meaningful activities.

The main aim of occupational therapy is to maintain, restore or create to match the ability of the person, the demands of their occupations in the area of self-care, productivity and leisure, along with the demands of the environment in which they live. The desired outcome is that the client achieves a satisfying performance and balance of occupations in the areas of self-care, productivity and leisure that will support recovery, health, well-being and social participation (Creek, 2003). Put simply, it is helping people do what they want to do (Wilcock, 1998).

According to Creek (2003), core assumptions of occupational therapists include:

- the drive to act is a basic human need
- engagement as the most important aspect of intervention – occupational therapy is most effective when there is a partnership between the client and the occupational therapist
- health can be expressed in terms of adaptation to the environment rather than freedom from disease/disorder
- the occupational therapist responds to a client's needs, values, interests and aspirations
- people who are unable to participate in their choice of occupations experience occupational imbalance, deprivation and alienation.

Occupational therapists work with all age groups, diagnoses and in a variety of settings, offering intervention on either an individual or group basis. As maximising occupational performance is a key aim of the occupational therapy intervention, assessment must take into account the person, their activity, their environment and the interaction between these.

The three fictional case studies that follow illustrate the breadth and scope of the role of the occupational therapist within a mental health trust.

Case studies

Case study 1: mental health for older adults

History

Stan was 76 years of age. He was born in inner-city South London into a White British family. He was the middle of three children. He described his childhood as a 'good one really'; his father worked on the docks and his mother worked as a cook. He attended school until the age of 14, after which he also went to work on the docks until he was forced to retire at 60, which was not his choice. He had met his wife of 40 years at a dance and they had a son and a daughter. He described his marriage as happy and his family as close. His wife had died 5 years previously. He had lived in the same home for 40 years and had a number of friends in the local area.

After the death of his wife he became low in mood and was referred to his local community mental health centre. He revealed that he and his wife had had an active social life together and he missed her. He was started on antidepressant therapy and was seen by the community mental health team on an outpatient basis. He did not take his medication and began saying he no longer wanted to live, that he was lonely, had lost motivation, had stopped caring for himself and the home, had lost weight, become socially isolated and overwhelmed with supporting his sister (who was physically unwell). He had also had a number of falls. His family were concerned about him; he was voluntarily admitted into the psychiatric ward and referred to occupational therapy for an assessment of his functional status.

Assessment

Stan reluctantly agreed to occupational therapy assessment and intervention. He was encouraged to attend the occupational therapy group room, where the therapist was able to observe Stan make his own drink, begin listening to music and play chess. His skills in daily domestic activity were assessed in the ward-based occupational therapy kitchen. A cookery assessment took place to determine his skills in the kitchen. It emerged that Stan had a limited repertoire of meals, with which he was bored, and this added to his feeling of being 'useless'. A home environment assessment revealed that his home was cluttered, and it was suggested that this may have contributed to his falls. He was finding it difficult to transfer on and off his chair and in and out of the bath. It also emerged that he had little structure to his week.

Goals for occupational therapy intervention included:

- extending his repertoire of meals for cooking at home
- with assistance of his family, clearing out clutter from home and installing equipment to help with transferring on and off chairs and into the bath
- helping Stan to develop a structure to his week.

Intervention

Stan was encouraged to attend the cookery group on the ward to develop his cookery skills and the 'moving on group' in preparation for discharge. A number of home visits took place in the presence of his family to help Stan to clear up his home and to install equipment to assist with transfers off chairs and into the bath. The skills that Stan learnt in the cookery group were then transferred to his home environment by means of a number of individual cookery sessions at home. The new recipes were written down and put into a file to compensate for some mild memory difficulties. For his trips home Stan at first used cabs to and from the hospital but later travelled by bus.

He was encouraged to go the hospital shop daily to buy a newspaper as this got him into the routine of getting out every day. He began to attend a woodwork group at the local day centre. It was agreed that a home carer would visit him upon discharge to assist with tasks in the home. In addition, Stan was offered bereavement counselling and social work support to enable him to help his sister.

Outcome

Stan was discharged from hospital to live in his own home. He continued with the routine of going out for the daily newspaper and was cooking a range of meals at home. After some time he joined a local men's club where he enjoyed playing pool and darts and generally socialising. He re-established his old social contacts, continued to support his sister and enjoy visits from his family. He was discharged from occupational therapy and followed up by his community mental health team.

Case study 2: mental health for children and adolescents

History

John was 15 years of age. He was born in London and had two full siblings and a step-sibling from his mother's subsequent relationship. His parents had separated before John began primary school. He had been a high achiever at school in his earlier years, and had a passion for sports. When in secondary school he began school refusing, did not sit his GCSEs and withdrew from his leisure pursuits after school. He was attending to his self-care but was taking up to an hour to get ready each morning. His concentration was good but he was taking excessive time to complete regular, day-to-day tasks and would become increasingly frustrated by this. He was becoming more engaged in compulsive behaviours, which was having an impact on his family as they were trying to work around them. He began using cannabis regularly. He began experiencing psychotic and obsessive features. He was referred to the child and adolescent community mental health team. With medication, his psychotic features subsided and a diagnosis of obsessive–compulsive disorder was made. He was then referred to occupational therapy for support with regards to his obsessive–compulsive behaviours and the impact they had on his occupational status.

Assessment

During assessment a number of points became clear. Again, there was a lack of structure to John's day; he was experiencing high anxiety and low self-esteem and was socially isolated. He was also concerned about the impact his recent difficulties were having on his family and about his non-attendance at school.

To gain a greater understanding of his presentation the occupational therapist then observed him completing a task using a standardised assessment. This revealed that it was John's processing skills that were having an impact on his functional status. He was rushing tasks, he was missing out parts of the task and was placing a huge amount of pressure on himself to remember things during the tasks.

Goals set for occupational therapy intervention included:

- transferring cognitive–behavioural techniques developed with a psychologist into day-to-day tasks
- creating a more fulfilling structure to his day
- developing peer relationships.

Intervention

Time was spent exploring the role the obsessive–compulsive features fulfilled. Benefits included having his own room in a home where there was little space and the attention he got from his mother. As occupational performance is the interaction of the person, their activity and their environment, the intervention was geared towards the home environment, namely the challenges presented by the space at home and John's relationship with his mum.

John worked at setting some mutually agreed achievable goals with regards to his leisure pursuits, his education and peer relationships, and these were graded into smaller functional objectives such as finding out the times and costs of local courses, attending an open day at the local college and re-establishing phone contact with a friend from school.

Outcome

After some months of working with the occupational therapist, John had re-established his sporting interests and was was participating in a range of sporting activities on a weekly basis. He began attending his local college with the view to sitting his GCSEs and was forming peer networks via college, old school friends and his new football group.

Case study 3: mental health for adults in the community

History

Iris was 39 years of age. She was born and brought up in a small village in the UK in a close, cohesive family. She is the middle of three children. Her parents worked hard in their small business. She enjoyed primary school, was able to make friends and enjoyed learning. At secondary school she was bullied, and noted that she was often unhappy. She managed to complete secondary school and was part way through college when she first became unwell at the age of 19, and was admitted to a psychiatric hospital with psychotic depression. After discharge, she completed an administration course in her 20s, and obtained a job as an administrator which she found enjoyable, but at times stressful. She had three further admissions to psychiatric hospital, the most recent 2 years ago, and had not worked for the past 7 years. She was stable at the time of referral, attributing this to taking medication and the support she received from her care coordinator, a registered mental health nurse who Iris would see weekly and phone between these sessions for support, which she did on average twice a week.

Her care coordinator referred her to occupational therapy for:

- anxiety management
- assistance with appropriately structuring her week.

Assessment

Iris was living alone in a rented flat. She was independent with all aspects of personal self-care. She would prepare and eat her own meals daily. She was able to budget and live within her means. She was in regular contact with friends, although she noted that they did not go out as often as they used to. Iris said that at times she felt lonely and panicky, and had learnt to manage this by 'keeping busy'. She also described finding it difficult to make decisions and to solve problems.

Her typical week largely consisted of attending a variety of courses at the local adult education centre over the 5 days, and she admitted that she would panic if this structure were not in place. Although she was able to identify clear benefits of attending these courses – which included meeting people, providing a structure to her day, increasing her self-esteem and stopping her thinking and becoming anxious – she also noted that she was doing too much, which made her feel tired and stressed, and which had been triggers for previous relapses.

Goals set for occupational therapy intervention included:

- being able to solve day-to-day problems without undue stress/anxiety
- having more structure in making decisions
- developing a more balanced weekly routine.

Intervention

In the first instance, intervention was geared towards developing alternative coping strategies for her feelings of panic, as she recognised her overactivity as a way of coping with them. Strategies for change included challenging beliefs about 'not being busy' and about mental health issues and stigma, and self-soothing and relaxation activities, including yoga and aromatherapy.

Once Iris felt able to manage these feelings of panic, she reflected on her week and noted that much of it was focused on leisure-based as opposed to productive or work-based activities, and she wanted to consider voluntary work at the next stage to provide a more balanced structure to her week and prepare/evaluate her readiness to return to paid employment. She was put in contact with an organisation that supports volunteers and obtained work in a local charity shop which supports the homeless.

Outcome

After a period of voluntary work, Iris went on to obtain part-time paid work as a receptionist in a hairdressing salon. She continued with her yoga class and took up swimming with a friend she made during her voluntary work. She maintained and built on her established friendships, and continued to participate in activities with them such as meals, and going to the cinema and theatre. She also reduced the frequency of her contact with her care coordinator.

Occupational therapy within a multidisciplinary team

The case studies show the breadth of occupational therapy and its interface with other members of the multidisciplinary team. In recent years there has been debate about and pressure from services for practitioners to work generically as mental health practitioners as opposed to using core occupational therapy skills only, but the profession has yet to reach a consensus on this. However, it is recognised that, particularly in the field of mental health, at times the role of the occupational therapist will overlap with the roles of colleagues and it is now common practice for occupational therapists to hold care coordinator roles under the care programme approach (Department of Health, 1990).

Occupational therapy and the legal aspects of detention

Occupational therapists have a working knowledge of the legal aspects of detention. Under the former Mental Health Act 1983 they did not have 'holding powers' but could be directly involved under Section 58. In such a case, a second opinion approved doctor (SOAD) would assess a client and certify whether the treatment proposed by the responsible medical officer should be given. Under these circumstances the SOAD, in addition to consulting with a nurse involved in the client's care, would also consult with one further non-medical member of staff. Occupational therapists working with the client could be approached by the SOAD for their comments on the nature of their contact with the client and the client's history. They could provide a unique insight into the mental state of the client through participation in occupation, in addition to the impact of occupationally focused interventions on the progress of treatment and their professional opinion of the proposed medical treatment.

The Mental Health Act 2007 offers scope for occupational therapists with the appropriate experience and training to take on the new role of approved mental health practitioner (which is based on the approved social worker role under the former Act) and potentially the role of responsible clinician (which replaces the responsible medical officer). The responsible clinician role may be particularly relevant with clients whose primary needs are best met by an occupational therapist focusing on rehabilitation and enhancing or facilitating vocational opportunities (Carr, 2007).

Future directions

Just as it is has been important to consider occupational therapy against a background of the changes in social and medical psychiatry, so too is it appropriate to consider the future of occupational therapy within these contexts. The social inclusion agenda is important in this regard. Adults with mental health problems are one of the most socially excluded groups in society (Office of the Deputy Prime Minister, 2004). They have the lowest employment rate of any of the main groups of people with disability and can be socially isolated – an important risk factor for deteriorating mental health and suicide. The current action plan to address social exclusion of mental health service users covers a number of themes: stigma and discrimination; the role of health and social care in tackling social exclusion; employment; supporting families and community participation; gaining access to decent homes; and financial advice and support. Occupational therapists are ideally placed to play a significant role in the social inclusion agenda for mental health service users because of their focus on and skills in enhancing occupational performance and considering the whole person in the context of tasks and their environment, with particular emphasis on employment, community participation and financial skills.

Mental Health: New Ways of Working was launched in April 2007 as a Department of Health initiative coordinated by National Institute for Mental Health in England. Evolving from the national conference for consultant psychiatrists in 2003, it is essentially a 'bottom-up approach with top-down strategy' and is linked with a range of organisational changes, reports and initiatives. It considers all parts of the system and is thus relevant to all professional groups. There are 13 cross-cutting themes within the document relevant to all mental health professionals. The profession of occupational therapy is set five key objectives within this document:

- to develop a strategy for occupational therapists working in mental health
- to explore new roles under patient group directives
- to explore new roles under the Mental Health Bill (now the Mental Health Act 2007)
- to establish occupational therapy secondment within the social inclusion unit
- to set out a career framework for occupational therapists, in terms of both generic and specialist functions.

It suggests a need to:

- embrace this agenda and embed its principles in practice
- form partnerships to facilitate service integration and the introduction of new roles and innovative practice

109

- identify what it is we need to do, and where and how we will continue to do it, in new and innovative ways.

There is a recognition that for occupational therapists to be integral to the 'fit for purpose' mental health workforce there is a need grasp opportunities to use their expertise in new roles and areas of work. The future of occupational therapy practice has been best summarised by the College of Occupational Therapists (2006): 'Occupational therapists will value recovery and will work within a socially inclusive framework to achieve goals that make a real difference to people's lives'.

Acknowledgements

I would like to acknowledge my colleagues in Lewisham Mental Health for Older Adults Occupational Therapy Service and Liz Evans, Senior Occupational Therapist in Croydon Adolescent Community Mental Health Team, South London and Maudsley NHS Trust, for their contribution to the case study material.

References

Carr, J. (2007) The introduction of new roles under the Mental Health Act 2007. *Mental Health Occupational Therapy*, 12, 99–100.

College of Occupational Therapists (2006) *Recovering Ordinary Lives: The Strategy for Occupational Therapy Services for the Next Ten Years (Core)*. COT.

Creek, J. (2003) *Occupational Therapy as a Complex Intervention*. College of Occupational Therapists.

Department of Health (1990) *Caring for People: The CPA for People with a Mental Illness Referred to Specialist Mental Health Services* (Joint Health/Social Services Circular C(90)23/LASSL(90)11). TSO (The Stationery Office).

Department of Health (2007) *Mental Health: New Ways of Working for Everyone. Developing and Sustaining a Capable and Flexible Workforce*. TSO (The Stationery Office).

Mayers, C. (2000). The Casson Memorial Lecture 2000: reflect on the past to shape the future. *British Journal of Occupational Therapy*, **63**, 358–366.

Office of the Deputy Prime Minister (2004) *Mental Health and Social Exclusion*. Office of Deputy Prime Minster.

Paterson, C. F. (2001) A short history of occupational therapy. In *Occupational Therapy and Mental Health* (3rd edn) (ed. J. Creek). Churchill Livingstone.

Ralph, R. & Corrigan, P. (2004) *Recovery in Mental Illness – Broadening our Understanding of Wellness*. American Psychological Association.

Wilcock, A. (1998) Occupation for health. *British Journal of Occupational Therapy*, **61**, 340–345.

CHAPTER 11

Mental health nursing

Richard Gray and Hilary McCallion

The National Service Framework for Mental Health set out a comprehensive vision for mental healthcare in the UK (Department of Health, 1999). Nurses form the largest part of the mental health workforce and have a pivotal role in delivering the National Service Framework. Mental health nursing is a profession that is patient centred, promotes evidence-based ways of working and values patients' aspirations and goals. It is concerned with patients' psychological, physical, social, cultural and spiritual needs, promoting good health, and treating ill health. These are the fundamentals of mental health nursing and are valued by mental health patients and carers (Department of Health, 2006).

In 2004 there were 96 269 mental health nurses registered in the UK. Although there has been a trend towards the treatment of mental illness in the community and a dramatic rise in the number of community mental health nurses, the majority continue to work in in-patient settings. Over the past decade mental health nurses have increasingly focused on working with patients with serious and enduring mental health problems such as schizophrenia and bipolar disorder. Mental health nurses are increasingly undertaking new ways of working: for example, as prescribers of medication, nurse consultants or cognitive–behavioural therapists.

The Chief Nursing Officer in England has recently led a major review of Mental Health Nursing (Department of Health, 2006). This has set the direction for mental health nursing for the next 10 years. The vision is that mental health nursing will deliver a range of evidence-based interventions that will improve patients' health and experience of healthcare.

Mental health nurses undertake a 3-year undergraduate degree or diploma. Their careers follow a variety of clinical, managerial and academic paths. Since December 2004, as with all other health workers with the exception of doctors, jobs have been graded using the nine-band 'Agenda for Change' system. It is expected that mental health nurses will continue to develop their clinical knowledge and skills through a process of lifelong learning and ongoing clinical supervision. Over the past decade the major innovation in post-qualification training for mental health nurses has been the 'Thorn' programme (Lancashire et al, 1997). This 18-month training programme equips mental health nurses to deliver a range of evidence-based interventions, including cognitive–behavioural therapy (CBT), family interventions and medication management for patients with severe and enduring mental illness.

Working in in-patient settings

Traditionally it is in-patient wards where newly qualified nurses 'cut their teeth' and consolidate what they have learnt in training. The downside to this is that the most inexperienced nurses are arguably working with patients with the most severe mental illness who have a greater need for skilled intervention. Over recent years in-patient care has received a great deal of criticism and attention, although there has been little policy guidance compared with acute care within the community (crisis resolution, assertive outreach, early intervention). In addition, there has been relatively little educational innovation for mental health nurses working in in-patient settings.

Qualified mental health nurses are supported in delivering nursing care by healthcare assistants who do not hold a professional qualification but may have completed a vocational qualification (e.g. an NVQ). From time to time 'agency' or 'bank' nurses – who are not permanent members of ward staff – may be used to cover sickness or vacancies.

In-patient mental health nurses provide care and treatment 24 hours a day 365 days a year. Nursing cover is generally organised on a shift basis, with nurses either working an 'early' (e.g. 7 a.m. to 3 p.m.), 'late' (e.g. 1 p.m. to 9 p.m.) or 'night' (e.g. 9 p.m. to 7 a.m.) shift. For a 20-bed unit there will be one or two qualified nurses on each shift, supported by up to three healthcare assistants. Nurses are involved in all aspects of in-patient care and treatment. It is the job of the mental health nurse working collaboratively with patients, carers and the rest of the multidisciplinary team to:

- ensure patients are actively involved in planning their care and treatment
- spend as much time as possible in face-to-face contact with patients
- provide a range of therapeutic (such as education on medication, health promotion) and occupational activities (such as cooking, art) on and off the ward.

Management of violence

In 1998/1999 the National Health Service (NHS) Executive reported about 65 000 violent incidents against staff in the NHS (National Institute for Clinical Excellence, 2005). For many mental health nurses much of their work is directed towards the management of violence. The National Institute for Health and Clinical Excellence (NICE) guideline on the management of disturbed/violent behaviour in in-patient psychiatric settings and emergency departments is an authoritative systematic review of the literature that was developed by the National Collaborating Centre for Nursing and Supportive Care. The guideline should guide mental health nursing practice in the prevention and management of violence, including risk assessment, de-escalation techniques, physical intervention, rapid tranquillisation and post-intervention reviews (National Institute for Clinical Excellence, 2005).

Mental Health Act, section 5(4) in England and Wales

Section 5(4) of the Mental Health Act 1983 allows a first-level registered mental nurse or a registered nurse for the mentally handicapped legally to prevent an informal in-patient who is receiving treatment for a mental disorder from leaving hospital. The nurse is able to hold a patient for up to 6 hours or until a doctor arrives. The Act also states that the use of section 5(4) is the nurse's decision and he or she cannot be instructed to exercise this power by anyone else. Section 5(4) is an emergency measure and lapses on the arrival of a doctor. In practice, however, nurses rarely use this power (Lovell et al, 1998). When it is used, patients are generally assessed within an hour, the most frequently observed outcome being the application of section 5(2). The mental health nurse's role in detaining patients under mental health law may be substantially increased if planned revisions to the existing legislation are introduced.

Working in community settings

An increasing number of mental health nurses work in community settings as care coordinators for people with serious mental illness in order to meet the requirements of the care programme approach. The main models of service delivery in the community are either case management or assertive community treatment. Early intervention and crisis intervention are also models of service delivery that involve mental health nurses. These have evolved from intervention research. Because the case-loads of community mental health nurses are limited (being typically between 20 and 30 patients), part of the role of a community mental health nurse is to deliver additional therapeutic interventions such as medication management, CBT or family work.

Interventions

Mental health nurses are involved in delivering a range of discrete evidence-based psychosocial interventions to patients with mental health problems.

The interventions that are central to the role of mental health nurses are:

- medication management
- cognitive–behavioural therapy
- family work.

Medication management

Medication is a central part of treatment for many mental health patients and has an important role to play in promoting recovery. Mental health nurses have traditionally administered medication. However, increasingly they are taking a leading role in helping patients manage their medication and in the future will be independent prescribers. Medication management involves the application of a range of interpersonal, assessment and process skills. Medication management improves patient outcomes by facilitating patient exploration of past experiences of medication, discussion of the positive and negative effects of medication, careful monitoring and management of unwanted side-effects and an exchange of information about medication and medication options (Nosé *et al*, 2003; Gray *et al*, 2004).

Cognitive–behavioural therapy

Cognitive-behavioural therapy has been used across a range of disease areas including anxiety, depression, panic disorder, chronic fatigue syndrome and schizophrenia. Mental health nursing has a very strong association and tradition with CBT, dating back to the 1970s and the establishment of the nurse therapy programme at the Maudsley Hospital by Professor Issac Marks. Some 250 mental health nurses have been trained as nurse therapists in the UK over the past 25 years, the majority working in the treatment of anxiety-related disorders and depression. More recently mental health nurses (and other mental health workers) have been trained to deliver CBT, specifically for psychosis, as part of the Thorn training programme.

Family work

As with CBT, family interventions and mental health nursing have a long tradition, spanning almost 20 years. Family work for schizophrenia has been a central element of the Thorn programme since its inception in 1992. Family interventions stem from work done in the 1970s which showed that if people with schizophrenia were from families that expressed high levels of criticism, hostility or over-involvement, they had more frequent relapses than people from families who expressed lower levels of these factors (Brown *et al*, 1972). Family interventions aim to engage families caring for someone with schizophrenia, provide information, reduce adverse family atmospheres, develop problem-solving abilities within families, help set realistic goals for patients, agree boundaries and limits to carer involvement, and reduce the expression of family anger and guilt (Pharoah *et al*, 2003). As with CBT, family interventions are an adjunct and not an alternative to medication.

Future of mental health nursing

Nurses are the backbone of mental healthcare and are able to deliver a range of effective evidence-based interventions in both in-patient and community settings. Future challenges include the development of new specialised ways of working and leading mental healthcare (e.g. nurse consultants), and the development of clinical skills in managing and promoting physical health in people with mental health problems. Mental health nursing is an exciting and evolving profession that is central to effective modern mental healthcare and treatment, and the delivery of the National Service Framework.

References

Brown, G. W., Birley, J. L. & Wing, J. K. (1972) Influence of family life on the course of schizophrenic disorders: a replication. *British Journal of Psychiatry*, **121**, 241–258.

Department of Health (1999) *The National Service Framework for Mental Health*. Department of Health.

Department of Health (2006) *From Values to Action: The Chief Nursing Officer's Review of Mental Health Nursing*. Department of Health.

Gray, R., Wykes, T., Edmunds, M., *et al* (2004) Effect of a medication management training package for nurses on clinical outcomes for patients with schizophrenia: a cluster randomised controlled trial. *British Journal of Psychiatry*, **185**, 157–162.

Lancashire, S., Haddock, G., Tarrier, N., *et al* (1997) Effects of training in psychosocial interventions for community psychiatric nurses in England. *Psychiatric Services*, **48**, 39–41.

Lovell, K., Gray, R. & Thomas, B. (1998) *The use of nurses' holding power in a large psychiatric hospital. Nursing Standard*, **12**, 40–42.

National Institute for Clinical Excellence (2005) *Violence: The Short-Term Management of Disturbed/Violent Behaviour in In-Patient Psychiatric Settings and Emergency Departments*. NICE.

Nosé, M., Barbui, C., Gray, R., *et al* (2003) Clinical interventions for reducing treatment non-adherence in psychosis: meta-analysis. *British Journal of Psychiatry*, **183**, 197–206.

Pharoah, F. M., Rathbone, J. & Mari, J. J. (2003) Family intervention for schizophrenia. *Cochrane Database of Systematic Reviews*, issue 4. Update Software.

CHAPTER 12

Social work

Alan Rushton

Although a universally agreed definition of social work has proved elusive in the past, progress is being made towards greater role clarity and it is generally acknowledged that social work sits at the interface of the person and the environment. The specialism of mental health social work is, therefore, concerned with the impact that people with mental disorders have on their environment and the impact the environment has on them.

The social work perspective, although recognising the genetic and biological contributions to mental ill health, emphasises the whole person and the wider social context of family and neighbourhood and the person's work, leisure and educational communities. Among other things, mental health social workers are concerned with the social capital of people with mental health problems (Webber, 2005). Social work is committed to the goal of incorporating the social component into psychiatric interventions in order to contribute to more socially improved, and not just symptomatically improved, outcomes. This more socially oriented model has as its aim helping people to lead more fulfilled lives, to manage better their behaviour and emotions, to help find solutions to their predicaments and to be connected to others, but also to be as independent as possible. It tries not to stress deficits (symptoms and poor functioning) but to emphasise strengths and to forge a working partnership with clients.

In the protracted journey towards establishing the professional credentials of social work, there has been a continuing wish to pull away from the powerful whirlpool that can draw everything towards a narrowly conceived medical model and to struggle to achieve a separate, more holistic view. Emphasis is placed on social inclusion, civil liberties and human rights, gender and race equality, and anti-discriminatory and culturally sensitive practice. Empowerment is the goal rather than welfare dependency. Social work practitioners and academics have pioneered these approaches and what was once thought radical is probably now mainstream.

This social work perspective has informed and driven the move towards a user-led approach; the creation of links to mainstream services such as general practice, and within local authorities to departments concerned with leisure, recreation, housing and regeneration; and also to initiatives that empower users such as direct payments, advance directives and crisis cards.

Much more progress needs to be made in integrating social work and health services. Professional relationships can be complex and at times fraught, and it is not always comfortable to be defending a minority social perspective in the face of a team unsympathetic to such a view. Social workers with good communication skills, tenacity and persuasiveness are able to keep the 'social' in the picture.

Having suggested that social work is anchored to a common value base, of course variations are to be found in the way mental health social work is practised. A variety of theoretical approaches and methods of intervention will be in evidence. Some social workers favour working at the more psychological end of the spectrum, concerned mainly with relationships, personal dilemmas, managing stress and anxiety (usually called 'clinical social work' in the USA). Other social workers focus on practical help with daily living, housing, finances and employment: factors that are all known to have a major impact on life stress and recovery from illness. Although personal/professional preferences are influential, in practice freedom is gradually being curtailed as the scope and boundaries of mental health social work are becoming more tightly drawn within the structure of the care programme approach. Consequently, limited latitude in decision-making and high rates of burnout and emotional exhaustion are commonplace in mental health social workers (Evans *et al*, 2006).

Having indicated some degree of consensus about the main elements of social work, what remains unresolved is whether the social orientation is 'unique' to social work or whether other professions would claim similar allegiances. If so, does the overlapping of roles obviate the need for separate professions? Rushton & Beaumont (2002) argue that this should be resisted because the independent social perspective would be at risk of dilution.

Qualifications and training

Over the years, social work training has become increasingly regulated, with a more prescribed curriculum and efforts to standardise assessments of competence. The new 3-year degree-level social work qualification should ensure that social workers acquire a sound value base, practice skills, knowledge of social science and a critical stance. Better-quality post-qualifying training should ensure a strong grounding in inter-professional and inter-agency work so that social workers can represent their views well in any mental health context: whether in crisis intervention and community outreach teams or in hospitals, residential care settings or court liaison schemes.

However, in depth, longer-term post-qualifying training in mental health social work at Master's degree level is still not widely available. An expansion of training opportunities of this kind is needed to develop the skills of intelligent interpretation of research findings and the ability to research questions pertinent to mental health social work. It is important that training adopts a life-span perspective so that, for example, social workers have both an understanding of the effect of children's psychological problems on their parents and of the parenting capacity of people with mental health problems.

Approved social worker role

The approved social worker role in mental health admissions, which derives from the 1983 Mental Health Act in England and Wales, requires the social worker to make an assessment and seek alternatives to compulsory admission where possible. The approved social worker programme requires 600 hours of training followed by assessment in order to gain the award. The successful candidate then needs to be appointed by the local social services authority before they can practise as an approved social worker, and they must be re-approved periodically to retain their authorisation. Other countries in the UK have similar training. These requirements for training are impressive compared with the those for the former mental welfare officers who were issued a 'warrant' virtually on walking through the door, without examined knowledge of the law and good practice.

It is has always seemed remarkable that UK mental health legislation has built into it the acknowledgement of a potential for conflict between psychiatrist and social worker. This tension can be constructively managed, although the imbalance in professional status can undermine the process. It is now envisaged that legal responsibility under new mental health legislation will be broadened beyond social workers to other mental health professionals. Anxiety is being expressed about the capacity of the new approved mental health professional to retain this independent role which is critical for civil liberties.

Social work and child and adolescent mental health

Whereas the term social work is currently being replaced by 'social care providers' and 'mental health workers', no parallel move is apparent in child care social work. The term 'child care social work' has been retained and a larger budget has been made available in order to build a stronger evidence base, to conduct more evaluation of the social work input and to make available more advanced training opportunities (Rushton, 2003).

Although social work may often be associated in the public mind with child protection failures, positive aspects can be noted in practice developments, such as intervening in complex family relationships and helping children where parenting is impaired because of mental health or substance misuse problems (Kearney *et al*, 2000). Progress is being made in supporting looked-after children with mental health problems and working with abused and neglected children placed in foster and adoptive homes and residential care.

The future

Several initiatives are in place to enhance the professional status of social work. All those working in social care will have to meet rigorous registration requirements and be bound by codes of practice: a procedure similar to that in teaching, nursing and the law. Through the new General Social Care Council, all qualified social workers must be registered. The General Social Care Council will also regulate social work education and training. Raising the educational standards and regulating the workforce are important steps in securing public confidence in social work, but will not alone guarantee more effective services. Although social workers are ceaselessly encouraged to inform themselves about recent research evidence, the kind of research that is directly helpful to the practitioner is still in short supply. Much more needs to be known about what is effective and what specific activities make it effective. Aside from some notable exceptions (e.g. Corney, 1981; Harrington et al, 1998; Huxley et al, 2003) there have been very few attempts to evaluate the impact of social work interventions using appropriate methodology. Randomised controlled trials in community mental health tend to examine the effect of the mental health team as a whole, with little reference to its composition and distinct professional contributions (see Johnson et al, 2005). More research is needed on the cost-effectiveness of specific, targeted social interventions and these proven methods should be more regularly employed. The newly created Social Care Institute for Excellence (SCIE) is charged with disseminating evidence and promoting knowledge about good practice through systematic research briefings.

Greater acknowledgement needs to be given to the beneficial influence of social workers on mental healthcare, especially their efforts to prevent psychological breakdown and to help with social integration. Social workers should play an increasingly valuable role in a range of key activities: as skilled practitioners, care planners, practice supervisors, policy leads, teachers and researchers.

References

Corney, R. H. (1981) Social work effectiveness in the management of depressed women: a clinical trial. *Psychological Medicine*, **11**, 417–423.

Evans, S., Huxley, P., Gately, C., *et al* (2006) Mental health, burnout and job satisfaction among mental health social workers in England and Wales. *British Journal of Psychiatry*, **188**, 75–80.

Harrington, R., Kerfoot, M., Dyer, E., *et al* (1998) Randomised trial of a home-based family intervention for children who have deliberately poisoned themselves. *Journal of the American Academy of Child and Adolescent Psychiatry*, **37**, 512–518.

Huxley, P., Reilly, S., Robinshaw, E., *et al* (2003) Interventions and outcomes of health and social care service provision for people with severe mental illness in England. *Social Psychiatry and Social Epidemiology*, **38**, 44–48.

Johnson, S., Nolan, F., Pilling S., *et al* (2005) Randomised controlled trial of acute mental health care by a crisis resolution team: the north Islington crisis study. *BMJ*, **331**, 599–603.

Kearney, P., Levin, E. & Rosen G. (2000) *Alcohol, Drugs and Mental Health Problems: Working with Families*. National Institute for Social Work.

Rushton, A. (2003) *The Growth of Evidence Based Social Work in Child and Adolescent Mental Health* (Occasional Paper). Association of Child Psychology and Psychiatry.

Rushton, A. & Beaumont, K. (2002) Social work in health care settings: turning full circle? *Child Psychology and Psychiatry Review*, **7**, 295–302.

Webber, M. (2005) Social capital and mental health. In *Social Perspectives in Mental Health. Developing Social Models to Understand and Work with Mental Distress* (ed. J. Tew) pp. 90–111. Jessica Kingsley.

CHAPTER 13

Chaplains in the psychiatric setting

Mark Sutherland

One of the greatest strengths of the National Health Service (NHS) is that from its inception chaplains, as practitioners of spiritual and pastoral care, have been seen as a constituent part of a complete provision of heathcare. This is a recognition that at times of major life crisis people need something more than the personal and private ministrations of their faith representatives. As the level of formal religious identity has declined in the general population, the number of chaplains has steadily increased. The work of a chaplain in healthcare is a sensitive and highly skilled form of religious, spiritual, and emotional support flexibly tailored to meet the specific needs of individuals regardless of whether they consider themselves 'religious' in any formal sense. Mental health is an area which raises the most difficult questions about spirit and mind, health and illness in terms of meaning, purpose and futility. The question for practitioners of psychiatry is why the contribution of chaplains is so poorly regarded, and why spiritual and pastoral care form at best, discretionary adjuncts to treatment?

Alongside the work with individuals chaplains also concern themselves with the quality of the healthcare culture. Working across all sections of healthcare, they position themselves at a series of intersecting boundaries within the healthcare institution and its culture. Chaplains work with patients in in-patient, out-patient and community settings. They support staff either individually, in teams or through groups, in areas such as work-related stress, ethical challenges and keeping personal and corporate vision alive. The absence of death and dying as a routine experience in the mental health setting deprives mental health chaplains (unlike their colleagues in acute and palliative care) of an undisputed area of operation. This affects their ability to develop a clear role and professional identity in relation to clinical mental healthcare services.

Finding the chaplain's voice

Chaplains find themselves outside the medical model of psychiatry. Consequently, they struggle to articulate a clear model of practice within a psychiatric culture dominated by explanatory models, which reduce the vicissitudes of human personhood to mere organic processes of illness. Chaplains arrive in mental healthcare already trained in other contexts. A glaring omission in their own general training (typically involving up to 5 years of graduate and postgraduate education) is that little consideration will have been given to the specific mental health demands of interfacing spiritual and emotional development. Unlike other healthcare professions chaplains have no NHS unified model of training and education. This, inevitably, weakens the establishing of a common chaplaincy identity and voice.

Chaplains are easily silenced in the face of a more dominant organic–medical discourse. For example, the strident cry for 'evidence-based' practice begs important philosophical questions about what is real. Psychiatry's increasing pursuit of organic explanative causes for mental disturbance reflects the distorting effects of psychiatry's uneasy relationship with the larger world of medical science. Consequently, psychiatry tends to confine its concept of what is real to the correspondence model (i.e. the real is what I can see and measure from the perspective of the objective observer). The difficulty here lies not in the model but in the minds of psychiatrists. Wedded to materialist explanation they have little acknowledgement for hermeneutic (the real is context related requiring journeying into another's experience) and metaphoric (the real is an intimation of the unseen, yet experienced) models of reality upon which chaplains rely (Chinen, 1996: p. 217).

Despite the lack of a common articulation of a model, chaplains can voice their approach to mental distress and disturbance. Some chaplains will employ a theological discourse, whereas others will employ a more psychological one. Yet, in my experience any tension between adherents of theology and psychology as the primary philosophy is more apparent than real. The emerging discourse of transpersonal psychology offers chaplains an approach towards the effective integration of spiritual and psychological approaches in the psychiatric context (Nelson, 1990).

Chaplains and clinical care

Chaplains are members of the multidisciplinary team, yet often find themselves outside the particular concerns of delivering clinical care. Freed from responsibility for delivery of clinical care, chaplains are able to address the more ordinary emotional and psycho-spiritual needs of the patient. The strength of being 'in-between' resulting from being deliverers of care, but not clinical care, enables chaplains to bring into clinical settings a more holistic approach which recasts the symptoms of mental distress in terms of a more general articulation of human pain and suffering. However, the absence of a curriculum of training for all chaplains within the NHS leads to difficulties with articulating their philosophy and approach to psychiatrists, in particular.

Hearing the chaplain's voice

The contribution of mental health chaplaincy to the wider psychiatric context can be defined under three broad headings: social justice, the centrality of relationality, and the language of the soul.

Social justice

Chaplains champion the struggle of the biblical poor, a reference from liberation theology used by Pattison (1997) as a symbol for the stigma and exclusion suffered by those with poor mental health. Mental health is central to any critical analysis of contemporary social experience. It is the one area where the lines of multiple social and individual deprivation intersect (Sutherland, 2000). Here, chaplains present a challenge to psychiatry's attempts to reify mental state through severing its connection with social and political factors. Currently, reification of mental state risks further colonising human pain and suffering, leading inevitably to a degree of 'psychiatrisation' of the human condition hitherto unparalleled (Rose, 2006).

Centrality of relationality

Relationality is a theological term for connection which includes but extends the concept of relationship. Chaplains challenge the marginalising of psychiatry's conversation with older traditions of emotional care, which espouse relationality as a significant element in the human being's quest for meaning and purpose. Relationship is the basis upon which human beings search for, and build, meaning. Breaches and abuses in relationship lie at the heart of the symptoms that psychiatric diagnoses attempt to categorise as illness. In emphasising relationality at the heart of their practice chaplains seek to relate to rather than explain symptoms as the disturbed cries of human pain and suffering. The particular concern of the chaplain is to engage with the human being through an exploration of the spiritual, emotional and social nature of disturbances to mental well-being. The basis upon which the chaplain seeks to do this is through the spiritual and pastoral care approach to relationship building, which employs the skilful use of human intersubjectivities (i.e. how your experience echoes through the evocation of elements in mine).

Language of the soul

Chaplains relate to older and widely established traditions of spiritual experience which evoke a language of both mind and soul. Increasingly, they are also interested in bringing this language into dialogue with the important language of brain. What both chaplains and psychiatrists share in the face of mental illness is that human experience is bounded within the:

'... complicated network of constraint that produces the kind of brain which humans happen to have – that is, a sufficiently large number of chemical and electrical reactions of the kind that are held within the boundaries of the brain' (Bowker 1995).

This is not to reduce mind and soul to brain. To do so is to create a category of confusion resulting from an essentially Newtonian view of causation (i.e. the brain as a machine directly causing behaviours). In contrast, spiritualities and theologies of mind and soul find an echo in a quantum mechanics view of the brain as fluid networks of communicative processes. The complexities of emotion (mental experience) and perception (spirituality) emerge from neural organisation of increasing levels of complexity. Both local (topographically adjacent) and non-local (topographically distant, yet operationally linked) neural processes communicate in response to the influences of external environment, which in most cases is expressed through the experience of relationality (Cozolino, 2002).

Disturbances to mental well-being have a complex and intertwined relationship with the upheavals of emotional and spiritual development. This is one of the key explanations for the presence of highly coloured if distorted religio-spiritual elements observed in psychotic states. Conversely, psychotic-like phenomena abound during phases of spiritual development/ awakening. It is safe to say that states of spiritual preoccupation and confusion abound so consistently in psychosis that the psychotic experience itself evokes a language of soul. Failure to use this language results either in the need to invent another to do justice to the data (Bowker, 1995) or, as is more commonly the case, to ignore the data completely.

A chaplaincy perspective views the psychiatric context as the place where we encounter our deepest fears of losing the attributes of human dignity and self-determination. For each of us our mental well-being is the area where the struggle for wholeness/holiness can seem most imperilled and precarious. Therefore, chaplains identify social justice, human relationality and the neurological structures displaying purposeful organisation (i.e. relationality of a different order) as the triple foundations for dignified personhood. In exploring the broad outline of the contribution of chaplaincy in psychiatry a crucial question remains unanswered – how might psychiatry make more effective use of what chaplains represent for the better service of their patients?

References

Bowker, J. (1995) *Is God A Virus? Genes, Culture and Religion.* Society for Promoting Christian Knowledge.

Chinen, A. B. (1996) Western analytical philosophy and transpersonal epistemology. In *Textbook of Transpersonal Psychiatry and Psychology* (eds B. W. Scotton, A. B. Chinen & J. R. Batista), 217–228. Basic Books.

Cozolino, L. (2002) *The Neuroscience of Psychotherapy. Building and Rebuilding the Human Brain.* Norton.

Nelson, J. E. (1990) *Healing the Split. A New Understanding of the Crisis and Treatment of the Mentally Ill*. Tarcher.

Pattison, S. (1997) *Pastoral Care and Liberation Theology*. Society for Promoting Christian Knowledge.

Rose, N. (2006) Disorders without borders? The expanding scope of psychiatric practice (transcript of the 18th Aubrey Lewis Lecture at the Institute of Psychiatry, London). *BioSocieties*, **1**, 465–484.

Sutherland, M. (2000) Towards dialogue: an exploration of the relations between psychiatry and religion in contemporary mental health. In *Blackwell Reader in Pastoral and Practical Theology* (eds S. Pattison & J. Woodward), pp. 272–282. Blackwell Publications. Oxford.

Part 3

CHAPTER 14

Personal safety

Michael J. Travis

It cannot be stated strongly enough that if you are ever in a situation that feels unsafe you should (a) try and exit that situation as rapidly as possible and/or (b) summon assistance as quickly as you can. Never put yourself in harm's way if this can be avoided.

When considering personal safety as a psychiatric trainee there are a series of factors that should be considered but which cluster around three main areas. These are: patient factors, environmental/situational factors and team/training factors.

Patient factors

These factors, which increase the risk of violence, will also be part of your risk assessment. They should, however, always be considered when approaching any patient and can be represented as questions for which you would like an answer, from an informant, relevant staff or the patient's notes.

Does this patient have a previous history of violence?

A previous history of violent acts is the best predictor of future violent acts. Generally speaking, the more serious the intent of the previous act and the less the remorse or understanding of the act, the greater the future risk. With time from last violent episode the risk is attenuated, but remains the only robust predictor of violence.

What is the patient's age and gender?

In general younger people tend to be more likely to commit violent acts than older people and males are more likely to be violent than females. It must be remembered, however, that even the elderly and females can be very violent, and other predictors are probably more important in judging the risk to personal safety.

Has there been a stated threat of violence?

People who are threatening violence will often act on their threats if their demands are not met. There is a popular misconception that threats of violence are in some way 'bluster', 'attention-seeking' or the patient 'working out their anger'; such threats are a clear warning, should be taken seriously and attempts should be made to explore them with the patient.

Does the patient have an association with a subculture prone to violence?

These subcultures sometimes involve street gangs or other violent subcultures with which the patient identifies. Again, the risk of violence is increased as the patient is more likely to express themselves through violence rather than verbally.

Is there a history of alcohol or other substance misuse, irrespective of diagnosis?

There is a marked additive effect for mental illness and substance misuse in terms of predicting violence and offending behaviour. In a community survey in the UK, patients with 'dual diagnosis' were over four times more likely than patients with psychosis alone to commit any criminal offence, three times more likely to be reported as being aggressive and eight times more likely to feel hostile. Swanson *et al* (1997) noted an increase in risk from over threefold to almost tenfold for patients with mental illness as a whole with comorbid alcohol misuse. Similarly, in a study of patients who had committed homicide, Eronen *et al* (1998) reported a risk of homicide for patients with schizophrenia of 7 times the average, and for patients with comorbid alcoholism this risk increased to 17 times. It is interesting to note that in the Swanson *et al* study the increased risk of violence associated with alcohol misuse alone was about 7 times and in the Eronen *et al* study it was about 10 times. Thus the increased risk associated with comorbidity of schizophrenia and alcohol misuse is additive rather than synergistic.

These data are reinforced by a prospective trial of involuntary out-patient commitment for patients with serious mental illness. Swartz *et al* (1998) reported that in their sample of 331 patients, the majority of whom had schizophrenia, substance misuse alone increased the risk of violence twofold, with an additive effect for non-adherence to antipsychotic medication.

Is it likely that the patient is currently intoxicated?

Any intoxicant that a patient has ingested will tend to make them impulsive and impair their judgement. In these situations it becomes harder to discuss situations rationally and there is therefore an increased risk of violence.

What are the patient's current core symptoms?

Important symptoms related to risk of violence include active symptoms of schizophrenia or mania, particularly if there are delusions or hallucinations that are focused on a particular person or if there is a specific preoccupation with violence. Although there remains some debate, delusions of control, particularly with a violent theme, appear to predict violence. In addition, agitation, excitement, overt hostility or suspiciousness driven by mental illness or drug use all increase risk.

Is the patient collaborating with suggested management strategies?

If the patient fails to listen to reasoned discussion in terms of removing themselves from an escalating situation or taking steps to try and calm down, agitation, confrontation and therefore violence can occur.

Is there evidence of antisocial, explosive or impulsive personality traits?

Patients displaying these traits are more likely to be violent in any given situation than patients without these traits.

Environmental/situational factors

What is the extent of this individual's social support?

This is less important in a hospital setting; however, with mental health services increasingly being delivered at home this is an area of growing importance. Although there is little empirical evidence, there does appear to be an increased risk of violence from individuals who are isolated or marginalised from society. It might therefore be supposed that better social support provides a framework within which an individual will be more likely to exert control over their behaviour.

What is the immediate availability of a weapon?

It must be remembered that many objects can be used as weapons. Care should be taken to try and keep the agitated patient away from such objects, which include:

- knives/any sharp implements (e.g. scissors, metal nail files, nail clippers, etc.)
- cigarette lighters and matches
- glass bottles
- canned/tinned items of any description, including aerosols and especially aluminium drink cans

- electrical leads/wires
- electrical equipment with telescopic aerials
- televisions
- metal cutlery or breakable cups or plates
- any solid objects that could be considered dangerous or likely to cause injury to another person.

If the patient is hospitalised, the unit/ward to which the person is admitted should have a clear policy on the possession of such articles. The ward staff should have a clear knowledge of the likelihood of the patient having a weapon. It is prudent to ask the patient if they have any weapons. This is especially the case when seeing patients in the community. It is essential that a prior history of weapon use should be sought, as this increases the likelihood that the patient will have taken steps to obtain/secrete a weapon. If there is a high degree of suspicion that a patient has a weapon or they have stated they have a weapon, the situation should be treated with extreme caution and the police should invariably be involved.

Patients should always be asked to put weapons down on the floor and move away. You should never ask a patient to hand over a weapon directly to you as this requires an unwanted degree of close physical proximity to an armed agitated individual.

What is your relationship to the patient?

There is a tendency to think that a previously good relationship with a patient may endow an individual staff member with a special skill at de-escalating a situation with that patient when they become more unwell. Although this may be the case in certain circumstances, this familiarity may also make the patient more likely to focus on known staff members in relation to any psychotic beliefs or attributions, and therefore increase the risk to those staff members. It must be remembered that in the general population acts of violence are more likely to be between two people known to each other than between strangers.

Is the area where the patient will be seen safe?

As a general rule, you should inspect any room where you are likely to interview a patient and look for the following:

- Does the door open outwards from the room? (This makes the door more difficult to barricade from the inside)
- Are there one or two entrances to the room? (Ideally there should be two, as this also makes barricading the room more difficult)
- Is there a way of observing what is happening in the room?
- Is the room in line of sight and hearing of the main clinical area?
- Is there sufficient space in the room to restrain the patient safely should the need arise?

- Is there anything in the room that could be used as a weapon?
- Is the furniture arranged in such a way that the patient can be seated furthest from the door?
- Is there a fixed alarm system in the room and does it work?
- Is there a mobile alarm system and, if there is, can you get a mobile alarm to carry? (See below).

Team/training factors

Do other members of the team know where you are and what you are doing?

This is one of the first rules of personal safety. If you are entering a clinical area and, especially, if you are seeing a patient alone, other members of the ward team should be aware of where you are, who you are seeing and the nature of the interview. This will ensure that should there be a deterioration in the patient and an alarm is raised, the staff are able to respond rapidly.

Have you been trained in breakaway techniques?

Such training is now mandatory in many healthcare organisations and usually involves a day or half a day of theoretical and practical training by skilled practitioners in techniques that can be employed should a patient grab or attack you. These techniques are predicated on the use of the minimum force necessary to prevent harm to you while 'breaking away' from contact with the patient and running to seek assistance. As these skills are rarely employed, they should be refreshed at least once a year.

Do you know how to summon assistance to the area where you will be seeing the patient?

If as part of your room/area check you find there is a fixed panic alarm, ensure that you know how to use it and that it is positioned close to you and away from the patient in such a way that you can activate it as you move towards the door of the room and away from the patient.

If interviewing a potentially violent patient alone, you should always ask if there is a personal alarm available. These broadly fall into three types:

- a simple alarm that when activated emits a very loud noise and alerts the rest of the team to a possible situation; the team moves towards the sound (it is policy in some hospitals that all staff carry these at all times)
- a personal alarm which is part of a system that when activated causes an alert to sound on the unit and gives an indication, usually by position lights, of the location of the incident
- a personal alarm which is part of a system that when activated causes

an alert to sound from all of the other alarms and displays the location of the incident on a screen on the alarms.

You should be properly trained in the use of any alarm system before trying to use it.

Is there adequate team support should the situation deteriorate?

The aim of interviewing any patient is to ascertain their problems and try to collaboratively devise a plan for managing them. When assessing an agitated patient, this type of interview is more difficult but should still be attempted. Before seeing an agitated patient you should discuss contingency plans with the team should the patient become more agitated and distressed. In most settings this will involve the use of an 'emergency team' of staff specially trained in de-escalation and safe control and restraint techniques. Depending on the level of violent risk from your initial assessment, you and the ward team may do one of three things (see Table 14.1).

In the absence of a properly trained emergency team you may need to ask for support from the police before interviewing a patient when violence is likely.

Conclusions

Much of the above with regard to safety appears to be common sense. Often, however, the nature of emergencies in psychiatry is such that practitioners are encouraged to enter situations before they have ascertained sufficient information or made adequate contingency plans. Most breaches of staff personal safety are secondary to foreseeable and correctable errors of judgement or information gathering. Always give some thought to the above before seeing any patient.

Table 14.1 Recommended action according to level of risk of violence

Risk of violence	Recommended action
Low risk	Ward team aware that emergency team should be called if patient becomes more aroused
Violence possible but patient likely to collaborate	Emergency team called to unit/ward but not directly involved in assessment. The emergency team is then available for immediate response should the situation deteriorate
Violence likely and patient not collaborating	Emergency team to be called to ward and interview/assessment to take place with team present in interview area/room. Clear plan for restraint formulated with team members

References and further reading

Anderson, T. R., Bell, C. C., Powell, T. E., *et al* (2004) Assessing psychiatric patients for violence. *Community Mental Health Journal*, 40, 379–399.

Beer, M. D., Pereira, S. M & Paton, C. (2000) *Psychiatric Intensive Care*. Cambridge University Press.

Buckley, P. F., Hrouda, D. R., Friedman, L., *et al* (2004) Insight and its relationship to violent behavior in patients with schizophrenia. *American Journal of Psychiatry*, 161, 1712–1714.

Eronen, M., Angermeyer, M. C. & Schulze, B. (1998) The psychiatric epidemiology of violent behaviour. *Social Psychiatry and Psychiatric Epidemiology* 33 (suppl. 1), S13–23.

Mills, J. F. (2005) Advances in the assessment and prediction of interpersonal violence. *Journal of Interpersonal Violence*, 20, 236–241.

Swanson, J., Estroff, S., Swartz, M., *et al* (1997) Violence and severe mental disorder in clinical and community populations: the effects of psychotic symptoms, comorbidity and lack of treatment. *Psychiatry*, 60, 1–22.

Swartz, M. S., Swanson, J. W., Hiday, V. A., *et al* (1998) Taking the wrong drugs: the role of substance abuse and medication noncompliance in violence among severely mentally ill individuals. *Social Psychiatry and Psychiatric Epidemiology* 33 (suppl. 1), S75–80.

Travis M. J. (2002). Drug treatment, compliance and risk. In *Care of the Mentally Disordered Offender in the Community* (ed. A. Buchanan), pp. 143–174. Oxford University Press.

CHAPTER 15

Managing violence

Michael J. Travis

The management of agitated and violent patients will be dictated by their clinical state and your assessment of their potential risk. This will be based on similar themes to those visited in Chapter 14. Decision on management strategies should, ideally, be made in conjunction with other members of the multidisciplinary team and when possible after discussion with a more senior colleague.

For patients at risk of agitation and violence who are already in hospital, the normal ward team should have a detailed crisis management plan in place. In general the choices are between non-pharmacological management, oral medication (an increase in current dosage or addition to current dosage) or parenteral medication, usually in addition to or instead of oral medication. In practice a combination of these three strategies is often employed.

Non-pharmacological management

Non-pharmacological management of aggression/violence falls into three categories as shown in Box 15.1.

Environmental

As already discussed in Chapter 14, it is important to try to interview the patient to gain insight into the reason for their agitation and to aid effective management. You should use reasoned discussion but remember to maintain

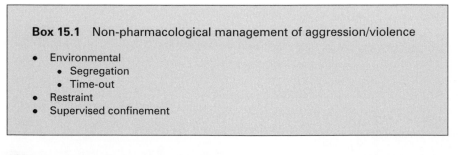

Box 15.1   Non-pharmacological management of aggression/violence

- Environmental
  - Segregation
  - Time-out
- Restraint
- Supervised confinement

distance from the patient. This distance is important to prevent the patient from feeling threatened as well as being good personal safety practice.

Segregation involves encouraging the agitated/violent patient to move to another area away from other people in order to reduce stimulation, allow further talking and hopefully help the patient to calm themselves. Segregation is generally without limit of time. The patient is allowed to re-integrate only when there has been a change in their presentation.

Time-out is different from segregation in that it is more likely to be part of a behavioural management plan than a crisis management tool. In time-out, a plan is devised such that if a patient exhibits certain behaviours they will be asked to go somewhere (e.g. their bedroom) to calm down for a specified period and then allowed to re-engage with ward activities.

Restraint

If the ward team is of the opinion that there is a serious degree of urgency and danger, either impending because of previous knowledge of the patient and non-collaboration or because of significant physical attacks, there may be a decision to restrain the patient.

Ideally this should be carried out by staff properly trained in appropriate control and restraint techniques, and there should be enough trained staff (usually an absolute minimum of four) to reduce the risk of harm to the patient and the staff from a restraint. A restraint is often the prelude to administration of additional medication or to placing the patient in supervised confinement (also known as seclusion). Please note that at the time of writing mechanical restraint is not used in healthcare facilities in the UK.

Supervised confinement

Supervised confinement is the restriction of a person alone in a low-stimulus environment (most often a specially designed room, which may be, and is usually, locked) for the protection of others from significant harm. Its sole aim is to contain severely disturbed behaviour that is likely to cause harm to others.

Supervised confinement is used to control, temporarily and immediately, a dangerous situation that cannot be managed in any other way. It should be used as a last resort when all reasonable steps have been taken to avoid its use, and is usually used only when violence is uncontrolled by any other means (e.g. medication, restraint). It should last for as short a time as possible. It should not be used:

- as a punitive measure or threat
- as part of a treatment programme
- because of shortage of staff
- to manage self-harm or threatened suicide.

Although local policies differ, good clinical practice would require that the use of supervised confinement is reviewed regularly and frequently by the multidisciplinary team and by senior members of the team as soon as practicable.

> **Box 15.2** Aims of pharmacological management
>
> - Immediate reduction in agitation, irritability and hostility
> - Immediate reduction of dangerousness
> - For patients with psychosis the long-term relief of positive psychotic symptoms
> - Lowest effective dose of antipsychotic
> - Lowest side-effect load (beware the paradoxical!)
> - Sedation and/or tranquillisation

Pharmacological management

The rationale behind the pharmacological management of agitation and violence is to provide an immediate reduction in agitation, irritability and hostility, thereby producing an immediate reduction in dangerousness (Box 15.2). Other aims include the long-term relief of positive psychotic symptoms using the lowest effective dose of antipsychotic leading to the lowest side-effect load. It is important within this to understand the difference between tranquillisation and sedation, as the two are not synonymous. Tranquillisation refers to the calming effect of medications, whereas sedation implies a reduction in the level of consciousness. Antipsychotics used to be called 'major tranquillisers' as they can produce tranquillisation without sedation, unlike medications such as barbiturates and benzodiazepines. The tranquillisation effect of antipsychotics is mediated primarily via dopaminergic D_2 receptor blockade as are the antipsychotic effects. Both immediate tranquillisation and longer-term antipsychotic effects can be produced by equivalent doses. Antipsychotics produce sedation by their blockade of histamine and alpha adrenergic receptors. The sedative dose of most antipsychotics is usually above their antipsychotic dose and increases the risk of side-effects. Current practice in the pharmacological management of agitation is therefore to use antipsychotics at doses that will be tranquillising and eventually antipsychotic, and to use adjunctive benzodiazepines to produce sedation.

Although evidence is generally sparse in this area, there are is enough to provide general guidance on the key areas outlined in Box 15.3.

Oral v. intramuscular medication

There was a tendency (in the 1970s and '80s) to try to use antipsychotics as if they were antibiotics or digoxin, with considerable use of 'loading doses'. Although these reports are old, they are worth reviewing briefly here. In an open-label study, Erickson *et al* (1978) compared both oral and intramuscular medication. Loading for 5 days with 60 mg haloperidol per day intramuscularly was no more effective than 15 mg per day of oral haloperidol. A double-blind study using fluphenazine indicated that 48.5 mg intramuscularly was no different from 7.5 mg given orally, with the greatest change in both groups occurring during the first 4–8 hours (Escobar *et al*,

---

Box 15.3   Key areas in the pharmacological management of agitation

- Oral v. intramuscular medication
- Intramuscular v. intravenous medication
- Older 'typical' antipsychotics v. newer 'atypical' antipsychotics
- Antipsychotics v. benzodiazepines – alone or in combination
- Benzodiazepines

1983). This result was replicated and extended by Coffman & Nasrallah (1987), who reported no difference between groups treated with either 16.3 mg of intramuscular fluphenazine or 7.2 mg of oral fluphenazine in the first 24 hours after initiation of treatment.

A more recent study reported similar results with 2 mg oral risperidone in addition to 2 mg oral lorazepam versus 5 mg intramuscular haloperidol in addition to 2 mg intramuscular lorazepam (Currier & Simpson, 2001). These data, taken together, indicate that there is little advantage to 'loading doses' of antipsychotics, and that if a patient can be persuaded to take oral medication this will be as efficacious as that given intramuscularly.

Older, typical intramuscular antipsychotics

When a patient must receive a short-acting intramuscular antipsychotic the standard medication they receive is haloperidol. There is extensive literature comparing intramuscular chlorpromazine with haloperidol and haloperidol with another butyrophenone, droperidol. Chlorpromazine is no longer used intramuscularly because of problems at the injection site and orthostatic hypotension. Droperidol was withdrawn completely owing to a high risk of cardiac complications.

In terms of dosing, most guidelines would suggest an initial dose of 5 mg haloperidol intramuscularly followed by a further 5 mg if there is no response with 30–40 min (McAllister-Williams & Ferrier, 2002; Allen *et al*, 2005; Taylor *et al*, 2007). Further doses may do little to produce a greater degree of tranquillisation but may increase the risks of akathisia and 'neuroleptisation' (gross Parkinsonian symptoms rendering the patient akinetic), which may be counter-therapeutic. This is illustrated in Fig. 15.1, which shows a combined analysis of trials of intramuscular haloperidol and indicates that the effects peak at a dose of about 12 mg.

Intramuscular v. intravenous administration

There have been no randomised controlled trials (RCTs) comparing the efficacy of these routes of administration. A review of the open trials carried out in the 1980s indicated an equivalence for the two routes, with the intravenous drug perhaps having a slightly faster onset of action (Thomas *et al*, 1992). Despite this, the use of intravenous antipsychotics in psychiatric emergencies is now

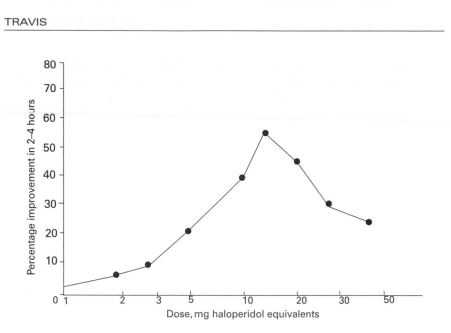

Fig. 15.1 Antipsychotic dose and early response according to Baldessarini *et al* (1988).

very rare. This is probably because intramuscular administration is easier. Intramuscular administration is also arguably safer and used appropriately is likely to lead to fewer extrapyramidal and cardiac side-effects. It might be suggested, however, that intravenous administration allows a better estimation of administered dose and possibly less chance for accumulation.

Older typical v. newer atypical antipsychotics

Two RCTs have compared intramuscular olanzapine (10–30 mg) with intramuscular haloperidol (7.5–22.5 mg). Both drugs proved equally effective in reducing scores on the Excited Component sub-scale of the Positive and Negative Syndrome Scale (PANSS–EC) at 2 hours in consenting patients (Wright *et al*, 2001; Breier *et al*, 2002). Similar results have been obtained with intramuscular olanzapine with lorazepam (Meehan *et al*, 2001, 2002) in consenting patients. The oro-dispersible formulation of olanzapine (Velotab) has never been evaluated in a randomised trial in acute agitation.

In consenting patients who accept oral medication, treatment with risperidone liquid concentrate and lorazepam appears to be comparable to intramuscular haloperidol and lorazepam (Currier & Simpson, 2001).

Intramuscular ziprasidone (10–80 mg/day), although not available in the UK, proved to be as good as intramuscular haloperidol (10–40 mg/day) in reducing agitation in consenting patients, even though it carries warnings about its use in patients at risk of QTc prolongation (Brook *et al*, 2000).

Antipsychotics v. benzodiazepines – alone or together?

A few RCTs compare intramuscular benzodiazepines with intramuscular antipsychotics in the treatment of aggressive and violent patients. In consenting patients, flunitrazepam alone (Dorevitch *et al*, 1999) or lorazepam alone (Salzman *et al*, 1991; Foster *et al*, 1997) are broadly as effective as haloperidol for the control of aggressive and violent behaviour, though there is a suggestion that the onset of action of benzodiazepines is more rapid. Moreover, benzodiazepines produce significantly fewer extrapyramidal side-effects.

Some studies also address the efficacy of combinations over single drugs. The combination of lorazepam and haloperidol has been consistently found to be more effective than either drug alone in consenting patients (Battaglia *et al*, 1997; Bienek *et al*, 1998), an advantage that may be generalisable to other combinations of antipsychotic and sedative drugs.

A randomised trial conducted in Rio de Janeiro in 301 aggressive non-consenting patients found that the combination of haloperidol and promethazine was as effective as midazolam in reducing agitation, but midazolam proved more rapid. The results of this study unfortunately do not generalise to the UK, where these treatments are rarely used in this way in these situations.

It must be noted that although combinations of intramuscular haloperidol and benzodiazepines may be recommended on current evidence, combinations of intramuscular olanzapine and benzodiazepines are cautioned against.

Benzodiazepines

The advantages and disadvantages of using benzodiazepines are shown in Box 15.4. Pharmacologically benzodiazepines all exert their effects by acting on the benzodiazepine receptors present on most GABA-A receptors. There they facilitate the inhibitory actions of gamma-aminobutyric acid (GABA) on neurons by prolonging the opening of the GABA receptor chloride channel after the binding of GABA.

The advantages of benzodiazepines are that their primary action is to produce sedation (which may be a wanted effect in agitated patients) and anxiolysis, and they do this relatively rapidly without a risk of extrapyramidal side-effects. Their effects on psychomotor performance are unlikely to be as great as those seen with haloperidol and, although dependence may be an issue with long-term benzodiazepine use, short-term use is not associated with dependence. In order to ensure a minimal risk of dependence it is essential that a clear management plan be drawn up at the time of commencement of benzodiazepines, indicating when and how they are to be withdrawn once the patient begins to improve. It is recommended that if regular benzodiazepine use has been for 8 days or less they may be abruptly stopped. Use for longer than this will usually involve a reduction in benzodiazepine dose of one-quarter to one-fifth of total daily dose every 3–14 days depending on the length of use and the half-life of the benzodiazepine(s) prescribed.

The only life-threatening side-effect of benzodiazepines is respiratory depression. Although the risk of respiratory depression is low, it is essential that if high-dose or parenteral benzodiazepines are to be used, the patient's respiratory rate, pulse and blood pressure are monitored frequently. Ideally there should be a continuous measure of the patient's oxygen saturation using

> **Box 15.4**   Advantages and disadvantages of benzodiazepines
>
> Advantages
> - Relieve anxiety
> - Sedation
> - Muscle relaxation
> - Few side-effects
> - Low overdose toxicity alone
> - Rapid onset of action
>
> Disadvantages
> - Sedation
> - Cognitive side-effects
> - Potentiation of central nervous system depressants
> - Psychomotor side-effects
> - Respiratory depression
> - Possible dependence and withdrawal syndrome

a pulse oximeter. If there are concerns that the patient might be experiencing respiratory depression, the drug flumazenil will effectively reverse the effects of any benzodiazepine. It must be remembered, however, that flumazenil may precipitate a worsening of the patient's anxiety/agitation and may precipitate seizures in patients who are tolerant to the effects of benzodiazepines. Flumazenil also has a relatively short half-life and therefore may need to be given as an infusion to patients who have received benzodiazepines with a long half-life such as diazepam.

Conclusions

It is clear that although non-pharmacological strategies are essential to the management of aggression and violence, especially as pre-emptive interventions, antipsychotics remain a central part of the management of the acutely agitated patient.

Despite received 'lore', high-dose/loading protocols have no advantage over minimal effective dosing, may produce short-term harm and in the long term may make patients less likely to accept a pharmacological intervention in the future. Although generally in psychiatry monotherapy is the aim whenever possible, current evidence suggests that combinations of antipsychotics and benzodiazepines may increase efficacy and reduce the total antipsychotic dose used or needed, and will almost certainly reduce extrapyramidal side-effects.

Key to the management of agitated and aggressive patients is the clear message that whenever possible oral medication should be offered before giving intramuscular medication. Not only does the current evidence strongly suggest that oral and intramuscular medications produce a similar level of calming, but offering oral before giving intramuscular medication at least allows some degree of 'choice' for the patient, will be seen as less punitive by the patient and will aid future discussions on management.

It can tentatively be suggested that the newer antipsychotics, particularly for those willing to accept oral medication, may offer even further benefits in the management of agitation or violence.

References

Allen, M. H., Currier, G. W., Carpenter, D., *et al* (2005) treatment of behavioral emergencies. *Journal of Psychiatric Practice*, **11** (suppl. 1), 5–25.

Baldessarini, R.J., Cohen, B.M., Teicher, M.H. (1988) Significance of neuroleptic dose and plasma level in the pharmacological treatment of psychoses. *Archives of General Psychiatry* **45**, 79–91.

Battaglia, J., Moss, S., Rush, J., *et al* (1997) Haloperidol, lorazepam, or both for psychotic agitation? A multicenter, prospective, double-blind, emergency department study. *American Journal of Emergency Medicine* **15**, 335–340.

Bienek, S. A., Ownby, R. L., Penalver, A., *et al* (1998) A double-blind study of lorazepam versus the combination of haloperidol and lorazepam in managing agitation. *Pharmacotherapy* **18**, 57–62.

Breier, A., Meehan, K., Birkett, M., *et al* (2002) A double-blind, placebo-controlled dose-response comparison of intramuscular olanzapine and haloperidol in the treatment of acute agitation in schizophrenia. *Archives of General Psychiatry* **59**, 441–448.

Brook, S., Lucey, J. V., Gunn, K. P. (2000) Intramuscular ziprasidone compared with intramuscular haloperidol in the treatment of acute psychosis. Ziprasidone IM Study Group. *Journal of Clinical Psychiatry* **61**, 933–941.

Coffman, J. A., Nasrallah, H. A., Lyskowski, J., *et al* (1987) Clinical effectiveness of oral and parenteral rapid neuroleptization. *Journal of Clinical Psychiatry* **48**, 20–24.

Currier, G. W. & Simpson, G. M. (2001) Risperidone liquid concentrate and oral lorazepam versus intramuscular haloperidol and intramuscular lorazepam for treatment of psychotic agitation. *Journal of Clinical Psychiatry* **62**, 153–157.

Dorevitch, A., Katz, N., Zemishlany, Z., *et al* (1999) Intramuscular flunitrazepam versus intramuscular haloperidol in the emergency treatment of aggressive psychotic behavior. *American Journal of Psychiatry* **156**, 142–144.

Ericksen, S. E., Hurt, S. W., Chang, S. (1978) Haloperidol dose, plasma levels, and clinical response: a double-blind study [proceedings]. *Psychopharmacology Bulletin* **14**, 15–16.

Escobar, J. I., Barron, A., Kiriakos, R. (1983) A controlled study of neuroleptization with fluphenazine hydrochloride injections. *Journal of Clinical Psychopharmacology* **3**, 359–362.

Foster, S., Kessel, J., Berman, M. E., *et al* (1997) Efficacy of lorazepam and haloperidol for rapid tranquilization in a psychiatric emergency room setting. *International Clinical Psychopharmacology* **12**, 175–179.

McAllister-Williams, H. & Ferrier, N. (2002) Rapid tranquillisation: time for a reappraisal of options for parenteral therapy. *British Journal of Psychiatry*, **180**, 485–489.

Meehan, K., Zhang, F., David, S., *et al* (2001) A double-blind, randomized comparison of the efficacy and safety of intramuscular injections of olanzapine, lorazepam, or placebo in treating acutely agitated patients diagnosed with bipolar mania. *Journal of Clinical Psychopharmacology* **21**, 389–397.

Meehan, K. M., Wang, H., David, S. R., *et al* (2002) Comparison of rapidly acting intramuscular olanzapine, lorazepam, and placebo. a double-blind, randomized study in acutely agitated patients with dementia. *Neuropsychopharmacology* **26**, 494–504.

Salzman, C., Solomon, D., Miyawaki, E., *et al* (1991) Parenteral lorazepam versus parenteral haloperidol for the control of psychotic disruptive behavior. *Journal of Clinical Psychiatry* **52**, 177–180.

Taylor, D., Paton, C. & Kerwin, R. W. (2007) *The Maudsley Prescribing Guidelines* (9th edn). Informa Healthcare.

Thomas, H., Schwartz, E., Petrilli, R. (1992) Droperidol versus haloperidol for chemical restraint of agitated and combative patients. *Annals of Emergency Medicine* **21**, 407–413.

Wright, P., Birkett, M., David, S. R., *et al* (2001) Double-blind, placebo-controlled comparison of intramuscular olanzapine and intramuscular haloperidol in the treatment of acute agitation in schizophrenia. *American Journal of Psychiatry* **158**, 1149–1151.

CHAPTER 16

Managing difficult clinical situations

Cleo Van Velsen

The fundamental tool of good psychiatric practice is the taking of a thorough and thoughtful history and describing a mental state. Initially when trainees start psychiatry, this can seem quite straightforward: there are areas of enquiry, plus associated questions, followed by a description of phenomenology, based on observation. There are many texts devoted to the art of history-taking and mental state examination, for example the *Maudsley Handbook of Practical Psychiatry* (Goldberg & Murray, 2002).

The importance of these skills cannot be underestimated. They require time, practice and patience, all of which can be jettisoned in day-to-day clinical practice. Any trainee (hopefully) can spot severe and overt psychosis, but learning how to elicit more subtle phenomena, such as encapsulated delusions or ideas of reference, can take time and thought, as can less tangible aspects of history. Untoward incident enquiries and clinical reviews often reveal that aspects of history and mental state were 'missed'.

I have chosen some common examples of situations where good clinical practice can be compromised. I will follow this with a discussion of so called 'difficult patients' and then certain types of encounters that can be problematic. I will conclude with suggestions for ensuring good practice.

Settings, situations and associated difficulties

Psychosexual history

In taking a history the trainee is exploring aspects of the patient's life, mind and experiences that are personal and sensitive. One difficult situation can be the enquiry into psychosexual history, including questions about whether or not the patient has experiences of sexual abuse. (Linked is the enquiry into sexual fantasies and practices when assessing personality.) If the trainee is too intrusive, awkward and obviously embarrassed, then the patient can be left with feelings of guilt or shame, and it can even lead to the patient having an experience of abuse all over again. If the area is avoided altogether (often rationalised in terms of time or it being a first meeting), the patient may experience this as a message that this is not an area about which the trainee wants to know. Thus, an important aspect of that patient's emotional experience may be left out, again increasing shame. Awkwardness of this kind can be increased by issues of age, gender and cultural difference between the trainee and patient.

Leaving it for the psychologist to do is not an option. The best way to manage is to acknowledge that it is personal and intimate, and demonstrate to the patient awareness of the possible impact. It can help to use the technique of normalisation, for example prefacing a particular question by a general statement regarding similar experiences of other patients.

Location

Interactions with patients take place in a variety of contexts, all of which can have an impact upon the quality and usefulness of the meeting. It is important that the clinical encounter is intimate enough, so that the patient feels engaged with the trainee, thereby reinforcing the therapeutic alliance. However, there also needs to be the establishment of good enough boundaries, so that both trainee and patient feel safe, and will not end up in a situation where important emotional and physical limits are transgressed to the detriment of both patient and trainee.

The campaign against the stigma associated with mental illness has partly been reflected in the move to community care and the closure of the larger psychiatric hospitals, plus change in language, such as referring to service users, etc. However, it is always important for the trainee to bear in mind their role within the system with regard to the patient. It is not the trainee's role to become a friend, although being friendly is important. Conversely, the trainee must not be so distant from the patient that no real engagement or alliance is formed (i.e. over-involvement v. under-involvement).

Out-patient clinic

This is the traditional location for the assessment of new patients and the treatment of known patients. Out-patient clinics are often chaotic with too many patients to be seen in too little time and frequent non-attendance of appointments. Such a setting can contribute to the process of objectification of a patient (i.e. where personal identity is lost to be replaced by a label, such as 'schizophrenic' or 'depressive,' rather than 'Mr A who suffers from schizophrenia'). Poor time-keeping, often by psychiatric trainees, not surprisingly leads to poor time-keeping by patients, as the patients feel that the trainee is not valuing the encounter.

Trainees can compound this difficulty by beginning a delayed interview by explaining that they have been held up at a meeting or another emergency. This just communicates to the patient that they should not protest and the patient should never be made responsible for the trainee's problems. Trainees need to prioritise appointment times with patients and to audit the out-patient clinics. If trainees find themselves relieved that several patients are missing their appointments, the out-patient clinic has ceased to be a therapeutic setting but has become anti-therapeutic.

Another difficult situation in the out-patient clinic is the constant change of trainee, often assigned to patients who have attended the clinic for many years. There is acknowledgement in current psychiatric practice of the importance of attachment in the engagement and management of patients, especially since psychiatric illness and disorder, by its very nature, attacks attachment. This difficult emotional situation is made worse when, because of institutional problems, patients never develop ongoing attachments to those who treat them.

Domiciliary visits

Domiciliary visits have become an increasingly important aspect of the assessment of new patients and the follow-up of existing patients. The advantage is that the patient is seen within their social system. In addition much information about clinical state can be gained from the state of the house or the flat, for example the amount of security, cleanliness, clutter, bareness, and the patient's capacity to manage basic skills.

What makes the domiciliary visit a potentially difficult situation is the element of intimacy once the trainee enters the patient's home. This can promote good communication at one level but it can also inhibit certain areas of observation or examination (e.g. psychosexual history). Also, does one accept a cup of tea or use the toilet?

It is important to complete a risk assessment prior to any domiciliary visit. This includes searching for problems of boundary distortions in the previous history.

Out-of-hours encounters

These are the clinical encounters in the late hours of the evening or the early hours of the morning, in a variety of settings (e.g. accident and emergency departments and police stations). A vignette for such an out-of-hours encounter is given in Box 16.1.

Box 16.1   Vignette for an out-of-hours encounter

A man of 26 was brought to an accident and emergency department by police because of an attempt to throw himself off a bridge. The admitting senior house officer learnt that he had absconded from a psychiatric hospital and she elicited paranoid beliefs regarding patients and staff at the previous unit. She noted that his suicide attempt was in the context of a wish to leave the previous unit and he was admitted to the local psychiatric unit. There was no full examination of his current suicidal ideation and shortly after admission, he jumped from a window and died.

People can present in a variety of states of distress, with self-harm, acute psychosis, suicidal behaviour or ideation, often complicated by intoxication from drugs or alcohol. The difficult task facing the trainee in such a situation is, to use Bion's (1961) metaphor, 'to think under fire'. Feelings of irritation, tiredness and anger at being woken need to be acknowledged but put to one side as far as possible. Full history-taking and mental state examination is often not possible (or appropriate) in such a situation, but investigating certain aspects of history and mental state such as suicidal ideation is essential. Appleby (2001) has shown that a significant number of patients who die by suicide have presented to services shortly before the suicide. The difficult clinical task of the trainee is to distinguish between what could be described as threatening behaviour ('admit me or I'm going to kill myself') and genuine distress. The risk is that a trainee will not base their assessment on a thoughtful examination but react to their own negative feelings, which the patient has aroused, and send them away.

Wards

Difficult situations on wards concern both patients who take up a disproportionate amount of time and energy and, at the other extreme, the 'forgotten' ones. All trainees will have the experience of one patient on a ward being the main topic of conversation over a sustained period in ward rounds, etc. Once again, these patients need to be understood, both from the point of view of diagnosis and of the system in which they are placed.

For example, people with a diagnosis of personality disorder are often not well placed on a general psychiatric ward, as the nature of the ward exacerbates various aspects of personality disorder functioning, such as reinforcing transfer of responsibility from patient to staff and reproduction of abusive or destructive dynamics from the patient's life. There can be unhelpful use of manpower (e.g. a patient being closely observed by two nurses for prolonged periods).

This situation can further lead to 'malignant alienation' (Watts & Morgan, 1994) as staff become exhausted, and then to dangerous acting out by the patient, both towards self and others. Appleby (1992) noted that 'the feature which most strikingly distinguished suicides was disturbed relationships with staff resulting in premature discharge.'

An example of a patient about which there is no discussion is someone with a diagnosis of chronic schizophrenia who has become depersonalised to the extent of being an institutional 'non-person'. The system, including the psychiatric trainee, has ceased to be interested and give meaning to the patient's experiences; a reflection of the process of schizophrenia, known for its effects on meaning and thinking systems. Many a patient described as 'settled' in their mental state, on further examination can be found to be most unsettled.

Trainees must always audit the amount of time being devoted to patients under their care on the ward instead of just reacting to what is there.

Understanding and managing 'difficult' patients

Hinshelwood (1999) suggests that the 'difficult patient is a label that does not connote a configuration of clinical signs and symptoms: it is not a DSM category but a way of describing the state of the professional during the encounter ... the professional does not like the patient or something about the patient; he suffers a disagreeable, or difficult feeling.'

Psychiatric trainees, and other mental health professionals, will often have a sense of unacceptability or guilt about negative feelings towards patients. Therefore, they can end up being unacknowledged, misunderstood and enacted in ways that can lead to unhelpful clinical situations, which can deteriorate rapidly.

It is essential for all psychiatric trainees to develop a model of mind with which to understand their reactions to patients. This includes the psychodynamic as well as other psychological models, as all address issues of patients' relationships to themselves and to their therapist. An example in which a trainee has not considered these factors is given below.

A trainee presents a patient whom he encountered in the accident and emergency department on several occasions. In conclusion he makes the diagnosis of a personality disorder. When asked from which personality disorder the patient suffered, the trainee is silent.

This interaction says more about the trainee's experience of the patient than his diagnosis. Personality disorder is a diagnosis with significant ramifications, and the example above describes how easily it can be assigned. In this way all difficulties are located within the patient whereas, in fact, they may lie in the interaction between the trainee and the patient. Such a negative therapeutic reaction between trainee and patient can be reflected in the system as a whole, leading to repeated and destructive acting out: both by the patient and taking a variety of forms, such as self-harm, absconding, violence to others, etc; and by trainees and others, for example being cruel in the name of being challenging, making moral judgements (based on unacknowledged dislike or hatred) and 'getting rid' of patients.

The rationale behind the Government paper, *Personality Disorder: No Longer a Diagnosis of Exclusion* (Department of Health, 2003) was based on a repeated scenario whereby patients diagnosed with personality disorder were denied services (including thorough history-taking and examination) on the grounds of 'untreatability' or being 'unsuitable' for community mental health services. The concentration on severe mental illness, it has been argued, is because of limited resources, but can also be a result of an institutional 'wish' not to engage with patients that are considered difficult and hard to manage.

The vignette in Box 16.2 illustrates warning signs that should alert any trainee to the possibility of being caught up in the dynamics described above. This includes use of particular words to describe a patient's behaviour:

Box 16.2 Vignette illustrating possible difficulties a trainee may encounter when assessing people with personality disorder

A patient with an established diagnosis of dependent personality disorder and alcohol misuse presented at the accident and emergency department with a friend who told the trainee that the patient had tried to hang himself and was interrupted by his friend. He had written a note and had also taken an overdose of ten temazepam tablets. The trainee decided that the patient was attempting to manipulate his admission to hospital, discharged him and 2 hours later the patient threw himself under a train.

---

namely 'manipulative', 'attention-seeking and 'behavioural' – all of which convey a negative judgement.

One answer to the management of a 'difficult' patient is not to locate all the difficulties within the patient but to examine the nature of the interaction between trainee and patient, bearing in mind that both are located within a particular political and social context. *The Response Aroused by the Psychopath* (Symington, 1980) highlights the importance of acknowledging and understanding the individual and systemic responses aroused by a 'difficult' patient.

Diagnosis and 'difficult' patients

Schizophrenia

Schizophrenia is the well-described illness within the field of descriptive psychiatry in which symptoms are highlighted. However, although 'psychotic patients ... exhibit certain symptoms clusters and personality patterns, how they arrived at that psychological place and how their fantasies and defences shake their current shape internal/external life is special to each case' (Waska, 2005). Reducing a patient to their diagnosis will reduce the meaning of the illness to the person, thereby inhibiting a therapeutic alliance.

Common features of schizophrenia include delusion, fragmentation of thought processes, acute disturbance, paranoia, chronic disintegration and isolation. An 'ideal response' once diagnosis has been made is containment (within a domestic out-patient or ward setting), treatment (including medication), plus practical help and advice on daily living skills. The aim is long-term rehabilitation and maintenance in an optimum situation.

What can actually happen is fear, leading to over-sedation or control or neglect as already described. In addition, there can be a change of diagnosis to personality disorder, which is sometimes appropriate but is sometimes a reflection of a process (i.e. a move from engagement and hope to despair and dislike).

Borderline personality disorder

The diagnosis of borderline personality disorder is associated with pervasive instability of mood and self-image and is expressed in problems in maintaining personal relationships (e.g. intense attachment followed by abandonment). There is impulsivity (expressed in a wide number of ways), suicidal behaviour and self-harm (e.g. self-cutting or multiple overdoses).

Main (1957) described patients with these characteristics who use up much time and energy and often create divisions among staff. Some staff may become 'over-involved', and want to bring increasing resources in order to help the patient. Others are excluded from such a view and tend to want the patient to be discharged. This conflicted situation leads to inconsistent treatment and the patient can 'disappear' between the split created. The trainee can be caught up in this complex situation and find themself caught on one side of the split or the other.

The ideal response with such a patient, individually and systematically, is to provide consistent care with clear boundaries and help the patient move from action to thought. The actual responses often described are chaos, disruption, arousal of feelings of love and hate, increased anxiety, inappropriate medication, abrupt discharge and in rare cases 'sexual healing', wherein an inexperienced trainee who perhaps has difficulties in his (usually) own life can be caught up in a sexual relationship with such a patient, leading to significant adverse consequences for both.

Antisocial personality disorder

This diagnosis is associated with increased aggression and violence, lack of empathy, cynicism, multiple relationships, impulsivity, etc. Patients with antisocial personality disorder are often very 'sensitive' in a paranoid sense when it comes to others' response to them, but instead of these being used in the service of understanding or compassion, they are 'corrupted' into cruelty and indifference. This makes the containment and treatment of such patients extremely difficult, both at an institutional and an individual level, as seen in a number of prison reports describing a culture of bullying, other delinquent behaviour and collusion by staff (http://inspectorates.justice. gov.uk/hmiprisons/).

Encountering a patient with a diagnosis of antisocial personality disorder who is aroused and angry is one of the most difficult clinical situations that a trainee can face, and the trainee's task is to avoid being caught up in the usual responses that the individual arouses (e.g. fear, anger and hatred). If the trainee cannot avoid these responses, they may get into a confrontation with such a patient, therefore escalating the risk of violence to self or others. Alternatively, the trainee might be 'bullied' by such a patient into prescribing drugs such as benzodiazepines.

In such a situation it is important that the trainee finds out whether the patient has been seen before in the accident and emergency department, and whether there are any other mental health staff that are familiar with them, and to consult with senior staff.

It is often helpful to make reflective statements to the patient such as 'I can see you feel rejected and angry', rather than ask too many questions. Such patients are used to a certain repertoire of responses, which the trainee needs to try and avoid. The aim is to enable the patient to leave in a less aroused state and with some plan of action in mind, without making threats or promises that cannot be kept.

Transference and counter-transference

This model, which is used to understand responses both from patients and therapists, derives from psychoanalytic theory but is relevant to all interactions. The transference describes the repeated pattern of relating to others, which is based on personality and previous life experiences.

The counter-transference reflects the responses a trainee (and other mental health professionals) will have to a patient, which are based on two components. The first is the particular life experience of the trainee. This is illustrated in the vignette described in Box 16.3.

Such responses are legitimate and can be therapeutic but they need to be understood as belonging to the trainee. What must be avoided is burdening the patient in a way that could leave them feeling that their psychiatrist is not robust enough to help.

Counter-transference is also a result of feelings and emotions being projected onto the therapist by the patient. An example of this is given in the vignette in Box 16.4.

What emerged in supervision when discussing the patient described in Box 16.4 was that the patient had experienced throughout her life feeling people being overwhelmed by and distancing themselves from her, and this had been repeated in the room with the trainee.

If this aspect of the counter-transference can be understood then it can be used as clinical information, which can enable the trainee to engage better with their patient. In the example described in Box 16.4 it was possible to

---

Box 16.3 Vignette illustrating counter-transference according to the life experience of the trainee

A trainee of 27 saw a female refugee of the same age. The patient was a doctor who had spent 3 years in prison in her own country, where she had been subject to consistent maltreatment and humiliation. The trainee found herself almost moved to tears in the interview which meant it was hard to think with the patient in the room owing to her own identification.

> **Box 16.4**   Vignette illustrating counter-transference as a result of feelings and emotions being projected onto the therapist by the patient
>
> A trainee was interviewing a patient with circumstantial speech. It was hard to interrupt and she found herself feeling trapped, disengaged and unable to make interventions. As the interview continued the patient spoke increasingly rapidly and loudly such that the feelings intensified and the trainee said less and less.

say to the patient that it seemed she had an experience all her life of not being listened to, and that was partly why she spoke and interacted in the way that she did.

Such a simple observation can help to clarify a situation and enable the patient to feel more understood. It also helps the trainee process difficult negative feelings rather than act them out.

Other difficult situations

One-to-one psychotherapy or other psychological treatment

Such a therapeutic encounter, by necessity, promotes a sense of intimacy which means that the boundaries and limits around the session need to be particularly secure. A situation where the boundaries for individual psychotherapy may not seem secure is illustrated in the vignette in Box 16.5.

What emerged in supervision was that both trainee and patient felt uneasy emerging from the session at 5.00 p.m. on a Friday afternoon when most people had gone home. It created an overwhelming sense of intimacy for the patient who therefore avoided the sessions. It further emerged that the trainee herself felt some relief as she had found herself fearful of the patient, as his uneasiness was communicated to her as a reflection of his own fear at being there with her.

> **Box 16.5**   Vignette illustrating insecure boundaries of individual psychotherapy
>
> A female trainee took on a patient for individual psychotherapy. The patient was a man of 35 with avoidant traits, who had never managed a close sexual relationship with a woman. The trainee had a slot open at 4.00 pm on a Friday afternoon and treatment commenced, but after three sessions the patient dropped out.

Generally such sessions should not be scheduled out of hours or just prior to a weekend. All details of arrangements, however seemingly trivial, must be discussed with the supervisor. A trainee should never take on such a treatment without regular supervision.

Gifts

It is probably quite simple to say that, on the whole, trainees should not give their patients gifts. However, the definition of 'gift' is a complex one (e.g. the patient might experience a trainee as giving them a 'gift' of their time or attention). In addition, when it comes to Christmas time, if the patient is on a long-stay ward it might feel appropriate to give a card, particularly as many of these patients have no family. Such acts, of course, should never be restricted to certain 'favourite' patients.

Most mental health trusts have a policy regarding gifts from patients to staff, but again the definition of gift is complex. Does this include a card from a patient expressing gratitude? What about a box of chocolates from an out-patient at the end of a period of treatment in the clinic?

For some patients part of their therapeutic progress has been the ability to develop a capacity to feel helped by the person treating them and, therefore, rejection of the gift could cause hurt.

A gift may, of course, be provocative (e.g. money) or aggressive (e.g. a pornographic magazine) and in this case should be seen as a violation of limits or boundaries, which needs to be explored with the patient.

This author is of the view that a hard and fast rule is difficult to enforce, and the trainee should consult with their supervisor, in order to understand the meaning of the gift in the clinical context.

Speaking to relatives in the absence of the patient

This is a delicate situation. There can be a tendency, particularly with patients who have conditions such as chronic schizophrenia or, conversely, those who seem agitated and aroused, to have a conversation with relatives without the patient present. The adverse consequence of this can be a loss of trust and a lack of engagement from the patient, which might in fact be collusive with their illness and disorder, rather than helpful.

Engaging with the family in the presence of the patient is, on the whole, to be preferred, but again the decision must be made with thought as to possible advantages and disadvantages.

Physical contact

The complex situation described in the vignette in Box 16.6 illustrates where a good intention to comfort, was later 'converted' into anger because the patient felt abandoned by the trainee who had moved on to another post. It is not helpful to say to the patient simply that physical contact is 'inappropriate', the trainee needs to describe why, considering the patient's

153

Box 16.6 Vignette illustrating potential problems following physical content between trainee and patient

A young woman, aged 27 with a diagnosis of borderline personality disorder began weeping in an interview with the male trainee as she was recounting her history of abuse, both as a child and as an adult in relationships with men. The trainee handed the patient a tissue and she took his hand and held it for 10 min. She told him later in the meeting that it had been very important to her that he had comforted her in this way as it showed she could trust a man. Ten months later the patient made an accusation of sexual assault against the trainee.

---

previous history, such an action is unhelpful (e.g. by showing the patient how other relationships in the past had repeatedly become experienced by her as abusive).

The same trainee helped an elderly woman in his next post, who was frail and fragile, by holding her by the shoulders and guiding her down the corridor. In this case physical contact demonstrated empathy and concern and the patient was unlikely to experience it as abuse.

The fundamental principle is that the meaning of certain actions to a particular patient are important to consider, both in the immediate and long term.

Secrecy v. confidentiality

It is always important to maintain confidentiality and to avoid disclosing out unnecessary details, but the decision needs to be a joint one between trainee and patient, not an imposed one. The example given in Box 16.7 serves to illustrate the difference between confidentiality and secrecy. Confidentiality promotes disclosure and therapeutic engagement whereas secrecy 'traps' the trainee into a relationship with a patient that can lead to acting out or collusion.

Box 16.7 Vignette illustrating the difference between secrecy and confidentiality

In his first interview with a trainee, a male patient, convicted of a sexual offence, said he would tell her about his childhood abuse but only if she agreed not to tell anyone else about it. The trainee agreed and found herself in the difficult situation of 'carrying' a secret that created a sense of intimacy and alliance with the patient that was uncomfortable.

Tools to help trainees manage difficult clinical situations

Experience of psychological therapies

In order to gain Membership of the Royal College of Psychiatrists, candidates are required to have some experience of psychological therapies: individual, group, family, and cognitive and/or psychodynamic. This is essential if some of the pitfalls described above are to be avoided. The aim is to develop a model of mind, which helps the trainee to recognise that they are never disembodied, entirely objective and neutral observers, but are participants in a complex, interpersonal interaction.

Thorough history-taking and mental state examination

The trainee must always make time for a thorough history and mental state examination. In almost every single inquiry, from an untoward incident to a homicide, lack of communication is cited as a significant difficulty. Such a lack of communication between professionals can proceed from a lack of communication between trainee and patient. Developing skills to recognise non-verbal communications and to explore verbal experiences in a less concrete way will increase the quality of communication.

Taking a detailed history is more than ticking the answers to questions: it entails relating the meaning of those questions to the particular patient's difficulties. If the trainee is working in a context where this is not possible (e.g. in an accident and emergency department in the middle of the night), then a note must be made and an effort made to complete a thorough history and mental state examination at a later date.

Avoidance of labels

Certain words and descriptions need to have a mental 'asterisk' next to them, requiring the trainee to rethink what has been said. These phrases and concepts include 'settled', 'manipulative', 'attention-seeking', 'behavioural' and stating that a patient 'lacks insight'. The first few of these have already been described.

Insight is a complex phenomenon which has been well examined by David (1990). Patients may demonstrate considerable insight into their own condition but not use the vocabulary of psychiatry. Trainees need to be sensitive about imposing a psychiatric discourse on the patient and, instead, use the psychiatric examination to draw experiences of illness from their patients.

Awareness of own emotions

Trainees need to be aware of their own emotions and responses that patients arouse: anger, love, hatred, hopelessness, despair, etc. It is often patients with the most complex psychopathology, within the realm of personality disorder, but not necessarily so, who arouse such feelings, creating a difficult clinical situation. Trainees need to ensure that they receive regular supervision from senior colleagues and peers and feel open to discussing their responses.

Awareness of increased suicide risk in personality disorder

Trainees must always bear in mind that people bearing a diagnosis of personality disorder can also suffer from an Axis 1 disorder. Self-harm for example is not a totally different phenomenon to suicidal behaviour. It is of note that patients with a diagnosis of antisocial personality disorder (Verona *et al*, 2001) plus those with borderline personality (Stone, 1990) have increased risks of suicide.

References

Appleby, L. (1992) Suicide in psychiatric patients: risk and prevention. *British Journal of Psychiatry*, **161**, 749–758.

Appleby, L. (2001). *Safety First. Five Year Report of the National Confidential Inquiry Suicide and Homicide by People with Mental Illness*. Department of Health.

Bion, W. R. (1961) *Experiences in Groups*. Basic Books.

David, A. S. (1990) Insight and psychosis. *British Journal of Psychiatry*, **156**, 798–808.

Department of Health (2003) *Personality Disorder: No Longer a Diagnosis of Exclusion*. Department of Health.

Hinshelwood, R. D. (1999) The difficult patient. The role of 'scientific psychiatry' in understanding patients with chronic schizophrenia or severe personality disorder. *British Journal of Psychiatry*, **174**, 187–190.

Goldberg, D. & Murray, R. (2002) *The Maudsley Handbook of Practical Psychiatry*. Oxford University Press.

Main, T. (1957) The ailment. *British Journal of Medical Psychology*, **30**, 129–145.

Stone, M. H. (1990) *The Fate of Borderline Patients: Successful Outcome and Psychiatric Practice*. Guilford Press.

Symington, N. (1980) *The Response Aroused by the Psychopath. International Review of Psycho-Analysis*, **7**, 291–298.

Verona, E., Patrick C. J. & Joiner, T. E. (2001) *Psychopathy, Antisocial Personality and Suicide Risk*. Journal of Abnormal Psychology, **110**, 462–470.

Waska, R. (2005). *Real People Real Problems Real solutions*. Brunner–Routledge.

Watts, D. & Morgan, O. (1994) Malignant alienation. Dangers for patients who are difficult to like. *British Journal of Psychiatry*, **164**, 11–15.

CHAPTER 17

Understanding and managing stress

Jerome Carson and Frank Holloway

Healthcare professionals have repeatedly reported high levels of stress and demonstrate an increased frequency of psychiatric caseness compared with the general population. It is clear that being a doctor can be bad for your mental health. The problem of workplace stress is taken very seriously by the Department of Health and NHS Employers (the umbrella organisation for the personnel function of NHS Trusts), partly because stress has been identified as the leading cause of absence due to sickness in the National Health Service (NHS) – up to 30% of the total. The Department of Health has elaborated policies aimed at decreasing stress and its causes in the NHS. These policies draw on broader work in this field by the Health and Safety Executive.

Among doctors, consultant psychiatrists report higher levels of stress than their general medical colleagues, despite objectively less heavy workloads (Deary et al, 1996a). Mental health professionals are confronted by many sources of stress in their jobs. Staff of all disciplines and at all grades identify as stressors: heavy workloads; increased paperwork and bureaucracy; lack of administrative support; the emotionally and physically demanding environment of the acute ward; dealing with difficult or violent patients; having a poor physical work environment; and having to take the blame when things go wrong (Sainsbury Centre for Mental Health, 2000).

In this chapter we consider the stressors that confront psychiatrists in general, the specific stressors of clinical training and the issue of how best to manage stress. We make brief mention of the issues faced by the doctor with a mental illness and say a little about the ways that the employing organisation can contribute to addressing the problem of staff stress. We start by framing the stress process within a particular model that better enables us to understand the complex set of factors that comprise the term 'occupational stress'. It is important to state that, despite the current moral panic surrounding it, stress is not necessarily negative. An optimal level of stress keeps us motivated and alert. Highly successful people in all walks of life positively embrace stress and most of us tolerate it well most of the time. However, excessive stress, particularly if it is prolonged, can result in mental and physical health problems.

The Health and Safety Executive (2001) defines occupational or work-related stress as 'an adverse reaction to excessive pressures or other demands'. This covers the physical and psychological consequences of stress and places the cause firmly in the workplace. General factors leading to work-related stress have been identified from the occupational psychology literature and include: the demands of the job; the individual's control over their work; the support received from managers and colleagues; relationships at work; the individual's role in the organisation; and change and how it is managed (International Stress Management Association, 2004). As we shall see, the stress process is rather more complex than this definition implies. One person's 'excessive' pressures may generally be quite tolerable to another person, but may become intolerable to that more sanguine individual when other aspects of their lives change. The organisational factors associated with staff stress are also rather different from the issues that people working in community mental health services have identified as being stressful (see Table 17.1).

The Whitehall Study followed up civil servants assessed on a variety of job-related and personality measures and explored the physical and emotional consequences of the workplace environment. These are not trivial. How we experience our job in terms of its demands and the latitude or control we have over decisions has a very significant effect independent of other risk factors on the occurrence of fatal coronary heart disease (Kuper & Marmot, 2003). High demand and low decision latitude are potentially dangerous to our physical health – and increasingly characterise the lot of the mental health professional!

Table 17.1 Sources of stress identified by members of a community mental health team[1]

Source of stress	Percentage identifying source
Administrative demands	79
Lack of resources	75
Work overload	58
Responsibility for patients	54
Patients relapsing	37
Fears of violence	33
Time management	33
Working with demanding patients	29

1. Data from Reid *et al* (1999).

A model of the stress process

There have been numerous attempts at developing a model of the stress process. The one we use here is shown in Fig. 17.1 and was developed by Carson & Kuipers (1998). This model identifies three distinct levels of the stress process: external stressors, moderating factors and stress outcomes. It provides a conceptual framework for examining the literature on the stress that psychiatrists experience.

External stressors comprise three elements: specific occupational stressors; major (external to work) life events; and the more innocuous sounding hassles and uplifts. Trainee psychiatrists are likely to face specific stressors linked to the relationship with their consultant supervisors and other members of the multidisciplinary team, their continual job mobility (which has its positive aspects as well) and the burden of studying for examinations. Adverse life events, such as relationship breakdown or the illness of a child, will take their predictable toll. Well-run teams seek to provide their members with regular uplifts.

The effect of external stressors will depend on the potential moderating factors that trainees are able to draw upon. These include self-esteem, coping skills, resilience, emotional stability, social support, sense of mastery

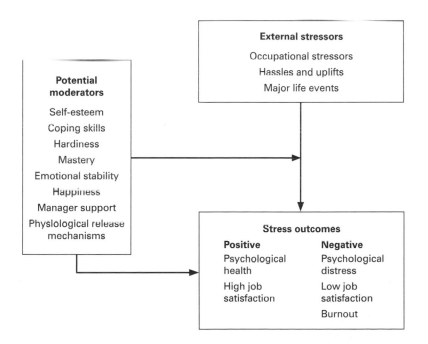

Fig. 17.1 The revised stress process model (after Carson & Kuipers, 1998).

and the 'ability to let off steam'. For instance, trainees with a more robust sense of self-esteem are less likely to be affected by work conflicts or untoward incidents involving their patients. Some of these moderating factors reflect one's temperament, others are consequent on contingent personal circumstances and yet others relate to readily modifiable domains of support, skills and experience. The better trained we are to face difficult situations and the better supported we are following them, the less likely they are to affect us adversely.

Stressors will have either positive or negative stress outcomes. Positive stress outcomes include psychological well-being and high job satisfaction. Negative stress outcomes include psychological distress, low levels of job satisfaction, occupational burnout (measured using a standardised measure such as the Maslach Burnout Inventory; Maslach *et al*, 1996) and overt mental illness. It will be clear that stress outcomes are by no means entirely determined by the demands of work. It is also worth noting that positive stress outcomes are common: most psychiatrists at all grades enjoy their job most of the time and find it a source of self-worth. There is also good evidence that on balance work is good for mental health.

Studies of stress in psychiatrists

Stressors

It is easy and potentially instructive to generate a list of what psychiatrists of any grade find stressful. The first study to look systematically at the specific occupational stressors confronting psychiatrists was undertaken in the USA (Dawkins *et al*, 1984). The main stressors the authors identified were 'a threat from a patient', 'unnecessary paperwork', 'being held responsible for substandard work performed by others' and 'provocative behaviour by a member of staff towards a patient'. Stressors were grouped into five main categories: negative characteristics of patients and their relatives (34% of items); administration and organisational shortcomings (25%); resource deficiencies (18%); staff performance (11%); and staff conflicts (10%). When old age psychiatrists were asked to list their main stressors seven major categories were identified: 'changes within the health service'; 'changes within community care'; 'personal stresses'; 'management issues'; 'resource issues'; 'lack of time'; and 'overwork' (Benbow & Jolley, 1998). Rather different factors were identified in a study of stressors experienced by psychiatrists in Wessex (Rathod *et al*, 2000). Out-of-hours duties, dealing with difficult or hostile relatives, long hours of work, paperwork, the demands of the job interfering with family life and 24-hour responsibility for suicidal and homicidal patients were noted as causing moderate to extreme stress by more than half of the sample. Patient suicide, which is uncommon but in adult psychiatry inevitable, is experienced as deeply distressing by the treating doctor (Campbell & Fahy, 2002).

Moderating factors

Potential moderating factors have been less well examined. There is some evidence that psychiatrists are both nicer and more neurotic than other doctors (Deary *et al*, 1996*b*), which may explain their higher perceived levels of stress despite their lower objective workloads. Cognitive styles that commonly help doctors deal with their jobs (e.g. developing an emotional distance from the patient) may be less well developed among psychiatrists. Having high self-esteem predicts good stress outcomes (Thomsen *et al*, 1998). Multidisciplinary team members report the support they receive from their colleagues within the team as being important in managing work stresses. Interestingly consultant psychiatrists have identified relationships with their colleagues as a significant source of stress (Guthrie *et al*, 1999)! Support from colleagues is particularly valuable in moderating the stressful impact of patient suicide.

One study has looked at the coping strategies used by psychiatrists to manage their stress (Rathod *et al*, 2000). The results will strike a chord with most psychiatrists. The most common reported positive coping strategies were getting support from your partner (56%), media entertainment (43%), exercise (32%) and socialising (20%). The most frequent negative coping strategies reported were worry (55%), getting angry and irritable (33%), blaming self (33%), driving oneself harder in career (31%) and losing sleep (28%). Use of alcohol as a way of managing stress is ubiquitous in our society and alcohol misuse is a major cause of doctors becoming unfit to practise. (The conceptual confusion surrounding the stress literature is underlined by the fact that most of these negative coping strategies can also be seen as adverse stress outcomes.)

Stress outcomes

Consultant psychiatrists work fewer hours than consultant physicians and surgeons, but report more emotional exhaustion and more depression as measured by the 28-item General Health Questionnaire (GHQ–28) than their colleagues (Deary *et al*, 1996*a*). A survey of community mental health teams found that psychiatrists scored highest in the burnout categories of emotional exhaustion (63.4%) and depersonalisation (47.5%) out of all the professional groups within a team (Onyett *et al*, 1997). This finding is not typical and more recent studies, which have also used standardised measures, have rather better news for psychiatrists. In an Anglo–German study psychiatrists had higher levels of job satisfaction than nurses and social workers, scored higher on the personal accomplishment component of the Maslach Burnout Inventory than other disciplines and had lower scores on the emotional exhaustion and depersonalisation components (Priebe *et al*, 2005). Social workers are currently the most stressed among mental health professionals, with psychiatric caseness as defined by the GHQ–12 double that of psychiatrists (47% compared with 25% – with a 17% rate in the general population; Evans *et al*, 2006).

Box 17.2 Professional and psychological facts about female psychiatrists

- They do not receive the same financial rewards (e.g. clinical excellence awards) as their male counterparts
- They are not equally represented in academic psychiatry
- They have lower professional status and hold proportionally higher numbers of staff grade posts
- In the USA, the ratio of complaints against female doctors is higher than against male colleagues
- Retirement because of ill health is higher
- They report poorer coping skills and more physical and emotional symptoms
- Women doctors are more likely to report stress, anxiety and depression

From Kohen & Arnold (2002)

Women doctors in general experience higher psychiatric morbidity and have a higher suicide rate than their male counterparts (Kohen & Arnold, 2002). The evidence for psychiatrists is contradictory: Guthrie *et al* (1999) failed to find a gender difference in stress outcomes, whereas Rathod *et al* (2000) found being female to be a robust risk factor for experiencing stress. What is clear is that women experience particular difficulties in pursuing a career in psychiatry (see Box 17.2).

Mental illness

Psychiatrists, like all other doctors, are at risk of developing overt mental illness that goes beyond GHQ 'caseness' and may ultimately affect their fitness to practise. Anecdotally doctors do not make good patients. The report into the death of Daksha Emson, a psychiatric trainee who killed herself and her young child in the context of a psychotic depressive episode, highlighted the problems within the NHS of treating the sick doctor (North East Thames Strategic Health Authority, 2003). Although there are rare high-profile exceptions, mental health professionals are reluctant to acknowledge their mental illness to colleagues and patients (ironic at a time when direct experience of mental illness is seen as an advantage for some elements of the workforce, such as the support time and recovery worker). This reluctance reflects continuing prejudice within the medical profession towards mental illness. There are also dilemmas for the sick doctor and the treatment team surrounding the requirement to balance the welfare of the doctor and that of their patients (Adshead, 2005). It goes without saying that mental illness per se should be no barrier to pursuing a successful career in psychiatry. There is a lack of dedicated resources for

---

Box 17.3 Resources and support networks for the sick doctor

- Psychiatrists' Support Service (Tel: 020 7245 0312)
- The Sick Doctors Trust (Tel: 0870 444 5163)
- BMA Counselling Service (Tel: 0845 920 0169)
- Doctors' SupportLine (Tel: 0870 765 0001)
  http://www.doctorssupport.org
- Doctors' Support Network (Tel: 0870 321 0642)
  http://www.dsn.org.uk
- MedNet for the London Deanery
  http://www.londondeanery.ac.uk/var/mednet
- National Clinical Assessment Service
  http://www.ncas.npsa.nhs.uk

---

treating the healthcare professional with mental illness, but resources and support networks do exist (see Box 17.3).

Stresses of being a psychiatric trainee

Is it more stressful being a trainee psychiatrist than a consultant? Certainly the structure of training imposes stresses on the neophyte psychiatrist. In 6-month training placements patients may be resentful towards trainees for a variety of reasons. First, they may be resentful that they are not seeing the consultant but a junior doctor instead. Second, they know the trainee will be leaving in 6 months and will hardly get a chance to know them. Third, how is it possible to make an impact on a patient who may already have had a long illness career? Research into other professions suggests that the training period may be especially stressful. For instance, a study of trainee social workers found a caseness rate of 64% on the GHQ–28 (Tobin *et al*, 1998). Cushway (1992) found caseness rates of over 50% in clinical psychology trainees.

The only published study to address this issue directly with psychiatrists is that of Guthrie *et al* (1999). Major stressors varied with grade. Consultants were most stressed by administrative difficulties, career threats and medical responsibility for suicidal and potentially homicidal patients. For senior house officers (SHOs) and specialist registrars, dealing with patients and managing personal problems were the most frequent stressors. Personal life events were felt to affect the ability to handle patients' problems. Senior house officers and specialist registrars reported significantly more stressors than consultants. Ward rounds, on-call, unexpected cover and academic work were all rated as more stressful for SHOs and registrars. SHOs and registrars scored significantly higher on emotional exhaustion and depersonalisation scales of the Maslach Burnout Inventory than senior registrars and consultants. Their GHQ–12 caseness rates were also higher: 37% for SHOs; 28% for specialist registrars; and 24% for consultants. Guthrie *et al* (1999) concluded that although the overall workload in psychiatry might be lower than in other medical specialties, the nature of the work is very different and it is sometimes personally threatening. How can trainees best manage the stressors of their work as psychiatrists?

Stress management for trainee psychiatrists

Although a great deal of research has been undertaken into the stress process, there have been very few systematic evaluations of stress management interventions for mental health staff. Virtually all trusts provide stress management courses as part of their in-service training. These courses look at ways of dealing with symptoms of anxiety, developing and enhancing coping skills, and changing perceptions and appraisals of work stressors using cognitive restructuring. However, as few trainee psychiatrists are likely to enrol for such courses, they will require alternative methods of dealing with occupational stressors. To help in this regard we offer some suggestions below.

Developing peer support networks

A wide body of literature shows the importance of social support in coping with occupational stress. During the training process, the support of one's peers is critical. These are the only people who are going through the same process. Although this can be sometimes harnessed in formal support groups, informal support is likely to be more important. Support from other members of the multidisciplinary team might be as helpful as support from one's own colleagues, particularly in the face of a shared difficulty such as a serious untoward incident.

Life–work balance

This is often mentioned in the popular press but is difficult to achieve. Studying is especially likely to intrude into personal non-work time. Trainee psychiatrists who are married and who have children will find it even harder to strike the right balance between work and home life. The NHS is, through the 'Improving Working Lives' initiative, committed to help its staff maintain a satisfactory work–life balance.

Lifestyle factors

The benefits of a healthy diet, exercise and moderate consumption of alcohol are all obvious and well documented. Excessive work stress can at times not unnaturally lead to comfort eating and binge drinking.

Professional socialisation

Relationships with consultant supervisors are critical and need to be worked on. Speaking to trainees who have worked with particular consultants before may highlight potential problem areas in advance. Supervision is an additional critical element in helping this relationship to develop.

Work routines

Sweeney *et al* (1993) suggested a number of practical ways of dealing with the stresses of the working day: first, making sure to take coffee and lunch breaks, preferably in non-treatment settings; second, planning in time for administration and report writing; third, having a cut-off at the end of the day to mark the transition from a work to a social role, such as a visit to the gym; fourth, spacing out rewarding and non-rewarding tasks; fifth, using skills such as time management, prioritising and limit-setting, and learning that sometimes it is alright to say 'no' to extra work demands!

Being aware of your own work limits

There are going to be times at work when you are unable to work effectively, not just because of physical reasons but sometimes for mental reasons. At times the pressure exerted from external life events, such as divorce or bereavement, may be so great that you need to take a few days off work just to recharge your batteries. Acknowledging that things are difficult can be painful but is likely to be ultimately helpful. Occasionally, you may need to seek external professional support to deal with a personal crisis.

Focus on your positive achievements and strengths

To have got to this stage in your career, you will already have achieved a lot. The American motivational speaker Jack Canfield (co-editor of the 'Chicken Soup for the Soul' series) suggests that we all need to keep a so-called warm and fuzzy file or a feeling good file. This can be a box file into which we can put appreciative letters or emails received from patients, carers, colleagues, friends or family. Over time these build up. When you are feeling down, that is the time to get out this file and read what other people have said about you. Not only will this help us see our achievements but it will also help us see the impact we have had on all these people. (The NHS appraisal process encourages us to do this.) We can also help our colleagues by thanking them when they are helpful or have done well.

Faith and spiritual values

Although the majority of mental health professionals find their own religious beliefs a difficult area to discuss at work, there is no doubt that having a strong faith or set of spiritual values can help tremendously at times of acute stress. This may, however, be something you have to share with people outside of your work setting.

Hobbies and interests

In contrast to what some academics believe, there is a life outside psychiatry! Developing hobbies and leisure interests can help us keep a proper perspective on our work.

Stress and the employer

A distressed workforce will be an ineffective workforce. The Health and Safety Executive (2001) identified causes of workplace stress and suggested strategies that employers and managers should be adopting: ensuring that job demands are reasonable; maximising people's control over their work; providing appropriate managerial support and encouraging peer support; addressing poor working relationships within teams; and managing change effectively. There is empirical evidence that support from management and colleagues, being able to participate in the organisation and good leadership improve stress outcomes for psychiatrists (Thomsen *et al*, 1998). The Disability Discrimination Act 2005 also puts specific responsibilities on employers in relation to staff with established illnesses.

Women now constitute the majority of psychiatric trainees. There are some obvious steps towards improving the personal lives, career prospects and job satisfaction of female psychiatrists (Kohen & Arnold, 2002). These include more opportunities for flexible training and part-time working, maternity rights and improved pension benefits for women.

Conclusions

There can be no doubt that psychiatry is a stressful profession. The trainee psychiatrist is entering a world where they have to deal with challenging patients, difficult relatives, consultant colleagues, the 'minefield' of the multidisciplinary team and health service managers. Furthermore, the general public have negative attitudes towards psychiatry and medication, as may other medical colleagues. The process of training may be more stressful than the lot of the consultant, although the transition from trainee to consultant seems to be particularly stressful. Mentorship schemes can be helpful for the younger consultant, who will benefit from the opportunity to discuss frustrations and difficulties with a more experienced colleague (Roberts *et al*, 2002).

In the absence of empirical studies which might demonstrate how best to help trainee psychiatrists deal more effectively with occupational stress, we have been forced to come up with a number of generalisations as to what might assist the trainee psychiatrist. Of the list of suggestions we have provided, establishing good peer support and good working relationships with consultant supervisors are likely to be the most critical stress management strategies available to the trainee psychiatrist.

References

Adshead, G. (2005) Healing ourselves : ethical issues in the care of sick doctors. *Advances in Psychiatric Treatment*, **11**, 330–337.

Benbow, S. & Jolley, D. (1998) Psychiatrists under stress. *Psychiatric Bulletin*, **22**, 1–2.

Campbell, C. & Fahy, T. (2002) The role of the doctor when a patient commits suicide. *Psychiatric Bulletin*, **26**, 44–49.

Carson, J. & Kuipers, E. (1998) Stress management interventions. In *Occupational Stress: Personal and Professional Approaches* (eds S. Hardy, J. Carson & B. Thomas), pp. 157–174. Stanley Thornes.

Cushway, D. (1992) Stress in clinical psychology trainees. *British Journal of Clinical Psychology*, **31**, 169–179.

Dawkins, J., Depp, F. & Selzer, N. (1984) Occupational stress in a public mental hospital: the psychiatrist's view. *Hospital and Community Psychiatry*, **35**, 56–60.

Deary, I., Blenkin, H., Agius, R., et al (1996a) Models of job-related stress and personal achievement amongst consultant doctors. *British Journal of Psychology*, **87**, 3–29.

Deary, I., Agius, R. & Sadler, A. (1996b) Personality and stress in consultant psychiatrists. *International Journal of Social Psychiatry*, **42**, 112–123.

Evans, S., Huxley, P., Gately, C., et al (2006) Mental health, burnout and job satisfaction among mental health social workers in England and Wales. *British Journal of Psychiatry*, **188**, 75–80.

Guthrie, E., Tattan, T., Williams, E., et al (1999) Sources of stress, psychological distress and burnout in psychiatrists: comparison of junior doctors, senior registrars and consultants. *Psychiatric Bulletin*, **23**, 207–212.

Health and Safety Executive (2001) *Tackling Work-Related Stress: A Manager's Guide to Improving and Maintaining Employee Health and Wellbeing*. Health and Safety Executive.

International Stress Management Association (2004) *Working Together to Reduce Stress at Work. A Guide for Employees*. http://www.hse.gov.uk/stress/standards

Kohen, D. & Arnold, E. (2002) The female psychiatrist: professional, personal and social issues. *Advances in Psychiatric Treatment*, **8**, 81–88.

Kuper, H. & Marmot, M. (2003) Job strain, job demands, decision latitude and risk of coronary heart disease within the Whitehall II study. *Journal of Epidemiology and Community Health*, **57**, 147–153.

Maslach, C., Jackson, S. & Leiter, M. (1996) *Maslach Burnout Inventory Manual* (3rd edn). Consulting Psychologists Press.

North East London Strategic Health Authority (2003) *Report of an Independent Inquiry into the Care and Treatment of Daksha Emson and Her Daughter Freya*. NELSHA. http://www.nelondon.nhs.uk/?ID=3119

Onyett, S., Pillinger, T. & Muijen, M. (1997) Job satisfaction and burnout among members of community mental health teams. *Journal of Mental Health*, **6**, 1, 55–66.

Priebe, S., Fakhoury, W., Hoffman, K., et al (2005) Morale and job perception of community mental health professionals in Berlin and London. *Social Psychiatry and Psychiatric Epidemiology*, **40**, 223–232.

Rathod, S., Roy, L., Ramsay, M., et al (2000) A survey of stress in psychiatrists working in the Wessex region. *Psychiatric Bulletin*, **24**, 133–136.

Reid, Y., Johnson, S., Morant, N., et al (1999) Explanations for stress and satisfaction in mental health professionals: a qualitative study. *Social Psychiatry and Psychiatric Epidemiology*, **34**, 6, 301–308.

Roberts, G., Moore, B. & Coles, C. (2002) Mentoring for newly appointed consultant psychiatrists. *Psychiatric Bulletin*, **26**, 106–109.

Sainsbury Centre for Mental Health (2000) *Finding and Keeping: Review of Recruitment and Retention in the Mental Health Workforce.* Sainsbury Centre for Mental Health.

Sweeney, G., Nichols, K. & Kline, P. (1993) Job stress in occupational therapy: an examination of causative factors. *British Journal of Occupational Therapy*, **56**, 89–93.

Thomsen, S., Dallender, J., Soares, J., *et al* (1998) Predictors of a healthy workplace for Swedish and English psychiatrists. *British Journal of Psychiatry*, **173**, 80–84.

Tobin, P., Gunnoo, V. & Carson, J. (1998) Stress and burnout in student health care professionals. In *Occupational Stress: Personal and Professional Approaches* (eds S. Hardy, J. Carson & B. Thomas), pp. 32–43. Stanley Thornes.

CHAPTER 18

Managing time: the key to professional success

Carl Gray

Managing time is a challenge to all doctors and healthcare professionals. The mastery of timetabling and the use of time to best effect are fundamental to successful professional life. Positive qualities in doctors – and attributes admired in trainee doctors – include being punctual, hard-working, efficient, reliable, calm, unflappable, good in a crisis, dependable, self-starting, completer/finisher and unhurried. These time-based qualities could and should apply throughout your career. Conversely, many failing professionals and unsuccessful trainee doctors have been blighted by failure to manage time.

This chapter discusses the nature of time, the usual problems with time, and introduces concepts of time management. This leads into discussion of time in relation to life as a whole and work–life balance. Most of this is common sense – but few of us are making the most of our time.

No one is perfect. Indeed, this chapter was submitted late and I was once late for a lecture I was giving on the subject of time management. However, rescuing wasted time from time-wasting activities is truly liberating – the time saved can be spent on more enjoyable parts of life and in delivering better care to patients with less effort. Relax, deliver more work for less effort and feel good about it. This chapter should underpin all the good advice in the rest of this handbook.

What is time?

Time is a complex phenomenon understandable in several different ways (Davies, 1995). Time governs all other areas of life, including activity and thinking. First, time is a physical parameter: one of the dimensions of reality and a fundamental property of matter and space. Pre-eminently a uni-directional process, the 'arrow of time' directs entropy, complex systems, chemical reactions and particle physics in irreversible directions (Coveney & Highfield, 1991). Reversed slow-motion films of flowers 'un-growing' and teacups leaping back unbroken from the floor are fun because they contrast so completely with known reality. Flowers do not turn back into seeds and teacup fragments just do not re-assemble themselves in our real experience.

Second, time is a parameter measurable by instruments: clocks and other timepieces. At the finest level, the time signals broadcast from Rugby and Frankfurt derive from atomic clocks based upon vibrating caesium atoms, accurate to tiny fractions of a second. Your wall clock or wristwatch will be accurate to a few seconds per day. People rarely need greater accuracy in measuring time.

Third, time is a physiological basis in complex organisms. Animals and plants run to multiple cycles, related by evolution to the daily and seasonal periods in the environment. The science of chronobiology covers a whole range of bodily functions which change with time, principally sleep, endocrine hormones, reproduction and hibernation. Moreover, over spans of years, ageing processes bring inevitable changes in individuals.

Fourth, time is a psychological experience. We are all as individuals aware of the passage of time in relation to internal events and external cues. Notoriously, the feeling of time varies over time so that our mental processes, and their relations to external events, give perceptual time which passes quickly or slowly in different circumstances. Sleep gives the passage of time, whereas, strangely, general anaesthesia is a period of unconsciousness without the perception of the passage of time: you go to sleep and feel that you wake up immediately.

Finally, and most awkwardly, time is a social construction. Almost all activities and interactions in civilised society are timetabled by minutes, hours, days, months and years. Occupation and behaviour are determined partly by age; activity generally depends upon the day of the week and the time of year. The worlds of shopping, travel, education, entertainment, religion, commerce, the media, politics and government, the law, manufacture and engineering, and even socialising are closely regulated by time. Most people have an appointments diary showing that on each day they should be at particular places doing particular things at particular times. People even regulate their leisure activities: cinemas and sports events have start and finish times, friends meet by appointment at pubs and restaurants. For the employed person, almost everything is timetabled, including work, leisure and rest. Step changes in activity, responsibility and function occur on particular days related to age: graduation, taking up a new job, marriage, becoming a parent, retirement.

Problems with time

Problems arise from the nature of time. Time is irreversible and we miss opportunities through failure of planning or of observation. You missed the train. The TV programme was half over when you switched on. The taxi went by before you waved. Our measuring devices – clocks, watches and calendars – may be lost, forgotten or inaccurate. Everyone has gone astray at some time because their watch has stopped. I once left my children at school on a day when it was closed; I had ignored the school calendar. Activity may lose synchrony with our body cycles: most people will have experienced oversleeping, crashing out with tiredness, falling asleep in meetings, or jet lag when travelling. Our perception of time may not be matched to external reality. The allocation of time for tasks is often underestimated. However, thinking and decision-making can be speeded up and the social and organisational demands on our person to be in certain places at certain times doing certain things are difficult to achieve in circumstances of excessive demand. Too much to do and too little time to do it leads to under-achievement against plan.

The usual time problems in medical life are:

- chronic lateness – attendance, replying to communications, delivering work
- taking on too much work
- underestimating the time required – work, travelling to a destination, meetings
- interruptions – consuming time by unexpected events
- procrastination – failure to start an unpleasant task
- perfectionism – never completing a task
- inefficiency – failure to deliver the expected workload in the planned time
- time-wasting – communications, distraction, laziness
- work–life balance – sleep, demands of parenthood, feeling tired
- conflict between morning and evening people.

In addition, some specific times of life and careers present special challenges for the use and management of time.

Concepts of time management

I visited this topic in my article in the *BMJ* 'Careers Focus' (Gray, 1998). If you visit the 'self-help' and 'management' sections of any large bookshop you will find numerous handbooks on time management. These have similar approaches and I recommend *Time Management from the Inside Out* (Morgenstern, 2000). Naturally, I have drawn on some of these published ideas in preparing this chapter. There are also 'time management consultants', who form a sub-branch of management consultancy dealing with 'executive coaching' and 'personal effectiveness'. If you were to consult these experts – instead of reading this handbook – you would spend good money on exploring the following techniques.

Diary exercise

The basic diagnostic approach is to undertake a diary exercise. Write down on a tabulated clipboard what you are doing in each of many subdivisions of the day. The subdivisions need to be about 5–15 min: longer periods are less informative. Unfortunately, the exercise is itself distorting and changes behaviour: a big sister is watching you and you tend to be better behaved under observation. Measuring any parameter in physics disturbs the system and alters the result; so it is in human activities. The very act of filling in the sheet is distracting and time-consuming, even if one refrains from entering, 'filling in this time sheet', every 5 min! No one enjoys completing time sheets for a whole day. The results are analysed by category. However you choose the categories, the results are usually informative. In most people's days, much time is wasted by waiting for things to happen, waiting for people to turn up, looking for lost paperwork, enduring delays for various internal and external reasons. Vast amounts of time are consumed by meetings, speaking on the telephone, gossiping and daydreaming. Actual working time is surprisingly small. People take longer coffee and lunch breaks than they say.

Informed by the results of the diary exercise, various techniques can be applied. These are all easily listed but are much harder to apply in practical detail. Recognise your own biological clock and use your most productive times of day for the most important tasks. Confine activity to what is worth doing and stop when it is good enough. Cease time-wasting activities. Communicate by the briefest methods. Adopt time-saving tricks. Recognise different types of demands upon your time and allocate the use of time in blocks that do not steal time from each other. Deal with interruptions economically. Speed up some activities, including studying, reading, writing and decision-making. Use electronic devices and computers efficiently. Use time-saving tricks in meetings. Travel efficiently. Organise an efficient timetable.

Biological clock

Your own biological clock is distinctive and permanent; it strongly influences your performance. The planetary rotation period is 23.93 hours and most human activity is entrained in daily cycles of 24 hours or multiples thereof. Unfortunately, humans have large interpersonal variations in diurnal cycles. People who like getting up early (larks) have diurnal cycles of 18–24 hours and are different from people who like staying up late (owls) who have diurnal cycles of 24–30 hours. Experiments that studied people isolated in caves without timepieces and external time cues found more owls than larks. In their important paper, environmental epidemiologists Gale & Martyn (1998) tested the validity of Benjamin Franklin's maxim: 'Early to bed and early to rise makes a man, healthy, wealthy and wise.' In over 1000 men and women aged over 65 years, the maxim was not supported. Owls were slightly wealthier than larks, but there was no significant difference in measures of health or wisdom. In my own paper on circadian rhythms and medical careers (Gray, 1999), I distinguished larks, owls, whales, ponies and hyenas. Wisely, I did not include psychiatry in the specialties allocated to diurnal types. Owls feel grim in the morning and do their best work in the afternoon and evenings. Conversely, larks leap out of bed early to do their best work and then deteriorate over the rest of the day. Obviously, where possible, one should arrange one's life to suit one's animal nature. A further fact of medical life that is neglected is sleep. Many under-performing doctors have had insufficient sleep. The planned week should include enough sleep (Howe, 1996) and time for catch-up sleep after deprivation.

Confine activity

Work itself must be regulated. Only take on what can realistically be achieved. Many activities are of little value and can be discarded or kept to a minimum. These include: preparing and reading minutes, filing paperwork, opening mail. Work should be prepared to the required standard and stopped when it is good enough. Many hours are wasted on perfectionism. The 'Eighty–Twenty' rule can be applied to most things: 80% of the value can be achieved in the first 20% of the time. Pieces of written work can be improved by periodical re-attention almost indefinitely if you let yourself. A final full stop must be written and the work sent off at some point. Handle and read incoming paperwork only once and send it to its destination – usually the wastepaper bin – immediately. Reply to letters by scrawling on the bottom and returning the sheet. This is much quicker than writing a new letter in reply.

Avoid time-wasting

Time-wasting activities must be addressed. Lack of punctuality in yourself and others wastes your time and that of others. Turn up on time or not at all. If others have not turned up, go away and do something else. Meetings deserve a chapter of their own. Many studies have shown that meetings are a large waster of time. They take too long, occur too often, waste time on formalism and minutes, have too little content and positively encourage bores to speak at length about themselves. At any time in a meeting most participants – using the word optimistically – do not know what they are doing: listening, deciding, speaking, thinking. Only the most ruthless chairmanship, an art that can be acquired by studying the greats, can confine business to less than an hour. Abolish a regular meeting, group or committee and you have saved hundreds of person hours per year forever.

Time-saving tricks

Organise your physical office space to be efficient and so that work flows naturally in space. Piles of papers on horizontal surfaces are obscure. Place things in vertical magazine racks for easy access. Keep very little and throw most stuff away. Keep patients' records in neat systematic enclaves. Put the usual phone numbers, codes and addresses on the notice board or sticky labels – why look them up every time?

173

Time-saving tricks do save time. Communications are a large time-waster. Most telephone calls are too long. Most of us receive too many emails and take too long in unnecessary replies. If you take out time spent on the telephone and handling email and snail-mail each day, hours are saved.

Prioritisation

Saying 'no' is the fundamental skill in regulating incoming work. This is not the simple 'no' of the 2-year-old child, but the reasoned 'no' of the adult worker. Does the boss want you to do this extra task rather than the one that consequently will be delayed or will not get done at all? The choice is his; the problem is his and not yours. Furious overworking is usual in British medicine. It is doing no one any good. Once you start saying 'no', you become more comfortable. Trainees do have to deliver some good work to remain in the good books of their superiors and should say 'yes' at least sometimes.

Prioritisation sounds easy: just do the most important things first. Unfortunately, we are timetabled to do a mixture of important, unimportant and useless activities all day. Urgent unimportant matters inevitably get attended to before non-urgent important matters. So allocate some time for the important things and postpone some less-important urgent things.

Doing it right first time saves extra remedial work and so saves time. To stop when it is good enough means reach the standard but do not perseverate into perfectionism.

'Flow activities'

Notoriously, the perception of time varies between people and within the individual at different times. 'Time drags with toothache but flees with a kiss' (Gray, 1998). Childhood summer afternoons seemed interminable because of boredom and insufficient content, whereas a person engrossed in an intense task or activity finds afterwards that the time has flown. The psychologist of everyday life, Csikszentmihalyi (1997), has defined the loss of perception of time when active as 'flow'. Flow activities are those with a challenging match between demands and skills requiring complete mental and physical concentration. The classical example is of athletes at the peak of their performance – which in sporting terminology is called being in 'the zone'. 'Flow activities' – including enjoyment of musical and entertainment events, watching a closely fought football match, types of religious fervour and indeed sexual ecstasy – represent peoples' happiest and most pleasurable times, and so gain corresponding attention in the pursuit of happiness.

Bringing flow to more mundane tasks, such as work, is a challenge but will be worthwhile. If thinking speeds up, then time spreads out into a wider, more comfortable space. Control of mental time is possible by training and practice, and books are available on, for example, speed reading. Perception of time is inversely proportional to the speed of thought. Train yourself in rapid reading, thinking and decision-making and you can get more done in the time available. The same techniques will deliver a step-improvement in study skills. If you are often bored, then you have insufficient mental activity going on, or perhaps repetitive activity, because of insufficient input and structure. Individuals may identify their own rate-limiting factors. Slow reading is a common problem, sometimes from unrecognised dyslexic traits. Inability to choose or decide is another – a problem based in personality. Identified personal problems can be addressed with expert help.

Avoid interruptions

Interruptions will feature in everybody's diary exercise as a time waster. But professional life will inevitably contain interruptions because unexpected things do happen unexpectedly. Of course, the unexpected is expected to occur – doctors on-call for emergency cases are expecting something – but its exact nature is unpredictable. Much of what is felt as interruption – incoming telephone calls, colleagues dropping by for a chat, patients turning up – is predictable and should be allocated a block of time. Perhaps one could deal with all telephone and other messages for an hour at 2 p.m. each day. At other times, the phone is not answered by yourself and your door has a 'Do not disturb' sign on it.

You can get rid of some work by delegation. Someone else can do it better and quicker. Trainees are often the recipients of delegated work, but you do have the possibility of sharing tasks within the wider team, including secretaries. You can also delegate upwards to your boss those tasks that really best lie in the bosses' domain.

Strategy saves time in the long run. Careful planning will ensure that you are doing the right work at the right time and are not distracted, interrupted, heaped upon, inefficient or burnt-out by overwork, or, even worse, overworking on the wrong or useless activities.

Diary control

The final and most important technique in time management is 'diary control'. Information technology offers techniques in communication and diary management. I have a diary screen which is available to myself and two secretaries and goes everywhere on my palm-top computer. However, I receive scores of emails everyday and must waste time dealing with them. Mastery of information technology is necessary for today's doctors, and as a minimum this must cover word processing, spreadsheets, databases, use of the internet and email, and presentations. Doing a computer course, such as the European Computer Driving Licence, is a good idea for trainees.

You should be the only person timetabling your own time. Modern electronic devices such as desk-top, palm-top and lap-top computers have some form of electronic diary which facilitates the planning of time, listing appointments, including recurrent ones, and irregular events. Different colours can light up different types of time, and flashing and audible reminders and alarms will remind you of impending actions needed and your partner's birthday.

Any form of diary planning depends upon allocation of blocks of time for different purposes. Use only a single diary system for all items including social, sexual and dental appointments together with the whole of work. Time allocation should use committed and uncommitted blocks to accommodate expected inroads of the unexpected. Uncommitted time can also be used for catching up on delayed items and doing creative activities. Occasionally, patients will fail to attend or a meeting will be cancelled. Have a supply of useful work with you that can be fitted in. If you do not control your diary, then it and other people will control you, and not sympathetically.

Time and life

Time management techniques should make an improvement in your use of your time, particularly at work. But how should you spend your next 946 080 000 seconds – a professional career lasting 30 years?

Doctors have notoriously overworked in recent decades, with a correspondingly poor work–life balance contributing to adverse effects such as burnout, mental illness, alcoholism and divorce. Nowadays young doctors, partly because of change in young professionals generally and partly by the design of modernised training programmes, have a healthier expectation of work–life balance.

But how can this be realised? Achievement comes from effort and yet work must now be confined to its proper fraction of life's time allowance. The phases of a medical career – medical student, trainee doctor, consultant, retired doctor – correspond with increasing criticality of time. Students have abundant time and seem to waste some of it by not having enough to do, though they do have to spend time growing up. Trainee doctors feel pressure of time with a full timetable and the pressures of on-call. Frequently, trainees have started their families and must balance work with family life.

Consultants in all specialties feel that they have responsibility for a wide range of urgent and important tasks, a full timetable of activities and abundant paperwork, with management, training, continuing professional development, appraisal and bidding for new staff and equipment. The NHS consultant contract is based on time: consultants are paid for their 'NHS time' assessed as 4-hour blocks (professional activities – PAs). For the NHS consultant, work is time and time is money. Consultants also have family lives. The retired doctor has to balance activity and rewarding pastimes with the sense that time is running out as illness and infirmity threaten. The poet Herrick wrote:

'Gather ye rosebuds while ye may, Old Time is still a flying.'

Young doctors have to establish the balance between life and work. Work is an important part of life and should be enjoyable and rewarding. Some work can legitimately be done at home (study, written work, reading papers, preparing presentations). The balance with family life and one's partner can be challenging. Increasingly, housework and child care are seen as matters for equal division between parents. The normal family timetable can be hectic; this stress is added to by the problems of child care during school holidays and from time to time by children's illnesses.

It is essential to allow realistic time for sleep, leisure activities, including exercise, socialising, and what used to be called 'romance' and is now called 'sex'. Finding, keeping and interacting with partners take time.

Some life events and activities have their own peculiar time demands. Preparation for examinations needs substantial blocks of time set aside for intensive study and preparation for at least 6 months ahead. This time has to be taken from other functions – principally leisure. Job applications and interviews also need time allocated for preparing the ideal CV, filling in the application forms, making visits and attending the interview. Before these late stages, time should be spent on more general activities in support of career development – visiting other hospitals, cultivating contacts, learning about training schemes, attending specific courses, reading *BMJ Careers*, *etc*. An attendance at any court or tribunal will inevitably mean wasting time, even whole days, on delays as the court decides when it wants you. Weddings seem to take up masses of time these days – time spent on wedding preparation will be to the detriment of other activities. Holidays bring their own time stresses. Booking, packing and preparation take time; the airport experience may be made more stressful by delays and the holiday time itself is more intense. Finally, a new baby makes the most demands on time. New parents underestimate the time that will be taken up by infants in their first year.

Conclusions

By the study of a diary exercise and the application of time management techniques, young doctors should become more efficient and so more relaxed in their professional lives. The passage of time is a passive, unconscious and strange matter until deliberately addressed as suggested above. Time paradoxes are commonplace. Going in to work later on some days may be more productive: an owl would have an extra hour's valuable sleep, it avoids the rush hour, giving a shorter time travelling to work, and the bird arrives feeling better and is more productive. But this would not suit a lark. Staying late seems to get more done but the work becomes poorer in quality and fatigue has to be redeemed next day. Staying late does not suit the bird who has already been up catching the early worm. Working at home can be productive and efficient. Some of what we do is unnecessary and therefore needs no time at all. Busy people are the most efficient at dispatching an extra job: 'If you want something doing, give it to a busy man', states the Yorkshire proverb. Longer holidays facilitate strategic thinking and save time in the long run. Deep sleep and keen approaches to leisure prolong active life. Early retirement from a full time job enables continued activity in a portfolio of part-time careers with elements of employment, voluntary service, creative activities and leisure.

Time management has been a struggle since ancient times: 'A time to get, and a time to lose; a time to keep and a time to cast away', and, 'To everything there is a season and a time to every purpose under the heaven' (Ecclesiastes 3,1). Wise doctors will take time out to think again about their use of their most precious resource; it is never too late to start saving time.

References

Csikszentmihalyi, M. (1997) *Living Well: The Psychology of Everyday Life*. Weidenfeld & Nicolson.

Coveney, P. & Highfield, R. (1991) *The Arrow of Time*. Flamingo.

Davies, P. (1995) *About Time. Einstein's Unfinished Revolution*. Viking.

Gale, C. & Martyn, C. (1998) Larks and owls and health, wealth and wisdom. *BMJ*, **317**, 1675–1677.

Gray, C. (1998) Time management. *BMJ Classified Supplement*, **316**, 4 April, 2–3.

Gray, C. (1999) Sleep and work. *BMJ Classified Supplement*, **318**, 30 January, 2–3

Howe, A. (1996) Jobs for sleep. *BMJ Classified Supplement*, **313**, 19 October, 2–3.

Morgenstern, J. (2000) *Time Management from the Inside Out*. Hodder and Stoughton.

CHAPTER 19

Negotiation skills

Peter Hill

You can negotiate when there is a conflict between what you want and what another party wants, provided that you both are willing to do so and have the freedom to adjust the demands and concessions you make in reaching an agreement. Each party shifts its demands and makes concessions until there is a balance to which both can sign up to. Both parties need to agree to a negotiation; it takes two to tango. Because there is a conflict of demands the process is competitive and each party will try to obtain as much as possible for themselves, and give away as little as possible to the other.

You may be negotiating with your colleagues about such issues as when you will be on call or about room facilities with a manager. You will not be negotiating about pass marks in exams or whether to apply the Mental Health Act, because there will be no freedom for you or another party to adjust demands. Negotiating is a skill that is useful for trainees but increasingly important for consultants because the consultant community is less of a hierarchy and essentially a community of peers which can not be directed by you. Consultants may also find themselves in a negotiation with managers who have little direct authority over clinical issues but control financial resources.

Negotiation is not the only way of resolving a conflict of demands. It may be that you or the other party have enough authority to impose a resolution, or that the situation has to be resolved by law or agreed procedures. Alternatively it may be that you both agree that a third party should arbitrate and you will be bound by their opinion; the jargon for this is 'binding arbitration'.

ORBits

If there is to be a satisfactory negotiation there has to be some overlap between each party's interests. These interests can be represented as a range extending from the maximum they can give away at one end to the most they hope to get in the exchange at the other. Knowing your negotiating range is critical; think of it as your negotiation ORBit, extending from the most you hope to gain – your **O**ptimal limit or top line – to what you absolutely must not give away – your **B**ottom line. Somewhere between these two limits is a **R**ealistic position that you think is likely to be obtainable.

If you have ever bought a second-hand car, especially from a private individual, you will recognise this. There is a stated price which both the seller and you know is optimistic – the seller's optimal position. You intend to buy for a certain sum – less than the stated price and a realistic position for you. There is a price that you absolutely cannot afford – your bottom line. Perhaps there is a chance that you will end up paying even less than your original decision – your optimal position. You haggle until there is a deal that both can sign up to.

This assumes that there is an overlap between your ORBit and the seller's ORBit. To put figures on it, let us assume you have an absolute maximum of £7000 but this would seriously stretch finances so there would be no skiing trip this year. This is your Bottom line. You would not feel comfortable about going much over a Realistic position of £6000, although you could if you really liked the car. There is a slim chance that you might beat the seller down to £5000 and you will open the haggling with that offer as this is your Optimal position. You now have your ORBit.

The seller asks £7500 (his Optimal) but in his heart knows that is not likely to work, given the car's age. He simply cannot go below £5500 (Bottom line) because he needs that for a deposit on a new car, which he has already ordered. He thinks most people will haggle and he will go along with dropping £500 off the price and £1000 if pushed (his Realistic).

The overlap of the two ORBits is shown in Fig. 19.1. Negotiation is possible and worthwhile for both parties, given that each is prepared to shift from an opening position. In this instance, the seller might well get what he thought was a likely price and you, the buyer, have a good chance of getting what you can realistically afford even though you may have to pay just a little more than you hoped. Would that it were always thus.

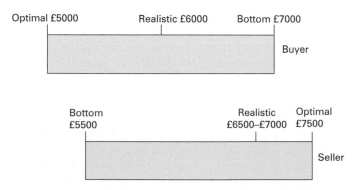

Fig. 19.1 Example of the overlap between ORBits of a buyer and seller.

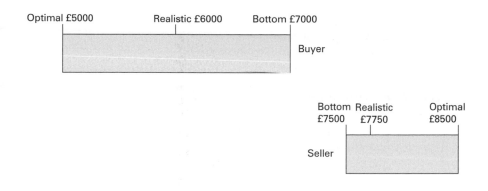

Fig.19.2 Example where the ORBits of buyer and seller do not overlap.

Let us consider a different scenario. It is probably easier to stick to buying a car, although most negotiations in medicine are about timing, physical resources or staff rather than money. You have an absolute maximum of £7000 to spend, would prefer to buy at £6000 and dream of a purchase price of £5000. You see a car advertised for £8500 and try to talk the seller down. Yet you do not yet know that he cannot possibly let his car go for less than £7500 and is looking for a price of £7750. Clearly this is not a negotiation that is going to work because your bottom line and the seller's do not overlap (Fig. 19.2).

What about the situation in which you hone your negotiating skills to the point where you start an offer (say £6000) at your Optimal position only to hear the seller agree, without haggling. What this reveals is that his ORBit is greater than you had imagined (Fig. 19.3). That is humiliating.

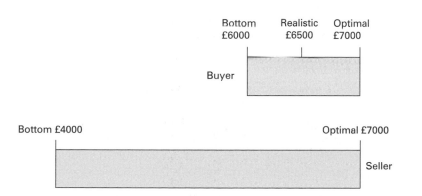

Fig. 19.3 Example where the seller's ORBit is greater than the buyer imagined.

Finding out

The obvious conclusion from the above examples is that you need to know what a realistic price is for yourself to pay, how much you can afford (your bottom line), and what the seller's bottom line is. In other words you should know your own economics, become an expert in the price of the particular car you want and, ideally, what the seller will drop his price to. The first two are not too difficult (although sticking to your bottom line is hard if you really want that car). The third is usually tough.

If you have ever tried to buy a carpet in, say, Morocco, you will know that the first question put to you as you enter the shop is 'Tell me, what is the most you can you afford … and I will find you the best carpet for that'. In an economy used to haggling to determine a price, the fundamental question of the customer's bottom line is the first objective and may be tackled directly. Yet obviously it would be crazy to disclose it. You would rapidly find yourself outsmarted and effectively in the third of the ORBit positions cited above. Nevertheless it is always worth asking the other party what their bottom line is; they may be unused to negotiating.

Essentially, most negotiation is competitive and secrecy/dissimulation is part of it. If they are canny and do not let you know their bottom line or you do not believe what they say, then you have a problem. It would pay to try and find out beforehand what the other side can afford to give away. If it is a room you are after, how many rooms are available and how many people are after them? What are the precedents for rooms being allocated? Did your predecessor have one? And so on. Do quite a lot of homework first.

Similarly, you can expect the other side to have done some homework in order to find out your ORBit, and specifically how much you can afford to give away. Generally speaking, do not disclose anything – especially in response to a suggestion like 'let's be grown up about this: you tell me what you can afford and I'll tell you what I can come up with …'. Politely acknowledge that it would be easy to do that but you wonder what the limit is as far as they are concerned.

The general process

Although the popular image of negotiation is drawn from industrial practice (bosses and unions) or complex financial deals (high-powered sales teams), includes ideas of smoke-filled rooms, confrontational exchanges, threats, business lunches and fast closure on deals, the reality is that in a National Health Service (NHS) setting, the process is more leisurely, quiet and there is more use of paper. There is time to find out, build one's case and actually negotiate.

Matters should start with a general discussion of the situation. Try to get the other side to move first (a general rule of negotiation is 'after you') by asking them to set out the situation as they see it. With luck they will say what they want you to do and what they are prepared to do. Try to get them to agree on principles ('Do we agree that patients need to be seen promptly?').

Eventually this will lead to you making a statement of your position, a reasonable account of your situation, the reasons for your demand and what it is. Almost certainly you will pitch your demand above what is realistic – about 20% is a good rule of thumb. Expect close questioning about this, particularly if you are dealing with a delegate or a relatively junior manager who may have to justify the eventual outcome to their more senior line manager. They may actually be sympathetic to your position, but by being a bit challenging they can learn how to justify your case and a final agreement to a higher authority who may be less sympathetic. That does not mean you can't stonewall, since this may enable them to say to their superior 'I made all the offers I could but nothing was acceptable'. But be a little careful about this as you can end up with a stalemate.

You will still be trying to find out what the other side's ORBit is. Generally speaking, asking questions works: 'How much can you afford?', 'When would a good time be?', 'What is the general policy on ...?' 'What happens elsewhere?' and so on. Listen for subtle signals of flexibility from the other side: 'I don't normally think it's appropriate ...', 'I can't help at this point in the financial year' or 'It would be difficult to agree at this point'.

Move in measured steps from your initial position, trying not to concede anything without getting something in return. In a face-to-face negotiation, perhaps about a hospital parking permit (it happens, believe me), the general pattern is to adopt an 'If you ... then I' mode. Ideally this is 'If you (specific), then I (vague)'. For instance, 'If you provide me with a parking permit for this year then I will see what I can do about getting the discharge letter situation sorted' (to which the response is likely to be a request for you to be more specific). This might lead to a counter offer of a priority listing for your permit if the discharge letter backlog is cleared by the end of the month; the symmetrical reverse of your tone – vague on their part, with a specific demand for action from you. You can then come back with a demand for a permit by the end of the month, converting their vague talk about priorities into a specific request. This can all be a bit tedious but it actually gives a glimpse of what the other side is prepared to give away.

Don't become aggressive, rude or angry. Keep a level head and a sense of humour. Stay friendly and use open body language – smiling and being relaxed. Don't belittle your opponent. Avoid histrionics. Never threaten what you cannot carry out. Stick to good humour with a hint of steel. Don't crow over minor victories. The same individual is going to be on your patch for some time and there is no point in making enemies out of opponents in negotiations. Nor is there any point in driving your opponent into a stubborn refusal to progress or adjust their position.

A face-to-face situation like this is not that common and it is much more likely that there will be a lengthier process of letters, phone calls, emails and discussions with various other people being drawn in. Nevertheless, there is a basic principle of making a series of proposals involving an exchange of demands and concessions.

What sometimes happens is that you find that you are negotiating a package. For instance, you need an updated computer, a colour laser printer and new software, but your manager is linking this to the suggestion that this requires an unaffordable secretarial upgrade which would mean sharing the cost of the secretary with another person. You are asked if you would be prepared to share the secretary. This is an isolated component of the package and you agree to it in isolation at your peril. It would be better to stick to the package as a whole, simply restating what you want, perhaps computer, printer and software and full-time secretary, just possibly hinting that the printer could be networked with one other secretary to reduce the running costs, so long as this does not inconvenience you. Don't agree separately to specific components of the package, although you can certainly adjust the mix of components and make another offer.

Remember that negotiation is only realistic if both parties agree to it. You may find yourself negotiating over something that is actually essential to your work (such as a parking permit) which is a waste of everyone's time. It would probably be better not to negotiate but to appeal to a higher authority who has the resources and sense to impose a solution, hopefully favourable.

Although books on negotiation all agree that you should never ever give anything away without getting something in return, this is practice derived from selling or industrial relations. Life in the NHS is a little different, as you may be working alongside your opponent for years and memories can be long. Sometimes, I suggest, it may be appropriate to be cautiously generous and generate goodwill. But don't bank on it and make sure it is publicly documented and acknowledged at the time.

Expert negotiators emphasise the importance of conceding what is of little value to you in exchange for something that you value without letting the other side know this. In practice this is difficult in NHS negotiations between managers and clinicians, since it is usually pretty clear what each side values. Between peers it may be very different. You may not mind doing Saturdays on-call because your partner at home always works Saturdays. Yet this may be a wonderful opportunity for your colleagues to avoid weekend duties. They may assume you are making a major sacrifice and you can, if you wish, extract an impressive price from them (they do two weekdays on-call for you in exchange for you doing their Saturday on-call, for instance).

Most importantly, never be tempted to breach your bottom line. If you genuinely decided that it was the point below which you could not go, then don't go below it. It is terribly easy to do so in the stress of a negotiation, especially a face-to-face negotiation.

The overall principles of the negotiation process are:

- to conceal your own ORBit while discovering theirs
- to obtain specific concessions in exchange for vague offers
- not giving away anything without getting something in return (unless you are not treating the process as a negotiation)
- sticking to a whole package and not agreeing to concessions on its separate components
- to offer what you can easily afford without revealing its value to you
- never ever going below your bottom line
- staying cool
- building power (see below).

Building power

Negotiation is not a logical process. The decision to end negotiating and agree with the other side has much to do with a perception that one is losing or winning so that now is the time to stop or jointly agree. You are able to choose this time yourself if you build power. You are also much more likely to have won important concessions if you are perceived as powerful.

There are several rather obvious ways to build power.

- Develop a commitment to your cause. You really want a good result and you know the issues in detail. This is particularly important if you are delegated to negotiate on someone else's part.
- Choose the place, yours rather than theirs.
- Choose the time to suit you or discomfort them (you may find yourself on the receiving end of power-building when invited to a pre-breakfast meeting).
- Force the pace ('I have a meeting to go to in 10 min and we need to wrap this up ...', 'Look, not much separates us now').
- Demonstrate your expertise or support ('I have read all the relevant papers', 'My colleagues are unanimous').
- From time to time summarise what you understand the position to be, perhaps biasing it a little in your own favour ('You have a problem with the waiting list and I need more secretarial support. Surely this is actually the same problem for both of us').

Of course, the other side will be doing the same. Usually it is best to ignore it but you may want to test their assertions ('Did you see the finance officer's response?'). If stuck, make a vague point ('Not everyone would see it the same way').

Don't be upset by emotional blackmail ('You may be creating difficulties for yourself by persisting with this ...'). Notice them doing it and realise that this is simply process, don't take it personally. At this point you don't have to compete, simply smile to let them know that you know what they are up to.

Best alternative to a negotiated agreement

Negotiation is a voluntary process. You don't have to do it and neither does the other side. If you sense you are losing and being driven dangerously close to your bottom line, consider stopping the process and breaking off. Similarly, if a negotiation is going on and on fruitlessly it may be wasting your time unprofitably. Don't get stuck in stubborn persistence unnecessarily; walk away.

But know what you are walking away into. In order to do this to your advantage, have in mind, before you start, what your best alternative to a negotiated agreement (BATNA) is. It might be to abandon the demand altogether. Or you may think it better to get someone to negotiate on your behalf. Or to carry out a coercive threat (industrial action). Consider each of these separately and know which is the best at any stage of a negotiation.

Agreement

More usually, negotiation proceeds until both parties feel that a reasonable exchange of concessions has taken place. One party will usually call a halt and it is up to the other to agree. Ideally this is a so-called win-win deal with both parties feeling reasonably satisfied. The difficulty is that there is usually a pressure to obtain an agreement – any agreement – because of time or pressure from other bodies. Be thoughtful at this stage.

If you agree too early, the risk is that the other side thinks that you have got away with something and they may stall. Conversely, dragging things out will sap energy. If you are offered a choice between two reasonable packages don't be impulsive but take time out to consider the options. Be very careful of using the term 'final offer'. Often it isn't really your final offer but means you are getting ratty.

If you have what appears to be a sensible agreement, agree on what you have agreed and make sure it is written down. It is wise to build in a review date in a few months to ensure that what you have both agreed is carried out and is workable.

Conclusions

Negotiation is a skill and people get better with time and practice. Psychiatrists are good negotiators and become better when they apply basic principles, as above. They often have an advantage because they can use clinical interviewing techniques such as active listening, adjusting their body language to the situation, inferring non-verbal communications, monitoring their own emotional responses and knowing their own typical responses to conflict. The only difficulty is that non-psychiatrists are sometimes vaguely aware of this and are wary. Don't overplay the psychiatric card.

CHAPTER 20

Presentation skills[†]

Kalyani Katz and Pramod Prabhakaran

'The whole art of teaching is only the art of awakening the natural curiosity of young minds for the purpose of satisfying it afterwards.'

(Anatole France, *The Crime of Sylvestre Bonnard*, 1881)

Presentation is a performance. A successful performance depends on good communication between a presenter and an audience. Most professionals are required to give a presentation at one time or another. Some, for example teachers and doctors, are expected to do so more often than others. Doctors, through their essential duties of training future generations, giving and explaining information to their patients and educating the general public about health issues, need to exercise skills in presenting information in an easily understandable and digestible form. Some doctors are born teachers; others have to learn, develop and master these skills. Once acquired, at a more senior level these can be of use in negotiating and planning the development of new services and in procuring funding in order to implement change.

The basic guidelines set out below should not only help trainee doctors, who are expected to take part in weekly academic programmes involving case presentations and journal clubs: they should also be of use to newly appointed consultants, whose responsibilities include teaching a range of professional groups, such as nurses, occupational therapists, general practitioners and social workers.

The precise style, mode and content of a presentation will depend on the type of meeting, the needs of the audience and the number attending. In all cases, the presentation must be educational, thought-provoking and entertaining. The audience must be made to feel further curiosity about the subject by the end of the presentation; this is a task for the presenter. It will be no great challenge to one who has both a passion for the subject and good communication skills, but, even with these, delivering the same talk

---

[†]This chapter was previously published in Bhugra *et al* (2007).

over and over again will make the task more difficult. It is essential to revise and update the material each time; there is always scope for improvement, as well as opportunities to incorporate new information. Remember also that communication is a two-way process; we often gain new ideas during the question and answer and discussion time, and we can ourselves learn through teaching others.

The kind of presentation we are dealing with here is quite different from a written article prepared for publication, although this, too, is a form of presentation. Reading aloud at a meeting a published article, or one that is prepared for publication, rarely makes a successful presentation. Changes will always need to be made to such material if it is to be easy for listeners to absorb and assimilate.

There is another basic rule that is often not adhered to. The presenter should never exceed the allocated time. We have all attended lectures where even the most passionate speaker has managed to put off an audience by being overenthusiastic and by speaking for too long. In our view, it is advisable to finish the talk even a few minutes early.

Let us now examine the different components of a successful presentation:

- preparation
- planning
- delivery.

Preparation

The first step in preparation is to collect all the relevant information about the nature and the theme of the meeting and about the topics being covered by other speakers. This is essential before any planning starts. Take for example a talk on depression in the elderly, delivered as part of a conference on healthcare for the elderly. If the talk is aimed at a wide range of medical and paramedical professionals, it will be different from a lecture given as part of an MRCPsych Part II course attended by trainee psychiatrists. It will be different again from a session aimed at helping general practitioners to identify early depression.

Proper knowledge of the particular context will help you to decide on the aims of your own presentation. Be sure to discuss and clarify your aims in advance with the organiser of the meeting. This will ease the process of planning. You may find a list of fairly common aims useful when thinking of the aims for your presentation:

- helping to spread new information (e.g. concerning the withdrawal of a product)
- improving awareness (e.g. of high rates of depression in the elderly)
- introducing change (e.g. the implementation of guidelines from the National Institute for Health and Clinical Excellence)

- inspiring action (e.g. incorporating the use of the 'single assessment process' to reduce the delay in the process of consultation for the elderly).

The second stage of preparation involves finding out more about your audience and how they intend to use your information. It may sometimes help to ask yourself the question: 'What would I wish to learn from this lecture if I were in the audience?' When analysing your audience, consider:

- the size of the audience
- their educational level
- their expectations and needs.

The presentation will not succeed unless your aims match the expectations and the needs of the audience. For example, community psychiatric nurses attending a lecture on suicide in psychiatric patients will want to learn how to assess the risk of suicide in patients. They will not be content to listen to your research findings on neurochemical abnormalities in patients who express suicidal ideas.

Knowing your audience will also help you to illustrate your ideas with relevant examples, ones that relate to their experience. In the long term, people tend to remember stories, rather than theory alone.

Some knowledge of the educational background of those in the audience will allow you to decide on the pitch of your talk; you must always avoid being condescending to those who come to hear you, but equally you must avoid speaking over their heads (if you do so, they will be unable to concentrate on your lecture and will 'switch off').

These days, through increasing media coverage and access to websites, the public has become more knowledgeable and more aware of health issues. It is not uncommon to find that a member of the audience has gleaned some new information from the media that you yourself have yet to hear through professional medical channels.

Planning

After the preliminary work of preparation, you can start thinking about exactly what you are going to say and how you will say it.

What are you going to say?

Start jotting down your ideas as soon as you have accepted an invitation to talk. You may find it useful to discuss your ideas with colleagues; constructive advice is often forthcoming, including suggestions of new reference material you may not have seen.

The next step in planning is to collect relevant material to support and illustrate your ideas. The Cochrane Library is the most comprehensive single source of information on the effects of healthcare interventions. It comprises a collection of databases. You can register for the 'Athens' password for the Cochrane Library at your local library or on the website of the National Library for Health (NLH) (http://www.library.nhs.uk). Registration allows access to various databases:

- Medline
- Embase
- PsycINFO
- Cochrane Library
- AMED.

These can all be accessed via the website for Health Information for London Online (HILO) (http://www.hilo.nhs.uk) or the NLH website. The internet is of course also a valuable source of evidence and information to draw upon for a presentation. The following are particularly recommended:

- http://www.hilo.nhs.uk
- http://www.library.nhs.uk
- http://www.rcpsych.ac.uk
- http://www.doctors.net.uk
- http://www.nice.org.uk

You may also consult a local librarian; in our experience librarians are always keen to help. Be sure to keep details of references.

Of course, you must decide when to stop collecting material and to start evaluating what you have collected. Resist the temptation to collect too much material; this can cause problems in both extracting and simplifying information. You need reliable evidence to support your ideas. To achieve this, evaluate and exclude information that will not stand up to scientific scrutiny. Allow plenty of time to arrange material in a coherent and logical scheme; this can be time-consuming.

The precise title of the presentation should become obvious at this stage. A bland title can be made more interesting through only a slight change. For example, 'Suicide prevention in the mentally ill' could be made to sound more engaging, and could make a more lasting impression on the audience, if the phrase 'An unachievable goal?' were added. But you must avoid using a glamorous title simply to impress; satisfy yourself that the title really does reflect the content of your presentation.

Be aware of 'political correctness' in expressing your ideas but do not be its slave.

How will you say it?

The mode of the presentation is dictated generally by the size of the audience. The smaller the group size, the easier it is to make the learning more interactive. The interactive model, which is generally thought to be more conducive to learning, cannot easily be used in a larger gathering. An ability to control the group is essential if you are to choose this method.

Despite the derogatory comments we often hear about the workshop model – for example, that it is a way of getting others to do your own work – it can bring advantages, such as spontaneity and audience participation. But there are risks. A presenter may feel exposed by difficult questions, or by encountering members of the audience with their own agendas.

The didactic model, best suited for larger gatherings, has not been popular of late. In a study comparing the interactive and the didactic methods of learning, the assessment of knowledge in postgraduate trainees did not reveal significant benefit in one system compared with the other (Haidet *et al*, 2004).

Whatever the mode of presentation, the use of visual aids is now the norm. There are several advantages in this. For example, visual aids help people to concentrate and they break the monotony of the speaker's voice. It has been said that people generally remember 20% of what they hear but 50% of what they see and hear (Treichler, 1967). Well-prepared visual aids, such as slides or PowerPoint presentations, summarise the text in a concise form and will help the audience to focus on and retain the information. Recently, PowerPoint presentation seems to have become the most favoured option. Previously, slides, acetates and flip-charts were in common use. It may help to have one back-up method in case of technical problems. The choice will depend upon the availability of technical equipment at the venue.

However, visual aids are no more than aids. Do not make them too fancy or gimmicky, or an end in themselves – they can also be distracting. Use key words or phrases for emphasis. If you download images from websites, check the copyright.

The clarity and visibility of projections is very important. Choose an appropriate font size and style, and avoid using block capitals. Each projection should contain a minimum of two and a maximum of five points. It is not a substitute for a detailed text. Avoid very 'busy' slides and avoid projecting those you intend to skip (unnecessary slides give an impression of inadequate preparation and lead to boredom in the audience). Exposure to too many stimuli – the phenomenon referred to as 'stimulus overload' – can raise stress levels and diminish learning ability (Mendl, 1999).

Allow roughly 2 minutes' talking time for each slide. This is a good way of getting the length of your talk right. A printed version of your slides will be useful as a handout, and will save the time you might have spent in preparing separate ones.

The final step in the planning is to arrive early at the venue, in order to familiarise yourself with the surroundings and organise your visual material. Late arrival in a state of panic can seriously affect the delivery of even a very well-prepared talk.

Delivery

It is through the delivery itself that a presentation will make a lasting impact; the delivery is therefore the most important element of the presentation.

The first few minutes of non-verbal communication are crucial in making a positive impression on your audience, and can also help to establish a good rapport. Once you have taken this opportunity, it will be easy to hold the audience's attention and interest; if you lose their attention it will be hard to regain it. It is, of course, advantageous to dress appropriately for the occasion and to walk confidently on to the stage.

Some famous speakers cultivate an image of untidiness and a chaotic personal style. We do not recommend this. Distracting dress may be able to seize the audience's attention, but will not be sufficient to sustain it. Excessive movements of hands, or pacing about on the stage or podium, can betray anxiety, and anxiety is infectious. The same may be said of excessively rapid speech, failing to look at the audience and rushing through the presentation. Smile and adopt a confident posture, for confidence is infectious too.

Make sure that you can be heard clearly by those furthest away from you and that they can see your slides or projections. Aim your delivery at the back row for at least a good part of the time, and certainly avoid speaking to your visual aids rather than to the audience. Learn to use appropriate pauses to emphasise certain points. If English is not your first language, do remember to speak slowly and to be conscious that your accent may be difficult to understand for those unused to it. This is one of the most common reasons why audiences lose attention. Practise speaking clearly and slowly, and ask a friend (a real friend, not just one who will flatter you) to comment honestly, or practise in front of a closed-circuit television to analyse your own performance.

A good introduction, followed by a statement of your plans for your allotted time slot, will help to gain the attention of your audience and keep them interested. It can be very effective to start with a controversial statement, or an event currently in the news, or perhaps an interesting real-life anecdote. It has been said that a good anecdote is worth a thousand pages of statistics. Better still is a good anecdote backed up by statistics.

Most people are averse to arrogance and appreciate some humility in the speaker. Occasional humour can lighten the atmosphere, and a relaxed atmosphere is more conducive to learning. Be cautious with jokes, however – they should be in appropriate taste and should actually be funny. A joke that fails to amuse can alienate an audience.

Dealing with anxiety

Knowing a few simple facts about anxiety should help you to overcome it. Any performance is likely to create anxiety or emotional arousal in the presenter. Performing at an optimal level in fact depends on some degree of

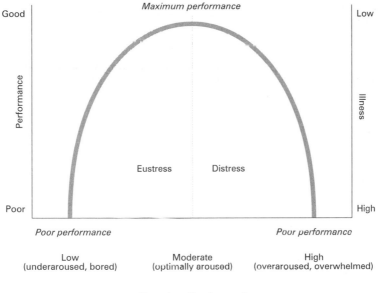

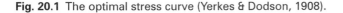

Fig. 20.1 The optimal stress curve (Yerkes & Dodson, 1908).

nervousness. Fig. 20.1, which depicts the well-established Yerkes–Dodson law, shows how performance improves up to a point, beyond which anxiety becomes an impediment (Yerkes & Dodson, 1908).

There are certain effective methods of controlling the more severe levels of fear. Use of alcohol, benzodiazepines, beta-blockers or excessive caffeine could be disastrous. Instead, try eating one or two bananas. It is not merely an old wives' tale that a banana has a calming effect. Good preparation and rehearsal are even more effective methods of reducing any apprehension that your performance will fail.

Just before you start, use some breathing techniques of the kind that are now widely familiar. The level of anxiety goes down once you begin. During the lecture, you should treat the audience as friends and try to create a relaxed and informal atmosphere in the room. Making eye contact with individuals certainly helps to reduce anxiety. Slow down and pause between sentences from time to time, in order to focus your thoughts. Use prompt cards or essential notes as a memory aid; under anxiety, it is easy to forget and lose your train of thought.

A common fear is that of not being able to answer questions after the lecture. Prepare yourself by anticipating the obvious questions and practise answering them. You need to remain in charge of the question and answer session. This session also gives you the opportunity to gauge whether the audience has understood your message and it enables you to clarify and emphasise your 'take-home' message. Before attempting to answer a question, it is very often necessary to rephrase it for the benefit of those in the audience who may not have heard or understood it. Entering into a dialogue with just one member of the audience is a common pitfall. To avoid this, direct your answers to the entire audience. If you do not know the answer to a question, do not hesitate to say so, but rather offer to research it and answer it at a later date.

Conclusion

Although all of this might seem like stating the obvious, we feel it is necessary to do so, having frequently sat through some very painful lectures. Richard Smith's article in the *BMJ* summarises the common mistakes that lead to a bad presentation (Smith, 2003). But to achieve success, prepare well, practise adequately, arrive on time, make contact with your audience and do not overrun your time. And try to avoid accepting the time-slot after lunch!

References

Bhugra, D., Bell, S. & Burns, A. (eds) (2007) *Management for Psychiatrists*. RCPsych Publications.

Haidet, P., Morgan, R. O., O'Malley, K., *et al* (2004) A controlled trial of active versus passive learning strategies in a large group setting. *Advances in Health Sciences Education: Theory and Practice*, **9**, 15–27.

Mendl, M. (1999) Performing under pressure: stress and cognitive function. *Applied Animal Behaviour Science*, **65**, 221–244.

Smith, R. (2003) How not to give a presentation. *BMJ*, **321**, 1570–1571.

Treichler, D. G. (1967) Are you missing the boat in training? *Film and A-V Communication*, **1**, 14–16.

Yerkes, R. M. & Dodson, J. D. (1908) The relation of strength of stimulus to rapidity of habit-formation. *Journal of Comparative Neurology and Psychology*, **18**, 459–482.

CHAPTER 21

Mental health review tribunals: reports and hearings

Kalyani Katz and Pramod Prabhakaran

It is often said that an after-dinner speech is like a lady's garment: it should be of the right size and style, and appropriate to the occasion. A report too must match its requirements in much the same way.

There has been a steady rise in the number of compulsory admissions of people with mental illness over the past two decades, and a proportionate increase in applications to mental health review tribunals by detained patients (Wall *et al* 1999; Department of Health, 2002). The tribunal rules require an up-to-date medical report. Most clinicians find that writing these reports in time, and giving evidence at the hearing, a tedious and onerous addition to their busy work schedule, especially if they are unfamiliar with these tasks and have not had sufficient training. Some guidelines are offered below in an attempt to make the task easier.

The introduction of the Mental Health Treatment Act in 1930 encouraged people with mental illness to seek help voluntarily. This was reinforced in the Mental Health Act 1959, which also introduced two radical changes: the decision to detain patients against their will for treatment became a medical, rather than just a legal, matter; and the Act highlighted the procedures and safeguards concerning compulsory detention and treatment. Furthermore, Parliament and European Law decree that any decision to detain patients be subject to an independent review. The result was the forming of mental health review tribunals, which have a responsibility to review the lawfulness of detention of people with mental disorders and thus safeguard the person's right to freedom from unjustified detention in hospital (Richardson & Machin, 1999).

No significant changes to the Mental Health Act 1983 were introduced in this regard before the remedial order of 2001, which addressed the problem of incompatibility with the law on human rights. This order shifted the burden of proof from the patient to the responsible detaining authority to show that the criteria defined in sections 72 and 73 of the Mental Health Act 1983 (described below) are not met, thus justifying continued detention.

It is now the duty of the responsible medical officer, as a representative of the detaining authority, to provide factual evidence in support of their clinical opinions justifying detention. It is no longer sufficient simply to express clinical opinions. Although the decision of the tribunal is legal, it is based on clinical information. The mental health review tribunal attempts to scrutinise subjective views and to provide objectivity in reaching decisions. In the absence of adequate objective evidence, the tribunal is obliged to rescind the section. In addition to its power to discharge the section and to reclassify the diagnosis, the tribunal's other powers are to recommend leave of absence, to recommend supervised discharge and to recommend transfer to another hospital. In restricted cases, the tribunal has the power to authorise conditional discharge.

It is a fundamental principle of the common law rules of fair process that all evidence that is likely to influence the outcome of a decision be made available to all parties. This principle applies in all contexts where the rights of individuals are at stake (Richardson & Machin, 2000). All reports submitted to the tribunal are therefore available for the patient to read. This has implications for those writing medical reports in which sensitive information is disclosed.

Writing the medical report

Before discussing the format of the report, we would like to consider the following.

- Who is the best person to write the report?
- To whom is the report addressed?
- What is the purpose of the report?
- What information should the report contain?

Who is the best person to write the report?

This should be the doctor who has the relevant information concerning the patient's illness, has sufficient knowledge of the Mental Health Act 1983 and is able to give adequate reasons to justify continued detention. A new or junior doctor with little knowledge and experience of the Act should not be given this responsibility without adequate supervision. If written by a junior member of a team, the report should be discussed fully with either the consultant or another senior medical member, and approved by this person. Preferably the report should be written by the person who is likely to give oral evidence at the tribunal hearing.

To whom is it addressed?

The tribunal report will be read not only by the patient and his representative but by all members of the panel, which consists of lay, medical and legal members. Medical jargon without full explanation is unhelpful. Excessive use of technical jargon can lead to significant difficulties at the hearing. It is worth pointing out that the usual practice of submitting a discharge summary in lieu of a proper report is therefore not appropriate. A discharge summary is aimed at professional colleagues familiar with technical language. It gives details of the patient's diagnosis, treatment and future care plans without requiring justification (as opposed to explanation) for opinions, its purpose is entirely clinical, unlike that of the medical report for the tribunal, which has legal consequences and requires justification.

What is the purpose of the report?

The purpose of the report is to justify continued detention of the patient in hospital. The report should address the criteria under section 72 as listed below (Langley, 1990).

- Does the patient have one of the categories of mental disorder, and if so, which?
- Does the original category under which the patient was detained need to be revised?

If the patient has a form of mental disorder, is the disorder of a nature or degree that warrants detention in hospital? If 'yes', then is the continued detention in hospital required for:

- assessment (section 2)
- treatment
- a limited or extended period (sections 2 and 3)?

Is continued detention in hospital justified in the interests of the patient's

- health or
- safety or
- for the protection of other persons?

If the patient is detained otherwise than under section 2, is there a likelihood of medical treatment alleviating or preventing deterioration in the patient's condition?

In the case of a patient with mental illness or severe mental impairment what is the likelihood of the patient, if discharged, being able to:

- care for himself
- obtain the care he requires or
- guard himself against serious exploitation?

The patient can be detained under four categories of mental disorder: mental illness, mental impairment, severe mental impairment and psychopathic disorder. The last three categories are defined in the Mental Health Act 1983. The lack of exact definition of the terms 'mental illness', 'nature' and 'degree' in the Act often causes difficulties when writing reports and attempting to justify detention. Some clarification of these terms will be useful.

Box 21.1   Guide to the symptoms associated with the legal category of 'mental illness'

The Department of Health defines mental illness as an illness having one or more of the following characteristics:

- more than temporary impairment of intellectual functions shown by a failure of memory, orientation, comprehension and learning capacity
- more than temporary alteration of mood of such degree as to give rise to the patient having a delusional appraisal of his situation, his past or his future, or that of others, or to the lack of any appraisal
- delusional beliefs, persecutory, jealous, or grandiose
- abnormal perceptions associated with delusional misinterpretation of events
- thinking so disordered as to prevent the patient making a reasonable appraisal of his situation or having reasonable communication with others

(Jones, 2006)

The reader may find the guide to the symptoms associated with the legal category of mental illness shown in Box 21.1 of benefit, although there have been some criticisms that these are either too restrictive or over-inclusive. It is clear that 'nature' is broader than diagnosis alone. In this context consideration of response and attitude to medication is critical. In determining the nature of the illness we are taking into account (a) the diagnostic category, (b) the chronology of the illness, (c) its impact on the individual, (d) response to treatment and (e) prognosis.

The 'degree' is generally accepted to mean the current manifestation of the patient's disorder and progress since admission.

The second limb of the section 72 and 73 criteria concerns the necessity of treatment for (a) the health of the individual, (b) the safety of the individual and (c) the protection of others. In the report it is important to give examples from the past to show how the risk to self/others would be affected if the patient were not detained.

It is not necessary to prove that there are risks in all three of these categories, but those that you do wish to establish should be borne out. In the case of risk to health through relapse, consideration should be given to the possible timing of the relapse. If it is likely to take place within around 6 months, this will be accepted as grounds for detention. Detention will be harder to justify if the period is likely to be longer.

To say that someone is a risk to others is a serious allegation. A patient swearing at staff, for example, would not be sufficient to support such a claim. Corroborating evidence could be adduced from old reports, but be sure that such information is accurate.

As for the patient's own safety, consider (in addition to any perceived risk of suicide or self-harm) other risks such as self-neglect, possible problems with road safety, vulnerability to exploitation, etc. But again, ask whether a propensity to self-neglect justifies detention when services may be available in the community to monitor and prevent it.

Desirability of treatment is not the same as necessity. The tribunal will rescind the section if the responsible medical officer's case is merely that it would be clinically advantageous (i.e. desirable but not strictly necessary) to keep the patient in hospital a little longer. No matter how 'desirable' it may seem, detention is a very serious measure which should be used only when necessary. To justify detention the test is not what is in 'the best interests of the patient' but rather whether the patient's health or safety, or the protection of others are seriously compromised at the time or in the foreseeable future.

What information should the report contain?

The core of the medical report as specified above must provide information that will allow the tribunal to answer the question 'is the continued detention of the patient lawful?'

The report must be succinct, and not over-inclusive. Avoid copying from previous reports without checking the accuracy of the information they contain. The essential structure of the report, and the guidelines for writing it, were agreed upon after consultation with the Royal College of Psychiatrists and are available on the Mental Health Review Tribunal website (http://www.mhrt.org.uk). We have incorporated these and some other guidelines (Brockman, 1993)about writing medical reports for the courts into our own format (Box 21.2).

In essence the report should contain answers to the following questions.

- What is the mental disorder? Give the ICD–10 diagnosis.
- What symptoms of the mental disorder does the patient currently manifest?
- Does the patient have insight?
- What impact has the illness had on the patient's daily life?
- What has been the response to treatment?
- Can this treatment be given in the community? If not, why not?
- Can the patient be relied on to accept treatment on a voluntary basis?
- What are the likely risks if the patient is not treated?
- What is the short- and long-term prognosis?
- What other factors influence the illness?

Of the above factors, 'insight' requires special comment. The patient's level of insight has a significant impact on the patient's prognosis. In our view, however, insight is not an 'all-or-none' phenomenon. We suggest you consider the following points.

- Does the patient accept that her/his experiences/beliefs are out of the ordinary?

199

Box 21.2   Report for the mental health review tribunal

Name

Date of birth

Address

Dates of admission and section

Date of the tribunal

Date of the report

Dates of previous tribunals

Sources of information

Diagnosis (ICD–10)

Circumstances of admission

Reasons for detention

Past psychiatric history

- Onset
- Number of admissions
- Reasons for relapses

Adherence to treatment plan in the community

Functioning in the community

Significant background information (relevant information only)

Mental state on admission

Progress since admission

- Symptoms
- Behaviour
- Insight
- Adherence to prescribed medication

Current mental state

Current treatment/leave arrangements

Reasons for continued detention

Provide factual evidence to support non-fulfilment of section 72/73 criteria but do not just repeat these

Relevant risk factors (you may submit risk assessment forms)

- Risk of self-neglect/self-harm
- Risk of aggression/violence
- Risk of absconding
- Substance misuse

Provisional discharge care plan

- Likelihood of its success if discharged

- Does s/he accept that s/he suffers from some form of mental illness?
- Does s/he accept the need for treatment, including medication and follow-up?
- If relevant, does s/he accept the impact of illicit substance misuse on her/his mental health?
- If relevant, does s/he accept that the criminal activity that led to the admission was associated with her/his mental disorder?
- Does s/he accept that there is a risk of recurrence of illness if s/he discontinues treatment?

Some of the above information, which could adversely affect the health/welfare either of the patient or of other persons, could be submitted in a separate document labelled 'not for disclosure'. Full reasons for doing so must be specified.

In restricted cases, if recommending conditional discharge, the tribunal finds it useful to have a list of conditions specified by the responsible medical officer.

The final paragraph of the report should summarise your concerns for the patient's health, for the patient's own safety and for the protection of others if the section were rescinded. It should give a provisional care plan in case the patient is discharged by the tribunal.

Above all, make sure that your report:

- is well structured
- is not unnecessarily long
- does not repeat details already described elsewhere
- is not full of medical jargon
- is submitted on time (within 3 weeks of the date of the application).

At the hearing

The tribunal considers both written and oral evidence before arriving at its decision. During the hearing, the tribunal will be rigorous in their testing of subjective medical opinions and will apply law impartially.

Tribunal hearings are not case conferences in which the responsible medical officer is the leader, nor are they occasions to humiliate clinicians. They are fact-finding courts in an informal setting (i.e. they are inquisitorial in nature and not adversarial). At times the rigorous cross-examination, where factual evidence is lacking, may feel adversarial. This can often be avoided by submitting a good report and being well prepared for the hearing.

Preparation

It is best practice to submit an up-to-date addendum report or to give one orally at the start of the interview. A full mental state assessment of the patient prior to the tribunal is absolutely essential to avoid embarrassing situations where the medical member of the panel has the most recent information, for example that the patient has been absent without leave for the past 3 days. Make sure you obtain all the relevant information from the nursing staff and other members of the multidisciplinary team.

We advise that you discuss the report and your findings with the patient before the tribunal. This can lessen any likely adverse effects the patient might have on hearing unpalatable information about their illness, and can prevent a consequent impact on the therapeutic relationship.

In summary, before a hearing you should:

- familiarise yourself with your report and any new information
- assess current mental state
- identify any difficulties likely to arise at the hearing.

Presentation

Although the tribunals are informal, you should follow the general etiquette of court proceedings while attending the hearing. The usual form of the hearing is that of questions and answers. The questions are, typically, probing; try to give short and clear answers. While giving evidence you should express within your areas of competence alone. Dignified responses are appreciated. Be aware of the difference between the interests of clinicians and those of the tribunal. The tribunal is concerned with the patient's freedom, whereas the clinician has clinical interests at heart. For the legal system clear polarities are important, such as legal/illegal and guilty/not guilty. This can create problems for clinicians who are used to the language of partial recovery or limited insight.

Finally, do not send an inexperienced junior trainee to give evidence without full prior training and some opportunity to observe one or two hearings (Nwulu, 2001). The most compelling witness is the one who understands the criteria for detention and expresses these clearly, both in writing and at the hearing.

References

Brockman, B. J. (1993) Preparing for Mental Health Review Tribunals: reports and dilemmas. *Psychiatric Bulletin*, **17**, 544–547.

Department of Health (2002) *Mental Health Review Tribunal Report April 1999 to March 2001*. Department of Health.

Jones, R. (2006) *The Mental Health Act Manual* (10th edn). Sweet & Maxwell.

Langley, G. E. (1990) The Responsible Medical Officer and Mental Health Review Tribunals. *Psychiatric Bulletin*, **14**, 336–337.

Nwulu, B. N. (2001) Medical representation at mental health review tribunal. *Psychiatric Bulletin*, **25**, 324.

Richardson, G. & Machin, D. (1999) A clash of values: MHRTs and judicial review. *Journal of Mental Health Law*, **1**, 3–12.

Richardson, G. & Machin, D. (2000) Doctors on tribunals: a confusion of roles. *British Journal of Psychiatry*, **176**, 110–115.

Wall, S., Hotopf, M., Wessely, S., *et al* (1999) Trends in the use of the Mental Health Act 1984–96. *BMJ*, **318**, 1520–1521.

CHAPTER 22

How to get published

Povl Munk-Jørgensen

Writing this chapter has a well-defined purpose: to help you get your research results published. There are a lot of books teaching you how to do this, and reading these books gives you the impression that publishing is easy. In a way it is easy, especially afterwards. But when you have had a manuscript rejected for the third time it definitely does not feel easy. When you are senior, with a long list of publications behind you, and journals invite you to write articles you will forget how difficult it is to publish a paper. Unfortunately, it is at this stage of your career that you start writing books about 'how to publish'. I promise I shall not tell you what to do, but instead try to remember some of my own troubles – and defeats – and honestly admit that it is difficult, but also a great thrill when you have your first publication in your hand.

I always completely lose interest in a research project at the very moment the analyses have been finished and the results established. Writing the manuscript presents an overwhelming psychological burden. However, because doing a research project without publishing the results is defined as unethical behaviour (almost as unethical as being an academic and not doing research) there is nothing but to write the manuscript.

Over the years, I have tried to set up some tricks to fool myself – more or less successfully – into writing, and more importantly writing in a way that leads to publication. These tricks, learned from experience over the years, have been supplemented by experience from editing scientific journals, from 1994 to 1998 as Danish editor of the *Nordic Journal of Psychiatry* and from 1998 onwards as editor of the *Acta Psychiatrica Scandinavica*.

Writing the manuscript

Writing to avoid being beaten up by your superego

A basic way to get things done is to be born Scandinavian. In Scandinavia we are raised and trained from cradle to nursing home to feel guilty, and our terrorist superegos help us get things done, in the case of manuscripts, especially if we have demanding co-authors waiting (but be wary of dynamic psychotherapy training – it can help you learn very useful ways to make your co-authors feel guilty but will eventually reduce the effectiveness of your superego in motivating you). However, as there are fewer than 25 million Scandinavians (and only a minority are psychiatrists, and only a very small number of those are researchers), the above-mentioned is poor advice for the international market. So here are some other methods.

Writing the manuscript before doing the research

The best way of getting a manuscript written, at least in my experience, is to write it before you do the research. It is possible to have more than three-quarters of the manuscript written before even seeing the very first patient for the pilot study. The secret is to write a high-quality protocol. Protocols are never a problem; during that phase of the process you are still interested, engaged, creative, energetic and innovative. By writing a good protocol the chances of performing an original study of high quality increases markedly. The spin-off product is that large (very large) parts of the protocol can be reused in the manuscript: the background for the protocol is the introduction of the manuscript. The only extra thing to be added is information from articles published in international journals while you are doing the study (you can be quite sure that when you have collected more than half of your proband patients for the study an article will be published reporting a study very similar to your own). Do not worry; that's life and there will always be room for a replication (yours).

The aims of the study in the protocol are exactly the same as the aims of the study in the manuscript. If they are not, you are carrying out another study than you thought – get the protocol right and copy the aims of the study in the manuscript.

A proper protocol will carefully describe the design, methodology, measures and the planned statistical analysis. This should be the same in the manuscript. So why not just copy the protocol to the manuscript? Of course some minor changes and additions are necessary, such as the number of drop-outs, kappa values, etc. It is also illuminating for the reader (and the editor) to be able to compare your power calculations from the protocol (now in the manuscript) with the report of what really happened.

Next is the results section. Is it possible to write this even before having seen the first patient proband? Yes, it is – partly. What can be done is to carefully plan the tables and figures to be presented and write these in the manuscript. For example:

Table 1 shows the sociodemographic variables for x probands and y controls examined during the period xx to xx.

Figure 1 shows a survival plot of the intervention group and controls from the end of the treatment period to relapse.

Table 2 shows bivariate analysis of correlation between independent variables and outcome.

There is a spin-off advantage of planning the results section in this way. When starting the analysis you know exactly what to do, which analyses to perform and how to present them. You, the editors, reviewers and your readers will avoid being presented with the creative results of a data fishing trip, mixed with an analysis of leftover data and strange factor analyses.

Computers are wonderful tools when you know what to ask them, but they will never ask questions. Therefore, the research question is the very most important part of the process when planning a project. The rest is nothing but technicalities – but that is another story.

Is it possible to write the discussion section of the manuscript before doing the study? Hardly. But what can be done is to write a project diary in which all the unforeseen events and mishaps are logged, besides those you knew already when designing the study. That makes it easy to write the section on the limitations of the study later, otherwise they are very difficult to remember when you sit down to write the manuscript.

Likewise, during the study it is advisable to continually identify publications from the existing literature and extract the information against which your findings shall be discussed. You had them at hand when writing the background to the protocol (the introduction of the manuscript). Do the same to the literature you identified during the study. If not, it is a demoralising uphill job to do it afterwards; researchers seldom carry the bookkeeper gene.

It should not be necessary to mention that the reference list wrote itself during the above process. This can be almost literally true if you use and update a bibliographic or referencing software such as Reference Manager (http://www.refman.com) or Endnote (http://www.endnote.com).

Now all that is left is to write the acknowledgements: 'The study was supported by the International Generous Grant for Important Matters' and thanking your spouse, 'without his (but more often her) loving support you would never had been able to do this study'.

And one final thing, please remember to agree upon the rank order of the authors the very first day (maximum second) you meet to discuss the possibilities for doing a piece of research together. Otherwise you are highly likely to loose good friends and colleagues.

How to get your manuscript published

It is said that every manuscript eventually finds its journal. This is not quite true. I kept a manuscript, or rather bits and pieces of a manuscript, for many years. It was never published, in fact it was never written, but if I had pulled myself together it would definitely never have been published because it was unoriginal, uninteresting and was not properly planned. Frankly, I have two of the kind.

The message is that if the research question is relevant, interesting and original, and the study well designed, well planned, well resourced and well staffed (and you remember to write the manuscript in advance), it will be well published, especially if you choose the receiving journal well (we will come to that now).

Where should I publish my fantastic paper?

This must be decided when you are discussing your idea for a research project with your colleagues and seniors, at the same time as you start writing (the major part of) the manuscript.

You should be regularly screening a handful or two journals that publish the kind of research you are doing. If you are interested in the course and outcome of schizophrenia, a journal specifically focusing on affective disorders is not among your priorities.

Think of the readers, not of your local research colleagues, not the editors and definitely not your boss. Identify your audience. Is it national or international? Is it the clinician or the scientist? Is your topic very specific or is it a topic of general interest?

If you are already a career researcher aiming at a professorship, then aim high and take impact factor into consideration. If you are a career researcher, you do not need to read this; if you want to be a career researcher and just are about to get started, please hang on.

Impact factor

The risk with impact factor-driven publication is that you may get a 'lucky' publication in a higher ranking journal but it may never be cited, never be downloaded and you may never get a reprint request, whereas the paper would have been widely read and discussed if it had been published in a national journal because it was handling a problem of great importance and relevance to local colleagues. However, some unlucky colleagues live in countries where research grants depend on impact factor points gained during the previous year (or two). The result is (at least it sometimes feels like this when editing a journal) that when these colleagues write their mother a letter they send her the copy and submit the original to the top journal on the impact factor list. When it is rejected, it is immediately submitted to the next on the impact factor list until it maybe reaches a journal to which it is relevant (e.g. *Grand National Mothers' Journal*) or a journal that lacks papers to publish. Sometimes it finally ends up in your mother's mailbox as a reprint and she does not understand why she should have this outdated letter once again.

So the take home message is make yourself familiar with the few, a handful or two, journals relevant to your research topic, define your audience and then choose the journal that is circulated to the audience you want to reach.

Language

'The language is a problem'. This is a common statement but the problem is not language; the problem is that most international journals are in English, edited by native-speaking English/North Americans, and reviewed by English and North American reviewers, who quite often have language problems, i.e. they speak no languages but English. However, a good editor and a good reviewer look at the substance of the manuscript, evaluate the research, the design and the methodology. Language is a minor problem. Most international journals will edit the language of manuscripts accepted for publication. In my capacity as editor I have met hundreds of reviewers who generously assist with language editing, some of them to such a degree that I think they deserve co-authorship.

If the study is interesting, well designed, original, etc. there is always a solution to the language question.

Message: language is not a substantial problem, it is a technical matter, but to make things run smoothly non-native English speakers should ask someone with English as a mother tongue to help them write the final version of the manuscript. It impresses editors, and there is no reason to hurt the feelings of those who 'have a language problem'.

Instructions to authors (or how not to hurt the editor's feelings)

The first draft of the manuscript is now ready, and you are preparing it for a specific journal. Now it is very important that you read the instructions to authors very carefully. Most journals publish a short version of instructions to authors on the inside of the back cover. On the home page of the journal you quite often find an extended and more detailed version. Be sure to prepare your manuscript in accordance with the instructions to authors in all details. Imagine an editor responsible for a journal with an acceptance rate never exceeding 15–20% (so at least four out of five manuscripts will be rejected). If you send signals to the editor that you do not care enough for your own manuscript to invest the time to prepare it properly for the journal, why should the editor care about it. You are tempting them to reject it right away. This is especially important when you have had a manuscript rejected from one journal and are now preparing it for submission to your second-choice journal. In this situation, it is as important to follow the instructions of the second-choice journal as when you submitted it to your first choice journal. When I receive a manuscript submitted to *Acta Psychiatrica Scandinavica* which follows the instructions to authors of one of the competing journals, the manuscript goes straight to the bottom of the priority list.

The optimum is to collaborate with a professional research secretary, she (and sometimes, however rarely, he) is normally much more skilled in this business than the researcher, so when you think you have done everything then ask the secretary to do it properly.

Finally, some journals have 'an instruction to authors' list' that covers an endless number of pages instructing you in minute detail. I myself never submit papers to these journals because I will not spend my time as an unpaid secretary for a journal and would definitely not ask the research secretaries of the department to waste their valuable time to do so. Furthermore, I think that papers loose something by being standardised to a degree that they all could have been written by the same person. However, this is a personal attitude.

As a basic rule: if you want to publish in a specific journal then follow the instructions to authors of the journal in all details.

Now the manuscript is ready for submission? No, it is not. You put it away for a week or two and try to forget all about it, then bring it out again and read it thoroughly, and all the mistakes and wrong messages, etc. will stand out clearly, so they can be changed and deleted (e.g. a conclusion sending the intelligent message that 'more research is needed' is now clear to you and must be deleted). Present me to the editor who wants to publish a paper concluding that more research is needed. Why should the paper be published? Why not wait for the next manuscript presenting the ' research that is needed'.

Is it now ready for submission? No, it is not. Now you send it to a senior colleague, someone you trust and who is willing to invest at least 2 hours of concentrated reading of your manuscript. This colleague's major task is to 'kill your darlings'. The younger you are, the longer your manuscript and the more detailed and meticulous the description, explanation and discussion, which are normally not needed. Your reader is familiar with reading scientific papers and is not interested in reading about all your 'beloved darlings'.

Submit the manuscript and forget all about it – for 4 months

Now submit it to the journal. Do not write a long accompanying letter when submitting to the journal, the manuscript should be able to stand alone and do not ask for special treatment of any kind. Every time you ask editors for something special, their time is taken away from editing the journal and handling your and other authors' manuscripts.

Then you start waiting. My advice is to forget about it but not any longer than 3½ to 4 months. Any decent journal should be able to handle your manuscript within 4 months and give you a qualified response. So do not waste your time worrying and speculating but get on with your research work. One little thing: if you have not received an acknowledgement saying that the journal has received your manuscript after 1 week, then ask for one. Information technology is a wonderful tool – when it works. If your manuscript has disappeared into cyberspace and never reached the journal you can wait forever. After 4 months, the journal has had its chance and it is now time to remind the editor (if your paper was submitted just before or during the summer holidays give them another 2–3 weeks). Ask politely:

Dear Sir/Madam,

Four months ago (17 July 2007) I submitted the manuscript [title] to your journal. I and my co-authors are now interested in knowing when we can expect a response from you.

Kind regards.

Yours sincerely,

Do not quarrel and do not blame the editor. If you write a very angry letter and it arrives on the editor's desk just as he is thinking about what to do about your manuscript having received two lukewarm reviews, you give him the best opportunity in the world to reject your paper. Always be neutral and correct, never be angry and never try to be charming.

Message: follow the instructions to authors in all details, check, double-check, ask someone to 'kill the darlings', submit the paper and forget all about it for 4 months.

The response from the editor

In principle, you may receive two kinds of responses from the editor. The first is a rejection. Some journals reject your paper right away when they can see that your manuscript has no chance of being published. This gives you the possibility for submitting to another journal very quickly; on the other hand, you get no professional feedback that would help you to improve the paper. Some journals have your paper reviewed even though the manuscript does not have a great chance of being published. This gives you the possibility to improve the manuscript but you waste several months before you can carry on with the next journal.

The second type of response is a good one: an invitation to revise the paper. In principle, there is a third kind of response, that is publication of your manuscript right away, but this outcome is extremely rare. For example, at the *Acta Psychiatrica Scandinavica* we receive about 600 manuscripts per year, and in the past 8 years we have had only one paper where neither of the two reviewers had any comments and both recommended it for immediate publication (one out of a little less than 5000 manuscripts).

The rejection

When a paper is rejected, it is rejected. Never start arguing with the editor. When the paper is rejected right away without having been reviewed it is simply because the editor (the journal) does not want the paper, and if you start arguing you run the risk of being told directly that they do not want it because it is not original, it is of low quality or something like that.

If your paper is rejected after having received two or three lukewarm to good reviews, do not start arguing/complaining to the editor. There are a lot of reasons other than quality for rejecting your paper: for example it might be on the periphery of the profile of the journal, the originality might not be sufficiently high, the journal might have recently published several papers with the same theme and is now giving room to other areas, the journal might have several papers like yours in the pipeline, or they might simply reject some extra papers to keep publication time down. Most international journals receive a lot more manuscripts than they can publish. For example, the acceptance rate of *Acta Psychiatrica Scandinavica* is between 15% and 20%, not because of low-quality papers being submitted but because of a limited number of pages for printing. This means that we have to reject a lot of very good papers, yours may be among those.

Fairness is a political concept which does not necessarily apply in publishing. When a paper is rejected you will never succeed in getting it published in that journal by victimising yourself, being a cry-baby, angry, threatening, mobilising the brigade of famous important colleagues, etc. The only thing you risk is having your name fixed at the back of the editor's mind, resulting in your having another paper rejected right away on a later occasion 'to prevent any problems like the last time'.

The revision

Receiving a letter from the editor encouraging you to revise your manuscript 'in accordance with the reviewers' comments and recommendations', together with a handful or two of the editor's own demands, is almost as cumbersome as having the paper rejected. You have forgotten about the paper, it is out of your mind, you had built up the illusion that you would never see it again except in print. Life is not so. So first of all, you have to bring the whole story back to mind, and what is next?

My own method is as follows. First, I run through the reviewers' comments – and the editor's – and think 'oh my God', 'this is terrible', 'do I really need the publication?', 'should we not simply dump the thing?' The next day I remember that it is unethical not to publish research results and then I read the comments once again, trying to identify specific messages, underlining them one by one, giving them numbers, identifying comments on the same items in the different reviews, finally ending up with a list: reviewer A, comments 1, 2, 3 and 4, etc.; reviewer B, comments 1, 2 (the same as comment 6 from reviewer A), 3, 4 (the same as comment 2 from reviewer C), etc.; reviewer C, comments 1, 2 …

Then I inform my co-authors and hope they are 'happy to leave the decision with you, Povl', giving me a carte blanche to make the changes. Then I make the changes, but if the reviewers' comments are based on a misunderstanding I prepare two versions of the revised manuscript, one in which all the changes are visible and one presenting the final product of the revision. The statement 'I prepare …' is a modification of the truth. If you have the privilege to work with an experienced research secretary, that individual should prepare the revision. The more professional the final layout the better. You are (hopefully) better at research than your research secretary and they are better at layout, spelling and punctuation than you.

A very important part of the response to the journal is the accompanying letter, in which you go through all the comments in order. For example, reviewer B, point 1 ..., authors' response, ...; reviewer B, point 2 (same as reviewer A, point 6) ..., authors' response, ...

An important point is not to follow a recommendation from a reviewer who has misunderstood something in your manuscript. The review process involves collaboration between the editor, the reviewers and the authors to obtain the best possible product. Do *not* lower the quality of your manuscript to please the reviewers/the editor, but in the accompanying letter explain why you have not made a change. Editors love these discussions. But please remember to explain yourself politely, do not use phrases such as 'the reviewer is an idiot', or the more moderate 'the reviewer has not understood ...', or even 'the reviewer seems to have misunderstood ...' The editor might send the whole thing to the reviewers and the final decision might depend on the reviewers' comments on the revised version. In any case, there is no need to criticise the reviewers – they are only human like yourself. Why not use phrasing such as 'as to point 3 reviewer B seems to have interpreted our formulations like ... We regret that our text has opened the possibility for misinterpretation, however, we have now revised other parts of the manuscript and this should make it more understandable ...'.

Another important point: all comments and recommendations for improving your paper should be followed. Do not try the following method which we sometimes see at *Acta Psychiatrica Scandinavica* (and is probably seen at all other journals) of trying to talk yourself out of the problem. For example, 'we feel we are right in this formulation ...', 'we think the original formulation gives the right meaning ...', 'it is our opinion that the presented analysis gives the complete answer although we have not re-analysed our data as suggested by the reviewer', etc. Editors have great experience in analysing accompanying letters and will reject your manuscript in the second round.

Another little trick: if (when) you have a manuscript rejected after review you should revise it in accordance with the reviewers' comments before you submit it to another journal. We are living and working in a small world and you will meet the same people time and time again. For example, as editor of *Acta Psychiatrica Scandinavica* I once rejected a paper after having had a response from one of the reviewers informing me that 'this is the third time I have received this manuscript, from three different journals; the authors have not changed it a bit since the first version, so I will not review it but ask you to refer the authors to the assessment I gave when they submitted the manuscript to the *Journal of Clever Thoughts*'. This is an example of a manuscript submitted to give the authors a line in their CVs and not to develop the science of psychiatry.

Finally, submit the revised version within the deadline given by the journal, and if the journal does not give you a deadline, give yourself one (1 month as a maximum). In this way you avoid the following situation. I took over the responsibility for *Acta Psychiatrica Scandinavica* on 1 January 1998.

In 2004 I received a 'revised manuscript' which I could not find in the files. After correspondence with the authors it became clear that they received an invitation to revise a manuscript from my predecessor in late 1996. The revision was not published.

About reviewers

Reviewers are colleagues; reviewers are humans; there are good reviewers and there are bad reviewers. Good reviewers are busy colleagues. If you are lazy or unqualified, colleagues, patients, journals and friends will never ask you to do a favour. If you are conscientious, qualified and up to date in your knowledge everybody will ask you. I received a message from a colleague to whom I had sent a manuscript asking for a review:

'Dear Povl,
I am swamped by manuscripts from different journals and I have now decided to do only one review per week. I therefore have to restrict myself to three to four manuscripts per journal per year, but should be happy to do this for your journal in the future'.

This is a wonderful colleague who realises that he is part of the scientific community. Being part of the scientific community you are at the same time an author, a reader and a reviewer. Therefore when you receive a request from a journal to do a review you should do it if you have the qualifications. I sent a paper to a colleague asking for a review and got the response 'I have no time'. This is fair and I found another. Six months later I sent another manuscript to the same person and got the same response. Fair enough, I found another. After another 6–9 months I tried a third time with a third manuscript and again got the reply 'I have no time'. I then deleted the person from the database but when sometime later I received a manuscript from the same person for publication I was very tempted to reject it right away because 'I have no time'. When you are in the publishing business as editor, author or reviewer you must act professionally, never emotionally, especially when you are an author. Being an author you are part of the scientific community, not only as author but also as reader and as reviewer, and you cannot gain the benefits without offering your expertise to the community.

There are expert reviewers and general reviewers. Many journals obtain a review from an expert reviewer and from a generalist reviewer. It can therefore be difficult to understand a rejection when one of the reviewers (the expert) is excited to have identified a colleague interested in the topic besides himself and the two he already knew about, but the rejection might be due to the generalist reviewer's response that 'the paper might be more relevant to a specialised journal'.

There are kind reviewers and there are rude reviewers. However experienced you become please remember that there is a person, sometimes a young person, at the other end of the process who has invested months/

years of their professional life (and maybe their private and emotional life too) in this project. As an author I myself have received many good and kind pieces of advice from anonymous senior review colleagues over the years. I have also received some from the rude end of the spectrum. Many years ago I submitted one of my first papers to an international journal, after waiting almost 9 months (a full pregnancy) I received three reviews, two very good and helpful, and one with only one sentence 'This is ridiculous'. The last has been very helpful, not in the immediate situation, but as a reminder to do my best, to behave politely, gently and professionally, and not to be nasty, rude or project stress and private problems onto colleagues under the cover of anonymity. As a young colleague receiving rude reviews, always remember to extract what you can use to improve your manuscript (if anything) and forget about the style.

The resubmission

Having resubmitted a revised version of the manuscript in which you have made all the changes carefully and meticulously and described them all in the accompanying letter, you will admit to yourself that the manuscript has definitely improved in quality. What can you expect from the editor? Sometimes the editor feels capable of making the decision and quickly sends you the message that your manuscript has been accepted. This is not what happens most often. In many cases the editor asks one of the reviewers (the most critical) to have another look, and in many cases there are still comments. After weeks/months you are asked for another minor revision. There may be another round and maybe even a fourth round – although this is quite rare. There is also the risk that your manuscript is rejected after the revision (or even the second or third revision), although this is very rare. What happens most often is that your manuscript is accepted for publication after the first or the second revision.

One of the best things in the professional life of a researcher is receiving the letter informing you that your manuscript has been accepted for publication. A message like that should be celebrated. In my own department we gather and acknowledge the author and mark the event every time one of us experiences the thrill of having been acknowledged in this way by the scientific community. I myself, even though I am 60 years of age and have over 150 peer-reviewed publications, still enjoy receiving the message 'Your manuscript has been accepted for publication'.

However, reading the second page of the letter of acceptance brings you down to earth very soon (therefore, please wait a day or two until you read the rest of the letter) because there are endless lists of what you have to do and what is forbidden: the copyright assignment, the need to collect signatures from co-authors and to declare once more that you have not been corrupted by industry, declarations of this and that, and lists of all the legal and other punishments that will rain down on your head if you do not behave. Read it carefully, sign it and act quickly.

Then you wait again. After some time you receive the proofs. The letter accompanying the proofs puzzles me every time. It is years since the process started and you designed your study. Perhaps it is not years but it is at least months since you submitted your paper to the journal, and you have been waiting and waiting for reviewers, editors and editorial secretaries, and now they demand you to read the proofs within 48 hours, no matter whether it is Christmas, Easter, frost or snow. Better do so, and do it carefully or even better ask a qualified research secretary to do it. My own experience is that you read proofs, and you read proofs and you read them once again, and you simply cannot find any more errors, and then when several thousand copies of the journal have been circulated the first thing you notice is an error. This is not a pleasant experience and we will not discuss it further in this chapter (the solution is called an *erratum*).

Most of the leading journals publish electronically as soon as the proofs have been approved by the author, by the editor and by the publisher. Being published electronically, the article is given a doi number, which will follow the paper even after it has received a regular reference number (year, volume, page) when the hard copy is circulated. This means that you can start citing a valid reference number for your paper immediately and frees you from citing it as 'in press'.

However, nothing can be compared to holding the wonderful smelling issue of the journal in your hand, with your article (now it is an article) on page 132: 'Professor Hübensprutz Schmeckenwasser, MD, The interesting study about important matters, from then to now.'

The journal might be rich and have sent you free reprints or you will have bought some yourself. What do you do with the reprints? I remember my first publication, I bought 50 reprints, sat down waiting for requests for reprints to come in (it was an article in a Danish journal). I gave one to my mother and one to my girlfriend, and kept the remaining 48, thinking they should not be wasted but be given to professional colleagues and researchers who asked for them. After another couple of months I sent another one to my mother – she called me to say she had already received one. Several years later when I cleared my office to change employment I found the remaining 47 reprints, kept one as a souvenir and dumped the other 46 in the paper recycling container.

So my advice to you: Send one to your mother and one to your spouse, one to the secretary responsible for the annual report and keep one in the department file. The rest should be sent immediately with compliments to members of the scientific community and active researchers within the field. This improves your odds of being cited and known for your research. Also remember the colleagues and staff within your own hospital/university, your own region and your own national scientific association. Do not forget the patients' associations and the public: write a short message in non-professional language and send it to local newspapers, to the local non-governmental organisations, etc. When all this has been done, the publishing process has come to an end.

Epilogue

So what to do now you have achieved publication? You have done all the right things, guided by wise seniors and mentors, so what will happen next? To be frank, unless you have discovered something equivalent to the double helix or *Helicobacter pylori* your publication will not lead to the hall of fame. On the contrary, it will be forgotten within a short while, if it was ever known. The majority of publications are nothing but part of the ongoing academic communication and discussion which is – it must not be forgotten – very important in itself. However, one piece of research or one publication is nothing, it is only valuable (except for something equivalent to the double helix or *Helicobacter pylori*) if it is part of an ongoing process. No single research project is sacred, it first becomes important when one project follows the other, one piece of research gives some results and generates some questions, which must be explored in a new research project, which must be followed by another research project, which must be followed by ... or a publication must be followed by a publication, must be followed by a publication ...; you are part of the scientific community.

But, however experienced a member of the community you become and however many publications you add to your CV, promise never to be so cold-hearted that you forget the thrill of receiving the letter from the editor:

'Your manuscript has been accepted for publication'.

CHAPTER 23

Mental health informatics

Martin Baggaley

Health informatics can be defined as the 'the knowledge, skills and tools which enable information to be collected, managed, used and shared to support the delivery of healthcare and to promote health' (http://www.nhscareers.nhs.uk/atoz.shtml#h). Mental health informatics applies to mental health services. Computers and the electronic transfer of information are part of normal day-to-day life and are increasingly important in health service delivery, including psychiatry. Psychiatrists need to understand the key principles of mental health informatics both to be able to work effectively now and also to appreciate the opportunities for more effective ways of working in the future.

Personal skills

To use information technology (IT) successfully requires a certain level of personal competency, although it is not necessary to understand the technology or how computer software is written.

European Computer Driving Licence

All staff working within the National Health Service (NHS) require a basic level of competence in health informatics. Basic IT skills are essential to support many healthcare practices. The European Computer Driving Licence (ECDL) has been adopted as the referenced standard for NHS staff and covers the basic use of information technology. It is widely used in 140 countries and is vendor neutral (i.e. it aims to cover skills independent of the software supplier). Most trusts offer free training to allow clinicians to study for and obtain the ECDL. Alternatively, courses are available in adult education centres. The syllabus includes:

- concepts of IT
- using a computer and managing files
- word processing

- spreadsheets
- databases
- presentation
- information and communication.

Effective use of email

Email is gradually replacing letters and written memos as the standard way of communicating. To get the most out of email it is important to understand how to use the software effectively and to be aware of the basic rules of etiquette, which unfortunately are rarely taught.

Microsoft Outlook

Most NHS personal computers have Microsoft Office as a standard suite of programmes, which includes Outlook as the standard email application. Outlook is like a postbox but it needs a mail system to operate. Many trusts will use an application such as Microsoft Exchange to distribute the email around the system.

NHS Contact

Contact is a fully integrated email, calendar and directory service for use by all NHS employees throughout their careers in the NHS. It allows for transmission of patient-sensitive data to another NHS user on contact using secure encrypted messages. It has a huge flexible database of contact details which, provided trusts and other NHS organisations keep it up to date, will prove to be a very useful way to contact other people in the NHS. Contact can be made from any personal computer that is connected to the internet (outside NHSnet) and it is compatible with Microsoft Outlook. Individual NHS clinicians can register to use Contact and over the next few years it is anticipated that all NHS organisations will use Contact instead of their own email server. The advantage of Contact is that it offers one address wherever anyone moves in the NHS and allows transmission of patient-sensitive information (within the system). One disadvantage is that email addresses cannot be as easily guessed. Most trusts currently use the format firstname.secondname@trustname.nhs.uk format, but Contact uses numbers to distinguish same names (e.g. john.smith99), which would not be known without having to look up the address.

Etiquette

Email is a very powerful tool but can easily be misused. It can be all too simple to send angry emails, copying them to everyone up to Chief Executive, which is soon regretted. It is sometimes possible to retrieve emails but do not rely on this to salvage potential disasters. It is a good rule never to send an email when feeling angry – better to calm down and review the matter the next day. It is also easy to appear rude when this was not the intention at all. There are many circumstances when a quick phone call is better than an email. Typing in capitals to indicate irritation is rude and should not be used. Avoid sending copies to everybody in the trust.

Email psychotherapy

There are some psychotherapists who provide psychotherapy by email. The regulation and ethical framework of such services is difficult to determine, especially when the therapist lives in a different country to the patient. Also, the efficacy of such treatment is not clearly demonstrated. Nevertheless, some service users appear to appreciate such contact and the impersonal nature of the interaction. Service providers charge per email or time taken over a case. Most internet psychotherapists are based in the USA, although it can be difficult to know exactly where they are based at times. In the UK, there are few services that offer internet therapy. However, there are a number of therapists and psychiatrists who use emails as a follow-up and as a way of monitoring the progress of patients they also see face to face. Email is much less intrusive than phone calls, and therapists and patients can read the message at their convenience. There are some web-based cognitive–behavioural psychotherapy treatment programmes, which have been demonstrated to be effective in the treatment of depression and other anxiety disorders.

Trust intranets

An intranet is effectively an internal internet. Users use a browser, such as Microsoft Explorer, to look at web pages that are not accessible to users outside the firewall (a firewall is software that prevents unauthorised access to individuals outside the trust). A trust can use an intranet to share information that might otherwise clog up the email system. For example, instead of sending out an email to all staff, notices of interest can be posted on the intranet.

Internet and NHSnet

The internet, then known as ARPANET, was brought online in 1969 under a contract let by the renamed Advanced Research Projects Agency (ARPA), which initially connected four major computers at universities in the south-western USA (University of California, Los Angeles, Stanford Research Institute, University of California, Santa Barbara and the University of Utah). The internet was designed in part to provide a communications network that would work even if some of the sites were destroyed by nuclear attack. If the most direct route were not available, routers would direct traffic around the network via alternate routes. Since then, the internet has expanded globally to become a key communication tool. Broadband is growing faster than ever and some areas had achieved 90% broadband penetration by the middle of 2007. Theoretically every clinician in the NHS has access to the internet through NHSnet. The NHSnet is a virtual private network that operates throughout the NHS and is inaccessible to non-NHS organisations. It provides access to both NHS-specific websites (prefixed nww.) and the world wide web (www.). Clinicians now have an enormous amount of clinically relevant material available at their desk, if they are able to access that material effectively. In addition, patients and carers have access to much of the same information through the internet, which means that the patient and carer may know as much or more about a particular topic as the attending clinician. One unresolved difficulty is communication to key stakeholders outside NHSnet, such as private providers and social services. It would be useful to exchange patient-sensitive data with such agencies but at present this raises difficult security issues.

Knowledge management

Clinicians are faced with an exponential growth of new knowledge, including new research and new guidelines and policy directives. This knowledge is available electronically, which allows clinicians to access this at their desktop, so that it is available as required when seeing service users. Many services can be configured to send out alerts when relevant research is published. Online searches can be performed and the relevant abstracts retrieved and saved to disk or printed out. Librarians are changing their function from managing books to becoming experts on electronic information management. It is possible simply to use an internet search engine to try to look up suitable material. However, it is usually more effective to access a site that can act as a gateway to relevant resources via hyperlinks. Such sites for psychiatrists might include the Royal College of Psychiatrists' website (http://www.rcpsych.ac.uk) and the National Library for Health mental health site (http://www.library.nhs.uk/mentalhealth).

National Library for Health

The National Library for Health is a digital library for NHS staff, patients and the public that allows access to other NHS agencies, such as the National Institute for Health and Clinical Excellence (NICE) and the National Patient Safety Agency (NPSA), and information resources such as Clinical Knowledge Summaries (which incorporate Prodigy advice on managing primary care problems) and Bandolier (evidence-based medicine). There are subject-specific specialist libraries, including one on mental health (http://www.library.nhs.uk/mentalhealth).

Athens account

All NHS employees can apply for an 'Athens' password, which allows access via the internet to a large range of electronic resources, including Medline, the Cochrane Library, and access to full-text versions of recently published original papers in the National Library for Health.

Map of Medicine

This product (http://www.mapofmedicine.com) is available via the NHS Care Records Service in England. Currently it includes over 380 patient journeys, with 1500 flow charts detailing clinical pathways, the equivalent of more than 6000 text pages. These journeys appear in the form of a unique graphical representation that enables you to follow a pathway more easily. These journeys also provide access to clinical thinking and process in digestible chunks, and allow retrieval of more detailed information as required.

Confidentiality and security

All medical data are potentially sensitive and information regarding mental health is especially so. The principles of confidentiality and security with regard to medical records are not fundamentally different for electronic notes compared with paper systems. However, the former cause greater concern because of the potential ease of browsing vast numbers of records. However, most electronic systems have the potential for being more secure than the paper equivalent (by for example having an audit trail of who has accessed what page). The National Programme for IT uses the principle of role-based access (i.e. access to data being dependent on nationally determined roles such as doctor, administrator, etc.) and having a legitimate relationship to the patient. Access is controlled by a Smart card and password, which is checked via the Spine (a national database of key information about a patient's health and care) once the individual logs onto the system. Other systems typically use password and user name access only. There is always a conflict between making information available so that it is useful to service users and clinicians and making it confidential. In general, the greater the control, the slower the access to the system and the greater the chance that the information is not available because the clinician has insufficient access rights. In order to reassure both clinicians and members of the public, the Secretary of State for Health issued what is known as the Care Records Guarantee (http://www.connectingforhealth. nhs.uk/crdb), which provides:

- that individuals will be allowed access to their own records
- that access to records by NHS staff will be strictly limited to those having a 'need to know' to provide effective treatment for a patient
- that information will not be shared outside the NHS unless individuals grant permission, the NHS is obliged to do so by law, or failure to share would put someone else at risk; any sharing without permission will be carried out following best practice guidelines

- that if individuals are unable to make a decision about sharing health information on their own behalf, a senior healthcare professional may make a decision to do so, taking into account the views of relatives, carers and any recorded views of the individual
- that where healthcare is provided by a care team including people from other services, the NHS and patient can agree to share health information with the other services, bearing in mind the effect failure to share might have on the quality of care received
- that individuals can choose not to share information in their electronic care records, although this may have an impact on the quality of care received
- a complaints procedure
- that individuals are entitled to check and correct mistakes in their record
- that the NHS must enforce a duty of confidentiality on their staff and organisations under contract to the NHS
- that the NHS must keep the records secure and confidential
- that the NHS must keep a record of everyone who looks at the information held in the service; individuals will be entitled to ask for a list of people accessing their records and details of when they looked at the records
- that the NHS must take enforcement action if someone looks at records without permission or good reason.

There is some discussion as to whether patients should opt in or opt out of having their data included in the Care Records Service. There is the concept of the so-called sealed envelope, where some information is not shared, for example with the Spine or other service providers. This is somewhat problematic in that if, for example, information about a depressive episode is kept from the Spine yet the service user is on anti-depressant medication, if information about medication was placed on the Spine, the information about anti-depressant medication would indicate depression. It is considered unsafe to leave out partial medication information and therefore it is the current position that all medication information would be omitted in such a case.

Data protection

The current UK legislation is the Data Protection Act 1998. This is a piece of complex legislation but contains eight principles regarding the handling of personal data. These state that all data must be:

- processed fairly and lawfully
- obtained and used only for specified and lawful purposes
- adequate, relevant and not excessive
- accurate and, where necessary, kept up to date
- kept for no longer than necessary

- processed in accordance with the individuals rights (as defined)
- kept secure
- transferred only to countries that offer adequate data protection.

Freedom of Information Act 2000

The Freedom of Information Act was passed on 30 November 2000 and gives a general right of access to all types of recorded information held by public authorities, with full access granted in January 2005. The Act sets out exemptions to that right and places certain obligations on public authorities. It requires all organisations in the NHS to set up and maintain publication schemes that tell the public what information is held.

Caldicott Guardians

Caldicott Guardians are senior staff in the NHS and social services appointed to protect patient information (Department of Health, 2006). The Caldicott principles and processes provide a framework of quality standards for the management of confidentiality and access to personal information under the leadership of a Caldicott Guardian. The name arises from the work of Dr Fiona Caldicott, a past President of the Royal College of Psychiatrists. Chief executives were required to appoint a Caldicott Guardian by 31 March 1999 and in 2002 this responsibility was extended to councils with social service responsibility. There are approximately 1000 Caldicott Guardians throughout the NHS and in councils with social service responsibility. *The Caldicott Report* (Department of Health, 1997) established a clear set of principles, reflecting best practice in the handling of confidential information.

Justify the purpose

Every proposed use or transfer of information within or from an organisation should be clearly defined and scrutinised, with continuing uses regularly reviewed by an appropriate Guardian.

Do not use patient-identifiable information unless absolutely necessary

Patient identifiable information items should not be used unless there is no alternative.

Use the minimum necessary patient-identifiable information

Where the use of patient-identifiable information is considered to be essential, each individual item of information should be justifiable with the aim of reducing identifiability.

Access to patient-identifiable information should be on a strict need-to-know basis

Only those individuals who need access to patient-identifiable information should have access to the pieces of information that they need to see.

Everyone should be aware of their responsibilities

Action should be taken to ensure that those handling patient-identifiable information, including clinical and non-clinical staff, are aware of their responsibilities and obligations to respect patient confidentiality.

Understand and comply with the law

Every use of patient-identifiable information must be lawful. Someone in each organisation should be responsible for ensuring that the organisation complies with the legal requirement.

Electronic patient records

It is intended that in due course all healthcare records, including those for mental health, will be electronic. Some general practices have become paperless, but few mental health trusts are close to such a position. Mental healthcare would particularly benefit from such a system, especially if the system is widely networked, given that mental healthcare is usually community based. This means that patients are liable to present at various sites, such as a community team base or an accident and emergency department or hostel. An electronic patient record provides the right information at the right time at the right place. There are important safety gains in implementing a full electronic patient record, particularly with electronic prescribing, which has been shown to reduce drug errors by 85%.

An electronic patient record also should improve the availability of information for both service users and carers, as it is possible to print off and possibly email copies of care plans, drug information leaflets, etc. to carers and services users.

As they move towards a paperless system, most trusts will still keep paper records for a transitional period. This requires careful management, and may in itself represent a risk as vital information may remain in the paper records while the community mental health team uses more up-to-date electronic information, unaware of the existence of relevant past material. A recent serious incident occurred at a trust with a well-used electronic information system when a patient was admitted to the in-patient unit. There were extensive electronic records going back 3 years which were used during the admission and the paper records were not examined. The patient carried out a serious assault which mimicked almost exactly one 4 years previously; this had resulted in a forensic assessment which was in the paper but not the electronic record. Had the existence of the assessment been known, the incident might have been avoided. Electronic patient records will inevitably change the way psychiatrists practise.

The practice of old-fashioned clerking will probably go, to be replaced by an electronic multidisciplinary assessment which will be updated and edited from already existing information.

National Programme for IT

The National Programme for IT, which is being delivered by the Department of Health agency NHS Connecting for Health, is bringing modern computer systems into the NHS to improve patient care and services. Over the next 10 years, the National Programme for IT will connect over 30000 general practices in England to almost 300 hospitals and give patients access to information about their personal health and care, transforming the way the NHS works. More information can be obtained at: http://www.connectingforhealth.nhs.uk/. Currently the National Programme for IT covers England only, but there are some similar initiatives beginning in Wales and Scotland. This is a vast ambitious programme which includes various smaller programmes.

Spine

Spine is a national database which will contain demographic information on the entire population of England. It is known as the PDS (patient demographic service) and will allow all electronic patient record systems that are deployed to use the PDS as their patient master index, rather than using a local patient master index. It will also contain key summary data, such as active problems or diagnoses, allergies, current medication prescribed, past medical history and the details of other clinicians involved in the patient's care. Potentially, this will be very useful in psychiatry, where it is common for patients to present to services other than their own. However, having a national database raises concerns about confidentiality issues. These are covered in what is known as the Care Records Service Guarantee 2007 (http://www.connectingforhealth.nhs.uk/).

Care Records Service

The Care Records Service is responsible for the provision of an electronic patient record. The country has been divided into three programmes: the North Midlands and East (NME), the Southern, and London. Each programmes has a local service provider, a large commercial company that is contracted to supply the service and a software supplier that is contracted by the local service provider to actually build the system. The plan is for the Care Records Service to provide an electronic patient record that allows clinicians with a legitimate relationship to access patient-centred information across all care settings. It should allow care pathways to be developed to support care across all settings and support the government initiative to move care from hospital to the community.

Electronic transfer of prescriptions

This programme is not for electronic prescribing but for the transfer of prescriptions electronically. Patients would be given a prescription which, provided they had nominated a chemist where they wished to collect the prescription, would be sent electronically to the chemist, who would dispense the medication. The invoicing by the chemist for the prescription would also be dealt with electronically.

N3

This is the programme to upgrade the network for the NHS to provide fast broadband access throughout England.

Choose and Book

Choose and Book (http://www.chooseandbook.nhs.uk) is a national electronic referral service which gives patients a choice of place, date and time for their first outpatient appointment in a clinic or hospital. The relevance of Choose and Book for psychiatry has yet to be determined as in England most services are related to general practice and require social service involvement. It is not possible to choose to receive services from one local authority in preference to another. It is therefore difficult to choose to refer a patient with schizophrenia to one of four community mental health teams.

UK Government policy

Mental Health Information Strategy

The latest strategy was published in March 2001 by the Department of Health. It was therefore written before the roll out of the National Programme for IT, but the principles that it covers have not changed. For more information visit: http://www.icservices.nhs.uk/mentalhealth/mh-is/pages/default.asp

Mental Health Minimum Data Set

The Mental Health Minimum Data Set (MHMDS) has been developed to improve information on mental health service usage and need. The dataset describes the care received by service users during an overall spell of care. It is person-centred, so that all the care received by individuals can be studied, and includes details of clinical problems, treatments given, outline aspects of social care and outcomes. Geographic markers allow analysis by any type of health, general practice or local authority administrative categories. The prime purpose of the dataset is to provide local clinicians and managers with better quality information for clinical audit, service planning and management. The dataset became mandatory for mental health service providers on 1 April 2003 and central collection of data provides improved national information, facilitating feedback to trusts and the setting of benchmarks. The MHMDS is an aggregated dataset, which should provide useful comparative information for service managers to compare how one service performs compared with another. It should be extractable from routinely collected clinical data, although in many cases the appropriate information system from which such data can be collected is not available.

Royal College of Psychiatrists

Informatics Committee

This is a College committee that works closely with the Mental Health Informatics Special Interest Group and reports to the English Policy Committee of the College. It meets on a bi-monthly basis and is able to advise the College and raise issues of concern to College members. The minutes of the meetings are available on the College members' pages of the Royal College of Psychiatrists' website (http://www.rcpsych.ac.uk). College members are required to register to use the site.

Mental Health Informatics Special Interest Group

This Special Interest Group of the College holds meetings, produces a newsletter and runs training workshops at College meetings for College members. Details are available from the College website (http://www. rcpsych.ac.uk/college/specialinterestgroups/mentalhealthinformatics. aspx).

The future

Mental health informatics is a rapidly developing field, driven by continuing technological advance, and is certain to change the way mental health services operate and psychiatrists practise in the future. Hand-held devices, perhaps 3G mobile phones, will allow electronic patient records to be accessible in service users' homes. Service users may be able to download their medical records to flashcards or access information via a website. There will always be differing levels of enthusiasm for such systems and progress will always seem slower than it might. However, if psychiatrists can understand the basic principles, they will be in a better position to obtain real benefit from developments rather feeling that technology is being imposed on them.

References

Department of Health (1997) *The Caldicott Report*. Department of Health.
Department of Health (2001) *Mental Health Information Strategy March 2001*. Department of Health.
Department of Health (2006) *The Caldicott Guardian Manual 2006*. Department of Health.

CHAPTER 24

Clinical governance

Rosalind Ramsay and Eleanor Cole

For the first 40 years of the National Health Service (NHS) there was an implicit notion of quality, with the assumption that providing well-trained staff and developing good facilities and equipment was synonymous with high standards (Halligan & Donaldson, 2001).

The arrival of the Thatcher government in 1979 saw the start of the first major reforms to the NHS. These initially focused on funding, management and organisational reform. From 1982 managers became accountable for output measures, at first concentrating on financial and workload concerns. In 1983 the Griffiths report (Department of Health and Social Security, 1983) described a lack of clarity in accountability at local level, and overturned consensus management, resulting in the appointment of general managers to lead healthcare units.

More service changes followed with the introduction of the internal market in the early 1990s, but these did not specifically look at how to achieve improvements in quality at a structural level. Quality continued to be seen as inherent in the system, sustained by the ethos and skills of the health professionals working in the NHS. Any quality initiatives tended to be insular activities, not integrated across a whole service.

Quality management ideas, which were developed in the Japanese car industry and taken up by business in the USA, crept into the American healthcare system in the 1970s, before arriving in Europe. New concepts included total quality management and continuous quality improvement, but these were not widely accepted. However, the rise of consumerism among the post-war generation was starting to challenge the traditional paternalistic role of healthcare professionals in general, and doctors in particular. Patients wanted more information, choice and involvement in decisions regarding their healthcare. This is illustrated in the rise of the service user movement and with the government's introduction of the Patient's Charter in 1992; shorter waiting lists, and the right to information and to complain were potential vote winners.

There were also questions about variations in practice as clinicians adopted the principles of evidence-based medicine, taking a more rigorous approach to their work. A series of high-profile service failures – an example being paediatric cardiac surgery in Bristol – raised concerns about professional self-regulation and doctors' accountability. These service failures prompted more urgent demands for change and attempts to address quality in a more systematic and explicit way.

Rise of clinical governance

The 1990 *National Health Service and Community Care Act* gave services a statutory duty of quality. Fuller development of this approach came with the first Blair government in the late 1990s. *The New NHS* (Department of Health, 1997) stated 'every part of the NHS, and everyone who works in it, must take responsibility for improving quality ... and it must be the quality of the patient experience as well as the clinical result'.

Clinical governance formalises this focus on the quality of services. *A First Class Service: Quality in the New NHS* (Department of Health, 1998) proposed that clinical governance would be the means by which NHS organisations could discharge their statutory duty to provide high-quality, safe and effective healthcare. It is 'the opportunity to understand and learn to develop the fundamental components required to facilitate the delivery of quality care – a no blame, questioning, learning culture, excellent leadership, and an ethos where staff are valued and supported as they form partnerships with patients. These elements have perhaps previously been regarded as too intangible to take seriously or attempt to improve. Clinical governance demands re-examination of traditional roles and boundaries – between health professions, between doctor and patient, and between managers and clinicians – and provides the means to show the public that the NHS will not tolerate less than best practice' (Halligan & Donaldson, 2001).

The commonly used definition of clinical governance is 'a framework through which NHS organisations are accountable for continuously improving the quality of their services and safeguarding high standards of care by creating an environment in which excellence in clinical care will flourish' (Scally & Donaldson, 1998).

Dame Janet Smith, chair of the Shipman Inquiry, wrote in the fifth report of the Inquiry that she did not find this definition particularly easy to understand and that the medical profession have been confused and uncertain as to what clinical governance means in practice (Shipman Inquiry, 2004). Having decided that it was impossible to define clinical governance she attempted to describe it as 'a system for improving the standard of clinical practice in the NHS and for protecting the public from unacceptable standards of care'. This system is made up of different activities within an integrated framework replacing what were 'previously disparate and fragmented approaches to the improvement of quality of care'.

A definition of clinical governance is given in Box 24.1.

> **Box 24.1** Definition of clinical governance
>
> Clinical governance is 'doing the right thing, at the right time, by the right person – the application of the best evidence to a patient's problems, in the way the patient wishes, by an appropriately trained and resourced individual or team. But that's not all – the individual or team must work within an organisation that is accountable for the actions of its staff, values its staff (appraises and develops them), minimises risks, and learns from good practice, and indeed mistakes' (Gray, 2005).

Developing a framework for clinical governance

A first-class service lists the main components of clinical governance as:

- clear lines of responsibility and accountability for the overall quality of clinical care
- a comprehensive programme of quality improvement activities
- clear policies aimed at reducing risk
- procedures for all professional groups to identify and remedy poor performance.

The New NHS (Department of Health, 1997) outlined structures that would support the development of clinical governance. These include the National Service Frameworks and the National Institute for Clinical Excellence (since renamed the National Institute for Health and Clinical Excellence) to set quality standards; the Commission for Health Improvement (since renamed the Healthcare Commission), the National Performance Framework and the National Survey of Patient and User Experience were to monitor standards.

Further legislation around the quality agenda came with *Supporting Doctors, Protecting Patients* (Department of Health, 1999a) with its proposals for professional regulation, and *An Organisation with a Memory* (Department of Health, 2000), which looked at learning from adverse incidents in the NHS. *An Organisation with a Memory* prompted the creation of the National Patient Safety Agency (NPSA) in 2001 to report and learn from mistakes and problems that affect patient safety.

Another element of the quality strategy is patient and public empowerment. Since 2003 NHS bodies have had a legal duty to involve and consult the public. New developments have included establishing patient advice and liaison services (PALS) and patient and public involvement forums in trusts as well as the independent complaints advocacy services. Another way to empower patients is to provide better information.

Underpinning strategies include information and information technology, research and development and education and training (Halligan & Donaldson, 2001).

Commission for Health Improvement and clinical governance reviews

The Commission for Health Improvement (now the Healthcare Commission) inspected clinical governance arrangements and provided feedback to local NHS organisations to inform development. Review teams assessed how well clinical governance was working throughout an organisation by making enquiries at corporate and directorate levels and in clinical teams about the different reviews areas, known as the seven components or 'pillars' of clinical governance (Box 24.2). The Commission for Health Improvement also described strategic capacity and the patient experience.

Standards for better health

The NHS Improvement Plan (Department of Health, 2004*a*) has continued the emphasis on the quality of services, with an increased focus on the individual service user, including patient choice, and also public health. At the same time *National Standards, Local Action 2005/06–2007/08* (Department of Health, 2004*b*) provides the framework for the NHS and local authorities until 2008. Within the framework are the *Standards for Better Health* (Department of Health, 2004*c*), which build on the work of the National Service Frameworks and National Institute for Health and Clinical Excellence. Standards are to be the main drivers for quality improvement and with fewer national targets there is greater scope for addressing local priorities. *Standards for Better Health* has tried to define the level of quality that all NHS organisations – including NHS foundation trusts and also private and voluntary sector providers of NHS services – need to meet to assure safe and acceptable services. This is through compliance with the mandatory minimum 'core' standards, and promoting service improvement by working towards the goals set in the 'developmental' standards. The standards aim to rationalise the existing standards and guidance into a single framework and are presented in seven domains (Box 24.3).

Box 24.2   The seven 'pillars' of clinical governance

- Clinical audit
- Risk management
- Research and effectiveness
- Use of information
- Patient and public involvement
- Staffing and staff management
- Education and training

> **Box 24.3** Seven domains of standards for promoting service improvement
>
> - Safety
> - Clinical effectiveness and cost-effectiveness
> - Governance
> - Patient focus
> - Accessible and responsive care
> - Care environment and amenities
> - Public health

As we can see, one of these domains covers governance, and of the remaining six, five are closely linked to the previous Commission for Health Improvement pillars of clinical governance: safety, clinical effectiveness and cost-effectiveness, patient focus, accessible and responsive care, and care environment and amenities.

The Healthcare Commission

The Health and Social Care (Community Health and Standards) Act 2003 replaced the Commission for Health Improvement with the Commission for Healthcare Audit and Inspection, generally known as the Healthcare Commission, in 2004. The Healthcare Commission has the overall function of encouraging improvement in healthcare and public health in England (with a more limited role in Wales). It pays particular attention to:

- availability and access to healthcare
- quality and effectiveness of healthcare
- economy and efficiency of healthcare
- availability and quality of information provided to the public about healthcare
- need to safeguard rights and welfare of children.

The Healthcare Commission aims to focus on service users and the public, to work in partnership with others and to be open and accountable for its actions. Its corporate plan for 2004–2008 (Healthcare Commission, 2004) made a commitment to reduce the existing system of multiple inspections.

The Healthcare Commission has developed criteria and an assessment process based on *Standards for Better Health* (Department of Health, 2004c). The new annual health check requires NHS trusts to make public declarations on the extent to which they meet the core standards, supplemented by comments from service users and the local community. The Healthcare Commission also regulates the independent healthcare sector and carries out improvement reviews of particular aspects of healthcare.

There has been sharp criticism of the standards on the grounds that they are 'inconsistent in depth, scope and specificity', whereas the domains have 'no apparent architecture ... or hierarchy' and do not match any existing conceptual models (Shaw, 2004). It remains to be seen how well the Healthcare Commission can develop its assessment processes. As Shaw commented, 'the Department of Health has misjudged the research, technical expertise and time needed to develop and test a fair and reliable process of external assessment. The burden will fall on the fledgling Healthcare Commission as assessor and on the early guinea pigs who are assessed.'

Integrated governance

Deighan et al (2004) have put forward the concept of integrated governance. They see this as a way of allowing governance to move out of its individual silos of clinical governance, corporate governance, research governance, information and financial governance so that trust boards can more easily agree a common set of objectives and set a high-level direction for the organisation.

Clinical governance in other parts of the UK

With devolution has come some differences in the development of clinical governance and its supporting structures. In Scotland, for example, the White Paper *Designed to Care* (Scottish Executive Health Department, 1997) introduced the term clinical governance to NHS Scotland. The following year clinical governance was defined as 'corporate accountability for clinical performance' with trust chief executives responsible for the quality of care provided by their organisations. NHS Quality Improvement Scotland (http://www.nhshealthquality.org) was set up in 2003 as the lead organisation to improve the quality of healthcare delivered by NHS Scotland. It works with the Scottish Intercollegiate Guideline Network (SIGN; http://www.sign.ac.uk), which develops national clinical guidelines containing recommendations for effective practice based on current evidence. NHS Quality Improvement Scotland describes clinical governance as the system for making sure that healthcare is safe and effective, that care is patient centred and that the public are involved.

Implementing clinical governance

Nicholls et al (2000) suggest we can understand clinical governance as 'a whole system cultural change which provides the means of developing the organisational capability to deliver sustainable, accountable, patient focused quality assured healthcare'. This reflects the view of *The New NHS*

(Department of Health, 1997) which recognised that 'achieving meaningful and sustainable quality improvements in the NHS requires a fundamental shift in culture'. Nicholls *et al* (2000) believe that clinical governance gives us a chance to find ways to move out of the comfort zone of the status quo to a more challenging culture with more active learning. They comment on the central role of the patient, with a real partnership between patient and professional being at the heart of clinical governance. They also remind us that staff are the key resource for health services.

Clinical governance requires changes at three levels – by individual professionals, by teams and by organisations (http://www.cgsupport.nhs. uk):

- Individual healthcare professionals need to embrace change – adopting reflective practice that places patients at the centre of their thinking.
- Teams need to become true multidisciplinary groups, where understanding about roles, about sharing information and knowledge, and about support for each other become part of everyday practice.
- Organisations need to put in place systems and local arrangements to support such teams and to assure the quality of care provided. Commitment and leadership from the board and throughout the organisation is clearly crucial.

Involving patients and carers in clinical governance

The NHS Institute for Innovation and Improvement's (2005) guide *Involving Patients and Carers* states that clinical governance reports should clearly describe how teams are developing continuous and effective patient involvement and how this has improved care as a result. One example they give involves discharge planning from a particular in-patient unit. The service users had reported being confused about who was looking after them, and had difficulty remembering contact telephone numbers, particularly at times of crisis. Users and carers received no written information on discharge. The service worked with service users and carers to set up a steering group which explored the views of service users about discharge planning information. The group adopted an idea from a user to create a crisis card the size of a credit card to give contact information about the care coordinator, general practitioner, social services and helplines. The local users helped to design the cards which are now used for all patients discharged from in-patient care. The service users felt more confident at times of crisis knowing that they could easily make contact with services when needed. There are plans to extend the use of the crisis card to other parts of the service.

Progress within trusts

Reviewing its findings from clinical governance reviews in mental health trusts, the Commission for Health Improvement reported a number of factors common to trusts that were performing well and to those that

Table 24.1 Characteristics of trusts according to performance in clinical governance reviews

Characteristics shared by trusts performing well	Characteristics shared by trusts performing poorly
Lower vacancy rates, particularly in psychiatry, or work to resolve vacancy problems, progress on improving working lives	Serious problems with recruitment generally in psychiatry and in-patient nursing, low morale, cultural and operational divide with social care staff
Good progress with developing NSF/NHS Plan services and the CPA	Limited development of new services and implementation of the CPA
Leadership cohesive, visible and well regarded by staff and partners	Staff see leadership as remote, weakness in executive/non-executive leadership
Strong relationships between clinicians and managers	Lack of engagement of clinicians in management
Cohesive structures between different parts of the trust	Disconnection between different parts of the trust
Strong structures to support clinical governance in directorates and sectors/ localities; understanding of relationship between the board and directorates, sectors and services	Limited structures below corporate level to support implementation and performance management of clinical governance, or structures to support clinical governance components
Well-developed clinical information systems and progress with performance management	Fragmented information systems and little development in performance management
Good progress on organisational and operational integration with primary care	Limited progress with organisational and operational integration with social care
Effective communication systems in place	Poor communication systems

CPA, care programme approach; NSF, National Service Framework.
Source: adapted from Commission for Health Improvement (2003).

had made less progress (Table 24.1). Generally trusts that were making progress in implementing clinical governance had made good progress in implementing the National Service Framework for Mental Health, developing integrated provision with their social care partners and implementing the care programme approach. The Commission for Health Improvement also found similar problems and characteristics in organisations that had been subject to investigation.

Barriers to clinical governance

A number of barriers to implementing clinical governance have been identified. Palmer (2002) refers to organisational culture, low prioritisation and lack of support. In spite of the rhetoric of a 'no blame' culture, many clinicians and managers feel there is a strong blame culture with fears, for example, that participation in clinical audit can lead to punishment of poor performers. Historically, clinical audit had a low priority and clinical governance may not be seen as central to an organisation's activity, and this is compounded by a lack of support for clinical governance activity.

Putting clinical governance into practice

Clinical governance was originally seen as being local in its orientation and operation. As a bottom-up mechanism it could inspire and enthuse, and create a 'no blame' learning environment with excellent leadership, valued staff and an active partnership between staff and service users (Degeling *et al*, 2004). However, government preoccupation with delivery and top-down performance management has undermined its developmental potential. Degeling *et al* (2004) argued that if clinical governance is to work it must reach every level of a healthcare organisation, including clinicians who are at the core of clinical work.

Can we redefine clinical governance as an integral part of everyday work, and express this in terms that relate to the improvement of patient care? Edwards (2004) commented that there are two preconditions for this to be possible. First, the notion of professionalism must include:

- using techniques to improve the safety and effectiveness of care
- standardising care
- taking responsibility for the financial resources required
- being accountable for quality and performance.

Second, policy makers and leaders must develop objectives and ways of working that will be meaningful to clinicians, supported by performance management and appraisal, and allow them to work more effectively.

Working with individual teams

In taking a bottom-up approach to implementing clinical governance, it is also essential to consider how individuals perceive it and their understanding of the concept. Murray *et al* (2004) used the Staff Clinical Governance Scale to explore staff knowledge of, attitudes towards and implementation of the seven pillars across three mental health/community trusts. They found considerable goodwill towards clinical governance, although over a quarter of responders had not heard of it. The majority of staff viewed clinical governance as useful, and as clear and welcome, although it was also felt to be complex and tiresome. One directorate that had put some effort into training and communicating about clinical governance had the most positive responses, suggesting the value of having a proactive approach to involving all staff in clinical governance.

Another mental health trust (Mynors-Wallis *et al*, 2004) has developed clinical governance portfolios for their teams to facilitate the recording of all the clinical governance activity a team does. The aim is to increase awareness of clinical governance, ensure that it is central to team activity, encourage clinical governance activity and monitor it. One member of each team acts as the portfolio coordinator. Review of the portfolios allowed the team coordinators to discuss their successes and difficulties in establishing clinical governance at team level, and to develop an action plan over the following year. The portfolios are linked in with other trust developments rather than being an isolated project. They have also enabled the spread of good practice.

Topic-specific clinical governance

Degeling et al (2004) recommended looking at clinical governance in a condition-specific way, encouraging staff dealing with a particular type of clinical work to define, describe, assess and manage what they do as a team.

Clinical governance and suicide prevention

We could also look at a particular topic, for example, suicide prevention, in this way. What can individual teams do to develop better practice in relation to reducing the risk of suicide among their users?

Suicide is the most common cause of death in men under the age of 35 and the main cause of premature death in people with a mental illness (Department of Health, 2002). The White Paper *Saving Lives: Our Healthier Nation* (Department of Health, 1999b) set a target to reduce the death rate from suicide and undetermined injury by at least a fifth by 2010. There is no single route to achieving this target as the factors associated with suicide are many and varied. Developing a coherent suicide prevention strategy needs the collaboration of a range of organisations and individuals.

The *National Suicide Prevention Strategy for England* (Department of Health, 2002) proposes six goals and objectives for action. What do these mean for practising clinicians in terms of quality of care? How can we conceive them in clinical governance terms?

Reducing the risk in high-risk groups

The identified high-risk groups include people who are currently or were recently in contact with mental health services as well as people who have recently self-harmed, young men, prisoners and groups in high-risk occupations. This means that for all individual teams and clinicians there are questions about training in suicide risk assessment and management.

What are the services for individuals in the immediate aftermath of an episode of self-harm? Is there a local implementation plan for the NICE guidelines (National Institute for Clinical Excellence, 2004)? The guidelines cover the first 48 hours after an episode of self-harm and recommend more sophisticated ways of trying to engage with service users and their carers, encouraging the notion of self-management as well recommending particular types of psychological intervention for which there is some evidence of effectiveness.

There is continuing concern about the evidence of increased risk of suicide in young men. This has caught the attention of the media. How are clinicians and services trying to engage with this group in their locality? Initiatives include a crisis helpline in some areas (CALM – Campaign Against Living Miserably), supplementing the work of the Samaritans and NHS Direct, and also work with substance misuse services to look at how they can improve the clinical management of alcohol and drug misuse in young men who self-harm.

The prison service suicide prevention strategy includes a number of plans to improve the screening and management of self-harm in this population by prison services, and also in collaboration with local mental health services. There are plans to improve the information flow into and across the criminal justice system concerning individuals known to be at risk of suicide.

A time of particularly high risk has been identified as the week after discharge, and clinicians need to make arrangements for early (7-day) follow-up for people at high risk as well as considering access to services at times of crisis (Twelve points to a safer service; http://www.medicine.manchester.ac.uk/suicideprevention).

Promoting well-being in the wider population

This is in line with standard 1 of the *National Service Framework for Mental Health* (Department of Health, 1999c), which aims to promote mental health for all and to combat discrimination against those with a mental illness. The strategy recognises the range of factors that may predispose to self-harm but goes on to take a narrower focus in addressing the needs of particular groups: young people; those bereaved by suicide; older people; people from Black and minority ethnic groups; and women in the perinatal period. The *National Service Framework for Children* (Department of Health, 2004d) and the *National Service Framework for Older People* (Department of Health, 2001) look at these issues further, and the Confidential Enquiries into Maternal Deaths (http://www.cemach.org.uk), which report every 3 years, continue to investigate these deaths and make recommendations.

Reduce the availability and lethality of suicide methods

Some of the recommendations might appear outside a health organisation's remit – including changes in car design and safety measures at identified 'hotspots' on railways and high buildings – but there may be scope for work with other agencies. For example, London Underground is working with local services to reduce the risks at 'hotspots' (Patrick Gillespie, personal communication, 2004). There are also questions about hanging, strangulation and asphyxiation. Estates and facilities departments will need to get involved by identifying ligature points such as non-collapsible bed and shower rails; clinical staff can look at the availability of other methods such as plastic bags. There are practice issues around the safe prescribing of antidepressants including the type of antidepressant prescribed and the number given in any one prescription. Clinicians can also ask users about unwanted medicines at home and look at their safe disposal.

Improving the reporting of suicidal behaviour in the media

There is guidance available from the Samaritans on suicide reporting in the media. Mind out for mental health, the Department of Health's anti-stigma campaign has tried to influence the ways in which the media report on mental health issues (e.g. providing workshops and training materials for trainee journalists). There is also scope for individual clinicians who have had training and feel confident about being interviewed by the media to give accurate and non-stigmatising information about mental illness and its impact on individuals and communities.

Promoting research on suicide and suicide prevention

There is evidence from epidemiological and clinical studies on risk factors associated with suicide, but no intervention studies in which suicide has been the main outcome because of the size of the sample needed. The strategy recommends research that focuses on high-risk groups, and intervention studies with more common outcomes that can be a proxy for suicide.

Improving the monitoring of progress towards the Saving Lives: Our Healthier Nation

There is already information available through the National Confidential Inquiry into Suicide and Homicide by People with Mental Illness (http://www.medicine.manchester.ac.uk/suicideprevention/nci) and the Confidential Enquiry into Maternal and Child Health (http://www.cemach.org.uk) on the progress towards the objectives of *Saving Lives: Our Healthier Nation* (Department of Health, 1999b). More detailed data may be available in the future to cover, for example, the occupation and ethnicity of individuals if coroners record these details.

Clinical governance and modernising services

Another way to consider and improve the quality of health services is through the use of modernisation tools and related training. The former NHS Modernisation Agency had aims shared with clinical governance: modernising services to improve the experience and outcome for patients. In 2005, the NHS Modernisation Agency merged with the NHS University and NHS Leadership Centre to form a new body, the NHS Institute for Innovation and Improvement. The NHS Institute is a special health authority in England. It has a number of functions: to identify best practice, develop the capability of the NHS for service transformation, facilitate local implementation, and promote a culture of innovation and lifelong learning for all staff. The Osprey Programme is a good example of a modernisation project to improve service quality throughout one healthcare sector.

Clinical systems improvement in South-East London (Osprey Programme)

Clinical systems improvement is a term used to describe the management of patient flow to improve the efficiency and quality of the patient's experience. The Osprey Programme combined with the Improvement Partnership in Hospitals was formed as part of a national pilot scheme involving a number of strategic health authorities, with assistance from the former NHS Modernisation Agency, to develop a spread programme for clinical system improvement in South-East London (Box 24.4). The project's aim was to build foundations and strengthen the infrastructure for improving patient flow through healthcare systems.

Clinical systems improvement engineers and flow redesign capability are the key components of the programme. The engineers support improvement work across the sector, developing innovative ideas to improve services. This is done by developing capacity for service improvement within the local health economy and through promoting coordination of this work.

Key objectives of the programme are:

- improving the way information is used
- building clinical system improvement skills and expertise locally at consultant and general practitioner level
- communicating and implementing flow management concepts in service design and planning
- linking funding decisions to service redesign.

Box 24.4 Improvement concepts in health service organisations in South-East London

- Queues are caused by a mismatch between capacity and demand
- Understanding how patients flow through health systems, with their bottlenecks (constraints), and understanding how reducing carve-out and implementing pooling stop this
- Understanding the true capacity and demand of the system and how to work towards limiting variation within the system
- Monitoring variation and improvement using Statistical Process Control (SPC).

The programme design is focused around dissemination of improvement concepts and measuring their uptake in health service organisations in South-East London.

Senior clinician involvement is crucial to the successful redesign of services and for sustaining any improvement. A key component of the programme has been the acquisition of skills locally at consultant and general practitioner level. Identified clinicians have taken part in a development programme that included training in service development and improvement methodologies. The programme provided funding for replacement sessions, allowing senior clinicians time away from their clinical responsibilities. Individual coaching with a system improvement engineer was also available. Clinicians selected a project that dovetailed with the priorities of their organisation. One of the authors has completed this programme as part of a local service improvement development. Understanding patient flow within the health economy was the overarching theme for the training programme (Box 24.5).

Clinicians completing the training served as an internal resource within their respective organisations, providing support and expertise to their peers. Participating clinicians were supported in this work by the engineers. Time commitment for the training programme consisted of a term of half-day introductory seminars and workshops. Subsequent monthly half-day learning sets provided an opportunity to test approaches, discuss problems and find solutions as a group.

An example of the work followed was examining bed management, a priority area for most of the participating trusts (Box 24.6). Bed management is an area where there is considerable scope for service improvement.

Clinicians can benefit greatly from being involved in service improvement work. The Clinical System Improvement project described is one very important way for clinicians to acquire the necessary skills and make a

---

Box 24.5   Content of the training programme

- Better understanding of flow
- Principles of demand and capacity
- Construction and interpretation of SPC charts[1]
- Process mapping and other diagnostic tools to identify problems with flow
- Understanding and improving the culture of organisations
- Understanding personal styles

SPC, Statistical Process Control.

1. SPC statistical method for measurement of improvement based on understanding of variation.

Box 24.6   Example of a project on bed management in an NHS trust

Aims

- Establish overview of patient flow through the trust
- Introduce improvements to reduce variation in flow
- Introduce improvements to increase predictability of beds needed for admission on a daily basis
- System to be as efficient as possible

Context

- Capacity exceeding demand for acute in-patient beds
- Numerous interfaces involved in patients' journey through mental health services
- New functional in-patient and community teams
- Pressures on staff finding beds for patients requiring admission
- Beds mostly being made available in response to bed pressures
- More efficient use of resources required

Outcomes

- No inappropriate admissions
- Reduced length of stay
- No sleepovers
- Reduction of staff stress
- Improved patient experience

Performance monitoring

- Top Level Analysis Trust Performance Indicators using statistical process control (SPC) charts to measure impact of any changes
- Total number of admissions to borough acute wards
- Total number of admissions to acute wards mapped to locality
- Number of patients in out-of-borough beds (sleepovers)
- Total number of discharges from acute beds
- Length of stay (80%, 20%)
- Percentage of patients seen within 7 days of discharge

Other investigations

- Audit of delayed discharges

Test targeted interventions

difference to healthcare quality. Trainees have many excellent opportunities to learn about and participate in clinical governance. Consultants are likely to be very pleased if trainees offer to get involved in audit projects. Similarly trainees can often attend clinical governance meetings at their hospitals and develop their knowledge of clinical governance. Special interest sessions can be used to shadow the medical director or other individuals involved in clinical governance within a hospital trust, or to develop a clinical governance portfolio.

Clinical governance provides a useful framework for service improvement but requires ownership by all clinicians, particularly those in senior positions. Mobilising a whole organisation to improve healthcare delivery remains an ongoing challenge and an exciting and worthwhile goal.

References

Commission for Health Improvement (2003) *What CHI has Found in Mental Health Trusts* (sector report). Commission for Health Improvement.

Degeling, P. J., Maxwell, S., Iedema, R., *et al* (2004) Making clinical governance work. *BMJ*, **329**, 679–681.

Deighan, M., Cullen, R. & Moore, R. (2004) *The Development of Integrated Governance* (NHS Confederation Debate 3). NHS Confederation. http://www.cgsupport.nhs.uk/PDFs/debate3.pdf

Department of Health (1997) *The New NHS: Modern, Dependable* (Cm 3807). TSO (The Stationery Office).

Department of Health (1998) *A First Class Service: Quality in the New NHS*. TSO (The Stationery Office).

Department of Health (1999a) *Supporting Doctors, Protecting Patients*. Department of Health.

Department of Health (1999b) *Saving Lives: Our Healthier Nation*. TSO (The Stationery Office).

Department of Health (1999c) *National Service Framework for Mental Health*. Department of Health.

Department of Health (2000) *An Organisation with a Memory*. TSO (The Stationery Office).

Department of Health (2001) *National Service Framework for Older People*. Department of Health.

Department of Health (2002) *National Suicide Prevention Strategy for England*. Department of Health.

Department of Health (2004a) *The NHS Improvement Plan*. Department of Health.

Department of Health (2004b) *National Standards, Local Action Health and Social Care Standards and Planning Framework 2005/06–2007/08*. Department of Health.

Department of Health (2004c) *Standards for Better Health*. Department of Health.

Department of Health (2004d) *National Service Framework for Children*. Department of Health.

Department of Health and Social Security (1983) *NHS Management Inquiry* (Griffiths Report). DHSS.

Edwards, N. (2004) Commentary: model could work. *BMJ*, **329**, 681–682.

Gray, C. (2005) What is clinical governance? *BMJ Careers*, **330**, 254.

Halligan, A. & Donaldson, L. (2001) Implementing clinical governance: turning vision into reality. *BMJ*, **322**, 1413–1417.

Healthcare Commission (2004) *Inspecting, Informing, Improving*. Healthcare Commission.

Khart, M. & Hart, R. K. (2002) *Statistical Process Control for Healthcare*. Duxbury Thompson Learning.

Murray, J., Fell-Rayner, H., Fine, H., *et al* (2004) What do NHS staff think and know about clinical governance? *Clinical Governance*, **9**, 172–180.

Mynors-Wallis, L., Cope, D. & Suliman, S. (2004) Making clinical governance happen at team level: the Dorset experience. *Clinical Governance*, **9**, 162–166.

National Institute for Clinical Excellence (2004) *Self-Harm* (clinical guideline 16). British Psychological Society & Gaskell.

NHS Institute for Innovation and Improvement (2005) *Improvement Leaders' Guides: General Improvement Skills. ILG 1.4: Involving Patients and Carers*. NHS Institute for Innovation and Improvement.

NHS Institute for Innovation and Improvement (2005) *The Clinician's Guide to Applying the 10 High Impact Changes*. NHS Institute for Innovation and Improvement.

Nicholls, S., Cullen, R., O'Neill, S., *et al* (2000) Clinical governance: its origins and its foundations. *Clinical Performance and Quality Health Care*, **8**, 172–178.

Palmer, C. (2002) Clinical governance: breathing new life into clinical audit. *Advances in Psychiatric Treatment*, **8**, 470–476.

Scally, G. & Donaldson, L. J. (1998) Looking forward: clinical governance and the drive for quality improvement in the new NHS in England. *BMJ*, **317**, 61–65.

Scottish Executive Health Department (1997) *Designed to Care. Renewing the National Health Service in Scotland*. Scottish Executive Health Department.

Shaw, C. D. (2004) Standards for Better Health: fit for purpose? *BMJ*, **329**, 1250–1251.

Shipman Inquiry (2004) *Fifth Report – Safeguarding Patients: Lessons from the Past – Proposals for the Future* (Cm 6394). TSO (The Stationery Office).

Wheeler, D. J. (2000) *Understanding Variation: The Key to Managing Chaos* (2nd edn). SPC Press.

CHAPTER 25

Lifelong learning and revalidation

Joe Bouch

Passing the MRCPsych examination is often seen as having arrived. When I passed the the exam in the mid-1980s my parents sent me a congratulations card (Fig. 25.1). A dog is pulling itself onto the top step of a steep flight of stairs. The dog is clearly exhausted, gasping and panting. Underneath was the legend 'you made it!' It was just how I felt.

I had reached the top step by my own efforts. The stairs had been steep. Many of my peers who had sat the same exam had not made it, but I had arrived. It was the start of a new life without exams. Not only did it represent a completion and an ending but also a passport to my future. I had reached the plateau and the journey from here would be an easier one – coasting, perhaps slightly downhill or with a following wind. There was a general feeling that passing the exam was the end of education rather than a stage along the way.

Current thinking about lifelong learning and revalidation represents a very different approach to education, learning and training, and a major departure from the educational culture of yesteryear.

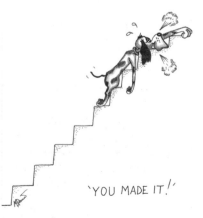

'YOU MADE IT!'

Fig. 25.1 'You made it!' (© Margaret Daniel).

Lifelong learning

Committing to lifelong learning is not a new suggestion. The Roman playwright and philosopher Seneca (4 BC to AD 65) proposed that 'throughout the whole of life one must continue to learn to live'. Such an idea has never been more relevant.

One aspect of living in the modern world is that change is rapid, with new knowledge, ideas, values and practices constantly emerging. There are few areas where this speed of change is more marked than in the medical profession. Our learning cannot be confined to undergraduate and postgraduate training. Afterwards we still need to keep up to date, learn new skills and adapt to changes in society. Our jobs change and we need to change with them. Cultural change must involve both learners and those involved in teaching and training. As an analogy consider recent thinking on doctor–patient relationships (see Chapter 29 by Rose).

Yesterday's doctor was an expert, who in a top-down way would dictate treatment with which the patient, in a passive–dependent way, would 'comply' (or not). Today's therapeutic relationship is characterised by 'concordance' (Marinker & Shaw, 2003). Doctor and patient are involved in a collaborative exercise to which the doctor brings professional expertise and technical knowledge and the patient brings their own values, experiences and understanding.

In a similar way the adult learner brings their experience and values. They have preferred learning styles. They are active rather than passive. Identifying gaps in knowledge and areas where development is required are primarily the learner's responsibility and they look to their trainer to point them to further resources for personal study. Assessments are staging posts allowing the learner to gauge their progress rather than hurdles to overcome. Instead of being isolated and in competition with their peers, the learner collaborates with them and is supported by them. The psychiatric trainee is an adult learner who does not come empty-handed to training.

Development

As I reflect on my own experience of training in psychiatry, both as a trainee and subsequently as a trainer, I have come to realise just how little time we spend on observing and being observed as we practise. The training I underwent was based largely on the acquisition of knowledge coupled with gaining experience. My work was supervised but not observed. Educationalists talk of three 'domains of learning': knowledge, skills and attitudes. It is my skills that are so important to how I practise. Imagine if as a trainee surgeon your trainer suggested that you go and perform an operation and then come back later and report how you got on. You would think he was joking! Yet this is how most of us have gone through our training in psychiatry.

In psychiatry some of us become expert in particular psychological treatments such as psychodynamic psychotherapy and cognitive–behavioural therapy where there is explicit focus on technique. Most of us work in a more general way. As psychiatrists we attach great importance to the therapeutic relationship: how we engage with our patients, talk to them but most of all listen (Shooter, 2005). It is our equivalent of the surgeon's scalpel. I believe that we focus far too little attention on developing and assessing these psychiatric consultation skills in our training.

'See one, do one, teach one' was the mantra of my medical student days. Although much criticised, it is probably only each 'one' that is the problem. Doing, most of all and then seeing are the two most powerful ways of learning and developing new skills. As Confucius said 'I hear and I forget. I see and I remember. I do and I understand' (Stratton, 2005). The evidence is that it is the learning that occurs in the workplace that is most likely to lead to improved practice (Davis *et al*, 1995).

Developing doctors' skills has become an explicit aim of training. In keeping with this, workplace-based assessments will look at how we perform in our jobs rather than merely testing our knowledge base (Norcini, 2003). Modernising Medical Careers (MMC) is a key National Health Service (NHS) initiative representing 'a major reform of postgraduate medical education' (http://www.mmc.nhs.uk). As part of this reform a 2-year foundation programme has replaced the old pre-registration house officer year. Four methods of workplace-based assessment methods are used.

Case-based discussion (CbD) is already familiar to us in psychiatry and involves assessing how we apply our knowledge to the assessment and management of our patients. It is essentially the same methodology as the long case in the MRCPsych part II examination, albeit of shorter duration.

The mini-clinical evaluation exercise (mini-CEX) and direct observation of procedural skills (DOPS) represent a departure. They are geared more towards assessing how doctors practise than testing what they know. Both involve observing how the doctor performs in real clinical situations. This is a step further even than the OSCE (objective structured clinical examination) of the MRCPsych part I, where doctors also have to demonstrate competency but in simulated encounters rather than real ones.

Multi-source feedback (MSF) involves asking the opinions of senior colleagues, peers, staff from other disciplines, patients and administrative staff about their perceptions of the doctor's performance (including their attitudes) as they do their job. A full description of these methods and how they are applied can be found at http://www.mmc.nhs.uk/pages/assessment.

Modified forms of these assessments are being used in psychiatric training (http://www.rcpsych.ac.uk/training/specialtytrainingassess.aspx). It is certainly not impossible that they might even come to be used as a part of revalidation procedures for career grade doctors.

Performance

Changes in educational theory have been, and continue to be, an important driver of change. Just as important though have been concerns about how well doctors are doing their jobs. In a number of cases of 'problem doctors' concerns about their competency and performance have been raised. A competency can be simply defined as what a doctor can do, whereas performance is what a doctor does do in practice.

Several high-profile cases involving senior doctors have highlighted these issues. One of the best known is of two Bristol cardiac surgeons who were found guilty of serious professional misconduct by the General Medical Council (GMC) in 1998. In two operations (switch procedures and correction of atrioventricular septal defects in infants) they were judged to have been operating outwith their area of competence. This case, which has come to be known simply as 'Bristol' represents a watershed for the medical profession. Its repercussions would be hard to overstate.

It has been determined that the structure, process and outcome of our training needs to be revised and 'modernised'. Our training must be appropriate to the jobs we are being prepared for. Assessments, including exams, should be 'fit for purpose'. This is the term used by the Postgraduate Medical Education and Training Board (PMETB), which became the main educational standard setting body in 2005 (Brown, 2005). It means that in our specialty we will be assessed on our competence to practise psychiatry rather than merely tested on our factual knowledge. We will need to demonstrate that after leaving training grades and throughout our careers we are maintaining our skills and improving our practice. It will be important for us, the regulatory bodies (most notably the GMC) and the general public to know that we are performing at a satisfactory level.

Continuing professional development, appraisal and revalidation

Continuing professional development (CPD), appraisal and revalidation are all mechanisms that have been established to tackle the twin concerns of our development and performance as doctors. They all deal with broad-based practice, which the GMC has categorised into seven areas in *Good Medical Practice* (General Medical Council, 2001; see Box 25.1). Although all three address both development and performance, they differ in the relative emphasis on each (see Fig. 25.2). Revalidation is most concerned with assessment of performance, whereas CPD is most concerned with development. Appraisal falls between the two, conceived as a formative process but also expected to form the basis of revalidation procedures. Figure 25.3 shows how the three processes interrelate, albeit that the final mechanism for revalidation has not yet been determined. The principles of revalidation are sound but their application is being debated at present.

> **Box 25.1** Domains of *Good Medical Practice* (General Medical Council, 2001)
>
> - Good clinical care
> - Maintaining good medical practice
> - Relationships with patients
> - Working with colleagues
> - Teaching and training
> - Probity
> - Personal health

Continuing professional development

The GMC defines CPD as 'a continuing learning process that complements a formal undergraduate and postgraduate education and training' (General Medical Council, 2004). The term CPD has gradually come to be preferred over continuing medical education (CME), as the latter is understood as having a narrower focus on clinical practice alone. CPD covers all aspects of our practice.

Our work is not only broad-based but also involves different 'levels of practice.' Southgate *et al* (1994) identified four levels of knowledge, skills and attitude that focus progressively from generic abilities through to those appropriate to the actual practice of each practitioner (see Box 25.2).

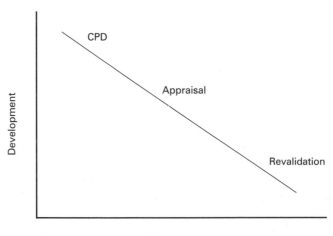

Fig. 25.2 Relative emphasis of CPD, appraisal and revalidation on development and performance.

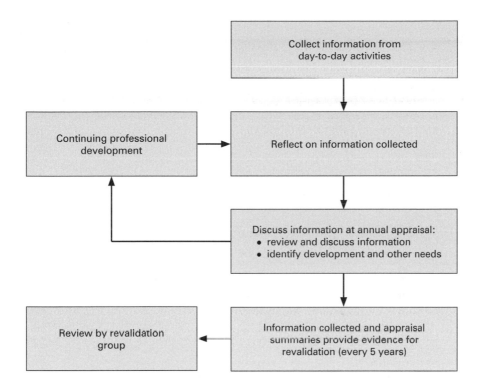

Fig.25.3 Appraisal and revalidation process (after General Medical Council, 2001)

Level 1 recognises that we all work as doctors. Teaching skills, presentation skills and basic medical procedures such as cardiopulmonary resuscitation are relevant to all doctors. Level 1 clinical skills should have been mastered by the end of foundation training.

Level 2 recognises that all doctors work within a particular specialty. For example, as psychiatrists we all need to know about the diagnosis and treatment of psychiatric disorders and the use of mental health legislation.

Level 3 relates to the sub-specialty within which a specialist works. As a general adult psychiatrist I need to know about the presentation and management of psychiatric disorders in adults and develop expertise in the relevant clinical services.

The focus of specialty training is on the development of Level 2 and 3 clinical skills. Achieving the Certificate of Completion of Training (CCT) will depend on having attained competence in these skills.

Level 4 relates to those aspects of our job that are specific to each of us. Specialists tend to have a number of roles over and above their main clinical responsibilities. These might include specific clinical interests, and managerial, educational and research roles. Much of the learning for these

---

Box 25.2   Levels of professional competence

Level 1

The common core of practice. The knowledge, skills, attitudes and psychosocial skills that all doctors who are engaged in any branch of the profession, including non-clinical specialties, should exhibit. The components are described in *Good Medical Practice* (General Medical Council, 2001).

Level 2

The core of practice appropriate to the broad specialty within which, and the level of responsibility at which, each individual practises. The components are described in *Good Psychiatric Practice* (Royal College of Psychiatrists, 2004).

Level 3

The core of practice appropriate to the particular sub-specialty in which each practitioner works. These are summarised in an appendix to *Good Psychiatric Practice* (Royal College of Psychiatrists, 2004).

Level 4

The actual profile of practice activities unique to each practitioner.

---

roles has traditionally taken place after specialist training but often in a less systematic way and without any assessment. It is likely that in the future 'post-CCT training' will have to meet the same standards as training for a CCT, and will play a much larger part in our working lives.

CPD is developmental – not just acquiring factual knowledge but developing understanding, skills and appropriate attitudes leading to changes in practice. CPD also concerns maintaining our existing knowledge, skills and attitudes and remedying any deficits.

Appraisal

The NHS appraisal process relates to all doctors working in the NHS. (An appraisal toolkit for career grade doctors can be accessed at http://www.appraisals.nhs.uk/ and http://www.rcpsg.ac.uk/cpdportfolio for Scotland.) There are similar arrangements in place for doctors working in private health organisations (which the GMC refers to as 'managed environments').

Most employment organisations have an appraisal system. Employees meet with their employers on a regular basis to consider aspects of performance, workload and development needs. The period since the last appraisal is reviewed and objectives agreed for the next period. In health organisations appraisals are conducted annually by medical managers – lead clinicians, clinical directors and medical directors (or those delegated to the role). As with CPD, a personal development plan (PDP) is agreed. Generally only one overall PDP is required, but it must take into account objectives identified as part of the CPD process and any additional objectives identified from appraisal (see Fig. 25.3).

As appraisal is an employer-led process the priorities are those of the organisation in which the doctor works. As CPD is based more on the individual it starts with our personal development as psychiatrists and includes our interests, aspirations and career progress.

The distinctions between CPD and appraisal are fairly subtle, as is how they relate to each other (Bouch, 2003a). CPD is best regarded as a support for and preparation for organisational appraisal. Most learning objectives will be determined during the CPD process, but others may arise from the appraisal process. Both appraisal and CPD are regarded as being primarily formative or developmental in nature. The relationship between appraisal and revalidation has a more chequered history.

Revalidation

Revalidation was proposed in 1998 by the GMC as a means of assuring the public that doctors were up to date and fit to practise. Revalidation would lead to a 'licence to practise' which would have to be renewed every 5 years. It was talked of being 'like an MOT test for doctors'. By April 2003 the mechanism identified for revalidation was that it would be based on five consecutive annual appraisals. Where a doctor worked in a managed environment (i.e. a quality-assured environment with clinical governance in place), in most cases no other information would be required for revalidation.

This decision was heavily criticised during the Shipman Inquiry (http://www.the-shipman-inquiry.org.uk), which was chaired by Dame Janet Smith and investigated the murder of over 200 patients by the general practitioner Harold Shipman. Dame Janet's criticism was that appraisal should not be equated with assessment of fitness to practise. She said that the purpose of appraisal is to support doctors' development not judge their competence. Therefore revalidation, whose purpose is to assess doctors' fitness to practise, should not be based solely on appraisal.

A heated debate followed but broad agreement emerged that revalidation is necessary (Norcini, 2005). The Chief Medical Officer Sir Liam Donaldson consulted the profession and other interested parties following the report of the Shipman Inquiry, and produced a report *Good Doctors, Safer Patients* (Department of Health, 2006). The report makes a number of recommendations concerning revalidation (the right to remain on the medical register), recertification (the right to remain on the specialist register) and periodic assessment during the whole of a doctor's career. These recommendations formed the basis of a government White Paper on the regulation of health professionals, which states that recertification will be based on 'a comprehensive assessment against the standards drawn up by that College' (Department of Health, 2007). These changes will be enacted through the forthcoming Health and Social Care Bill.

The Royal College of Psychiatrists and lifelong learning

The Royal College of Psychiatrists has responded to the changing educational landscape with a number of key developments (Bouch, 2003*b*):

- the CPD scheme – the practical aspects of which are described below (Royal College of Psychiatrists, 2001)
- *Advances in Psychiatric Treatment*, a journal for CPD which has been published since 1994
- CPD Online, which was established in 2004 to provide online educational modules
- the College Education and Training Centre, which was established in 2005 to develop a more systematic approach to the College's educational provision and develop training courses to meet the learning objectives of the Membership.

The College CPD scheme

In April 2001 the College introduced PDPs as the mechanism for achieving CPD objectives and moved from an individual, retrospective points counting exercise to a prospective peer-group-based activity centring on individuals' learning objectives.

Peer groups

The first step for the psychiatrist who moves from a training post into a career grade is to find or form a peer group. Although peer groups can comprise two to eight individuals, there are some practical reasons why three is generally a good number. For larger numbers it is more difficult to put diaries together and each individual has less 'air time'. Having as few as two members puts the group at risk of becoming too cosy. If meeting for an afternoon, a group of three allows 1 hour to be spent on each member. In the model devised by Harold Bridger of the Tavistock Institute can be used whereby one member takes the role of reviewer, another of reviewee and a third of observer and consultant to the process, the roles are rotated in turn.

CPD peer groups meet at least twice a year. They comprise colleagues with whom we feel comfortable (or at least not uncomfortable) and who we will work with to support us in the identification and meeting of our objectives. Some psychiatrists are in peer groups where members are from the same sub-specialty and are of a similar level of experience. If our peer groups are more diverse, however, new perspectives will be brought to bear and the conformity of 'group think' will be avoided.

The peer group system was initially conceived as a means of providing both support and accountability. Some groups have gone a stage further by developing into 'action learning sets' (Laverty, 2004). They use a problem-based approach to either meet or at least identify the means to meet specific learning objectives within the group.

Personal development plans

Personal development plans (PDPs) are simply statements of educational priorities for the year ahead. The form currently used in the Royal College of Psychiatrists' scheme asks us to list key aspects of our jobs and the roles we have, to specify related learning objectives and consider how we might best meet them. Realistically PDPs cannot be comprehensive. For a start what we learn will not necessarily be planned in advance. Nevertheless it is best to prioritise four or five areas for development from a broad range of practice and then set specific learning objectives.

Learning objectives should be specific, measurable, achievable, resourced and time-limited (SMART). Audit has shown that many of us are quite vague in the objectives we set (Bouch & Jackson, 2005). For example, 'psychopharmacology' is frequently given as an objective. Better might be 'to update my knowledge of drug treatments in treatment-resistant schizophrenia'. We also confuse aims and means. Hence 'to attend postgraduate meetings' and 'to read *Advances in Psychiatric Treatment*' are not learning objectives but may be good ways of meeting them.

Outcomes are important. How one's practice will change is key. Educationalists are increasingly using the term 'intended learning outcomes' as an alternative to 'learning objectives'. Learning outcomes have been defined as both what a learner knows, understands or can do as a result of learning and how a learner demonstrates the results of their learning.

Having set our learning objectives we need to consider how best to meet them. Each of us has preferred learning styles that may be relevant. Hence some enjoy working online whereas others prefer to read text. What we are trying to learn is also important. For example, developing cardiopulmonary resuscitation skills is better achieved by attending a workshop and practising on a 'Resus Annie' than by personal study.

CPD process

The College's CPD process (Royal College of Psychiatrists, 2001) is an annual cycle involving the following steps (see Fig. 25.4).

1   Reflect broadly on one's job and one's different roles. Select what appear to be key areas for developing, maintaining or remedying deficits in one's practice.
2   Prepare provisional learning objectives for the forthcoming year.
3   Develop and review one's learning objectives with a few colleagues in the setting of a peer group.
4   Complete a PDP with learning objectives, agreed by one's peer group.
5   During the year undertake a minimum of 50 hours of recorded CPD activities supplemented by a (recommended) minimum of 100 hours

of personal study, such as reading and research. This activity should help to address the learning objectives that have been chosen.

6   Collect evidence of recorded CPD activities as they happen.
7   Retain this evidence in a portfolio. It will be required for appraisal, revalidation and if randomly audited as a part of the CPD scheme.
8   Meet with one's peer group halfway through the year to review everyone's progress.
9   Meet with one's peer group at the end of the year to determine whether each person has fully or partially met their learning objectives.
10   Complete the review form, which is then returned to the College.
11   Start again, carrying through any partially met learning objectives to the next PDP.

Recorded activities comprise internal meetings, external meetings and some online study. Internal meetings such as journal clubs, case conferences and audit meetings occur in the workplace with our own colleagues. External meetings involve participating with colleagues from different disciplines, specialties and sub-specialties or workplaces. Online study

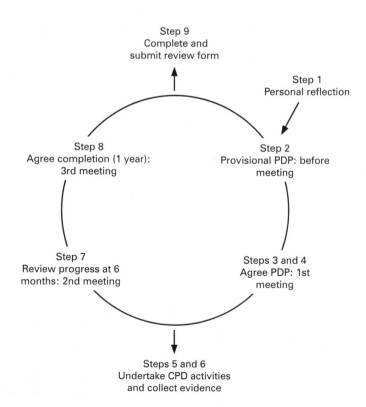

Fig. 25.4   Annual cycle of the CPD process.

involves completing modules that are timed and/or certificated. All of these should be backed up by 'evidence'. This is not 'proof' but rather an indication of the activity and the time spent, which can be retained in a portfolio and provided for the purposes of appraisal, revalidation or the College's CPD audit process (Bouch & Jackson, 2004). Evidence may be a certificate of attendance or probably more helpfully a programme that indicates the content of the activity.

Conclusions

Much is changing. CPD, appraisal and revalidation have all come at the same time. They represent an aspect of the increasing regulation of the medical profession. Although there are teething problems, they are here to stay. Other developments – notably MMC, the European Working Time Directive and PMETB – are changing fundamental aspects of medical training. Nothing is sacred. The structure, process and content of training, our training schemes and how they are approved, and assessment methods including the MRCPsych examination are being scrutinised. New standards are being set. There are different sets of hoops to jump through, forms to fill out and boxes to tick. As in any time of great change there is a danger of us, individually and collectively, taking a passive stance, becoming resentful and being driven by external forces.

It is possible to take an altogether different view, however, and to see the changes as something for our patients, for us as individuals and for the profession as a whole. The changes are making it clear that maintaining and developing our skills is central to our jobs rather than a peripheral aspect which we do in our spare time and is funded if we are lucky. This requires resources – both time and money – for personal study, attending courses and meetings. Our development has been put centre stage as being essential for good patient care. Taking this view we can participate in lifelong learning and revalidation in an internally driven, productive and creative way.

References

Bouch, J. (2003a) Continuing professional development for psychiatrists: CPD and regulation. *Advances in Psychiatric Treatment*, **9**, 3–4.

Bouch, J. (2003b) Continuing professional development for psychiatrists: CPD and learning. *Advances in Psychiatric Treatment*, **9**, 81–83.

Bouch, J. & Jackson, R. (2004) CPD audit policy. *Psychiatric Bulletin*, **28**, 30–31.

Bouch, J. & Jackson, R. (2005) Continuing professional development: the College and the members. *Psychiatric Bulletin*, **29**, 154–156.

Brown, N. (2005) The Postgraduate Medical Education and Training Board (PMETB) goes live. *Psychiatric Bulletin*, **29**, 431–433.

Davis, D. A., Thompson, M. A., Oxman, A. D., *et al* (1995) Changing physician performance: a systematic review of the effect of continuing medical education strategies. *JAMA*, **274**, 700–705.

Department of Health (2006) *Good Doctors, Safer Patients*. Department of Health.

Department of Health (2007) *Trust, Assurance and Safety: The Regulation of Health Professionals in the 21st Century*. Department of Health.

General Medical Council (2001) *Good Medical Practice*. GMC.

General Medical Council (2004) *Continuing Professional Development*. GMC.

Laverty, S. (2004) Helping doctors to solve problems. *BMJ Career Focus*, 329, 59–60.

Marinker, M. & Shaw, J. (2003) Not to be taken as directed. *BMJ*, **326**, 348–349.

Norcini, J. J. (2003) Work based assessment. *BMJ*, **326**, 753–755.

Norcini, J. J. (2005) Where next with revalidation? *BMJ*, **330**, 1458–1459.

Royal College Of Psychiatrists (2001) *Good Psychiatric Practice: CPD* (Council Report CR90). Royal College of Psychiatrists.

Royal College of Psychiatrists (2004) *Good Psychiatric Practice* (2nd edn) (Council Report CR125). Royal College of Psychiatrists.

Shooter, M. (2005) The soul of caring. *Advances in Psychiatric Treatment*, **11**, 239–240.

Southgate, L., Jolly, B., Bowmer, I., *et al* (1994) Determining the content of re-certification procedures. In *The Certification and Re-certification of Doctors: Issues in the Assessment of Clinical Competence* (eds D. Newble, B. Jolly & R. Wakeford), pp. 178–186. Cambridge University Press.

Stratton, P. (2005) A model to coordinate understanding of active autonomous learning. *Journal of Family Therapy*, **27**, 217–236.

CHAPTER 26

Mentoring and shadowing

Koravangattu Valsraj and Cecilia Wells

This chapter sets out how mentoring can be used as a tool to support continuing personal and professional development. The concept of mentoring is particularly relevant in the development of staff in a multicultural workforce such as the National Health Service (NHS). There can be significant difference in career progression between Whites workers and those from other racial groups, and mentoring can reduce the negative career progression and enhance conditions that foster the upward mobility of professionals from Black and minority ethnic groups (Thomas, 2001). We also consider how shadowing can provide an opportunity to gain a broad overview of organisational structures and understanding of management roles in complex organisations such as the NHS.

What is mentoring?

Mentoring can be said to have a long history. Odysseus asked his friend Mentor to guide his son's development while he was away fighting the Trojan War. Mentoring is broadly defined as the process by which one person (the mentor) actively encourages the development of another person (the mentee) outside the normal line-management relationship, for the benefit of both individuals (and the organisation for which they work). The mentor guides, supports and enables the mentee to grow and develop in a role and in their career. Both parties benefit from the relationship.

A good mentoring relationship is one in which the mentor and mentee enjoy a mutual respect and value the joint opportunities for personal development.

Peer mentoring is a variation of mentoring. It is different because both people take on the mentor/mentee roles, as they are peers or colleagues or friends.

A mentoring relationship lasts until the mentee has achieved all the goals set within it: most continue for about 1 year.

The role of the mentor

A mentor:

- has a mentee
- treats that person as an equal
- promotes the mentee's self-learning and development
- is willing to learn from the mentee
- is committed to development
- is an active listener
- provides positive and constructive feedback
- is willing to share learning and experience
- encourages the mentee to explore different options
- challenges the mentee to think differently.

The range of mentoring roles

The mentor has a range of roles, from confidant to career advisor (Fig. 26.1). No two mentoring roles are the same. The best relationships are those in which there is a clear and mutually acceptable understanding between mentor and mentee about what the mentor will and will not do, and what the mentee will and will not expect. Whatever the type of relationship the mentor will invariably have to be flexible to get the best out of the mentee. There are many ways in which the roles can be described. The mentor will continually combine and switch roles to adapt to different circumstances.

Confidant

The mentor plays a more passive role in a trusting relationship in which the mentee feels confident to share problems. The mentor is non-judgemental, allowing the mentee to relieve the burden of their work-related or other concerns.

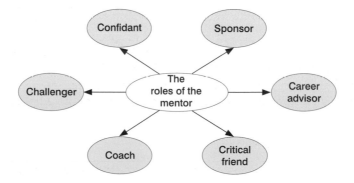

Fig. 26.1 The roles of the mentor.

Sponsor

This mentoring role is one in which mentors use their own network of contacts to provide opportunities for their mentees' development. This might simply be through introducing other colleagues or providing appropriate access to other functions or parts of the organisation.

Careers advisor

The mentor provides first-hand advice and widens the network of the mentee, enabling them to make informed career decisions.

Critical friend

Assumptions and perceptions are challenged in a non-threatening way. The 'critical friend' creates an environment in which the mentee can be challenged without malice and with the knowledge that it is being done for their own benefit.

Coach

The coaching role focuses more on the mentee's personal development, actively encouraging self-development by providing support, advice and information to allow the mentee to 'discover' the best way of doing their job and to learn and progress within the organisation. The coach also acts as a role model, displaying the skills and attitudes required to progress.

Challenger

The mentor challenges the mentee's assumptions. This requires the mentor to instill a proactive approach in the mentee, who should be actively encouraged to seek new and increasing challenges.

Mentoring and specialist coaching

Individuals may be able to decide themselves whether a mentor or a specialist coach would be more appropriate for their goals. Nevertheless, many of the skills and approaches of mentors and of specialist coaches are similar. In their coaching role, mentors share expertise with the mentee and provide feedback on different suggestions and approaches to work. A specialist coach focuses on a single area of expertise and teaches the person how to become more effective in a particular area of work or in using skills.

Mentoring and supervision

There are clear guidelines for supervision in clinical practice and it plays a major role in career development. It is important that there is an understanding of the key differences between mentoring and supervision.

The role of mentoring occurs outside the line-management relationship. The mentor has no power over the career of the mentee. Unlike supervision, mentoring can carried out both formally or informally.

Psychotherapy, counselling and mentoring

Mentoring needs to be differentiated from counselling or any form of psychotherapy. Therapeutic (psychological) interventions are usually focused on personal problems. Although the therapist and person in therapy do focus on solutions, these are not centred on the career or professional development of the individual. A mentor may help a mentee to identify that they need to seek counselling for a personal problem but would not act as therapeutic counsellor. Acting as a therapist may place the mentoring relationship on an unequal footing and shift the power balance to the mentor, which is not what is intended in a developmental role.

The role of a mentee

A mentee:

- has a mentor
- has an awareness of their own developmental needs
- is someone who wants to progress
- is someone who has aspirations
- is willing to learn and acts on learning
- takes personal responsibility for their learning and the mentoring relationship
- enables the mentor to learn also
- shares learning
- makes a commitment
- is willing to receive feedback.

The relationship between the mentee and mentor is an equal one. Both enter the relationship voluntarily. It is the mentee who steers the agenda and is in charge of their own learning. The mentee is a learner and has clear objectives about what they want to achieve. Both mentor and mentee need to be able to engage in dialogue and to understand each other.

Mentees will take increasing ownership for their development as the relationship and their career progress. The mentor will be there to assist, encourage and guide, but the responsibility for learning rests solely with the mentee. To get the best out of the relationship the mentee needs to be:

- proactive
- committed to the mentoring relationship
- clear about objectives
- clear about their personal development needs
- aware of their mentor's other commitments
- realistic about their expectations of their mentor.

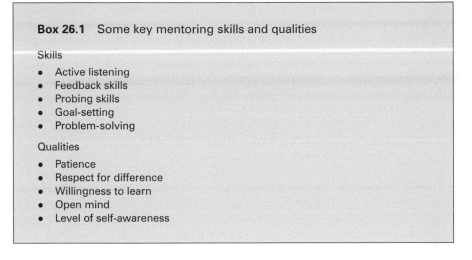

Box 26.1   Some key mentoring skills and qualities

Skills

- Active listening
- Feedback skills
- Probing skills
- Goal-setting
- Problem-solving

Qualities

- Patience
- Respect for difference
- Willingness to learn
- Open mind
- Level of self-awareness

Mentoring skills and qualities

Many of the core skills and qualities required for a mentoring relationship are essentially those required for effective management. Box 26.1 lists some of these (this list is not exhaustive).

Effective v. ineffective mentors

Applying the key skills and qualities could make the difference between an effective and an ineffective mentor. Box 26.2 compares and contrasts the two.

Benefits and challenges to professional mentoring relationships

As with any process getting the best from mentoring means being aware of both its benefits and challenges (Box 26.3). These apply to the mentor and mentee as well as to the organisation in which the mentoring relationship is taking place.

Benefits of mentoring to the mentee, mentor and organisation

Benefits for the mentee

The mentoring relationship focuses on the mentee's individual personal and professional development needs.
Benefits include:

- rapid and more accurate understanding of the culture, ethos and structure of the organisation

Box 26.2 The qualities of the effective and ineffective mentor

The effective mentor	*The ineffective mentor*
Is well prepared: • arranges meetings in advance • knows the mentee as a person, how he or she sees the world	Is poorly prepared: • works from his/her feelings about the mentee
Uses an agenda to give structure to the meeting – and sticks to it.	May or may not use an agenda. May run out of things to say
Allows enough time and does not allow interruptions	Rushes and allows him/herself to be interrupted
Listens well. Asks lots of open questions	Talks a lot
Uses reflection to get the mentee to expand on points	Always rushes onto the next point or skates over the surface
Summarises and tests understanding	Does not summarise or check for understanding, endures misunderstandings
Looks for opportunities to offer recognition – supports the mentee's strengths and successes	Offers insincere praise or none at all
Seeks the mentee's views of his or her goals – and is able to confront supportively where necessary	Offers own view of the mentee's performance – exclusively poor or, often, exclusively good. Confronts personally
Lives with the silence	Feels embarrassed by silence
Helps the mentee to find as many of his or her own solutions as possible	Offers advice too readily
Focuses on the future – on areas that the mentee can address and change. Keeps changes to a minimum at any one time	Focuses on the past. May get into too many areas or areas where the mentee cannot change (quickly)
Follows through. Does what he or she promises to do – and monitors the outcome in preparation for the next meeting	Fails to follow through: forgets to do what he or she promises, does not monitor the outcome in preparation for the next meeting
	Becomes too emotionally involved

- development of interpersonal, problem-solving and strategic skills, which in turn improve self-confidence
- access to a wider network of professional and general career advice
- improved individual performance and regular coaching and feedback on personal progress

<table>
<tr><td colspan="2">Box 26.3   Benefits and challenges to mentoring relationships</td></tr>
<tr><td>Benefits</td><td>Challenges</td></tr>
<tr><td>Transfer of knowledge and expertise (knowledge management)</td><td>For professionals, being mentored may be viewed as a sign of weakness</td></tr>
<tr><td>Proactive development and increased contribution to the role</td><td>May be viewed as a challenge to supervision</td></tr>
<tr><td>Innovative problem-solving</td><td>Culture not responsive to change</td></tr>
<tr><td>Changes in the organisational culture</td><td rowspan="2">Mentor is not at the right level in the hierarchy</td></tr>
<tr><td>Improved organisational competence</td></tr>
<tr><td>Retention and development of people</td><td>Choosing the right mentor</td></tr>
<tr><td></td><td>People may acquire the skills and leave the organisation</td></tr>
</table>

- a challenging environment in which the mentee is encouraged to think through and find answers to NHS issues, in a supportive and open relationship
- an understanding of the wider NHS environment
- development opportunities that are focused on matching personal and organisational NHS needs.

Benefits for the mentor

- Satisfaction in assisting someone to gain confidence, to the benefit of that individual and the wider needs of the organisation
- An opportunity to improve their own people skills and enhance their line-management role
- Increased responsibility for helping others to develop as part of their own career aspirations
- Opportunities to seek alternative opinions and gain a broader insight into issues from different perspectives
- Benefits from being challenged and discussing new or innovative ideas
- Enhanced reputation among peers and other mentees
- Increased motivation and improved performance of those who have been mentored.

Benefits to the organisation

- Increased performance and competency of the organisation
- Transfer of expertise to others

- Staff feeling valued
- Shared learning and development
- Enhanced image of the organisation.

The mentoring life cycle

Getting off to a good start

During the first months of a mentoring relationship both the mentor and mentee are getting to know each other and building trust. The first meeting is important in setting the tone for the way in which the relationship will operate. Preparation for the first meeting is essential and it is useful to agree an agenda in advance. Typical items might include:

- discussions about the mentee's background and mentor's career path and experience
- agree a mentoring contract and ground rules
- discussion of the mentee's strengths, areas for development, opportunities and threats to progress
- discussion of the mentee's aspirations
- clarification of the mentor/manager/supervisor boundary and roles
- setting of broad objectives about what is to be achieved in the mentoring relationship.

The mentoring contract

A mentoring contract sets the ground rules for the relationship and fosters commitment and trust. Below are listed a number of suggested areas for discussion, which you might like to include in a mentoring contract.

- What will be the boundaries of your discussion?
- What means will you use for communication? For example, will discussions mostly be face to face, by telephone or using other means?
- How often will you have a discussion? This should satisfy the needs and commitments of both mentor and mentee.
- How often will you review the way the mentor–mentee relationship is working, and what method will you use to do this? For example, you may decide that, once every 3 months, each of you will give the other feedback using the 'do more/do less' format.
- How long will the relationship last in the first instance?
- What kinds of behaviour do each of you find helpful and unhelpful in other people?
- What are the rules on confidentiality?
- How will the mentor manage the boundaries between mentoring and being a manager (if the mentor is internal)?
- What does each of you hope to get from the mentoring relationship?
- What are the responsibilities of the mentee?
- What are the responsibilities of the mentor?

Getting the best out of the relationship

Direction setting

Having established some broad ground rules and aims in the first meeting, the relationship will be most effective if the mentee has a clear direction. As the relationship progresses and the mentee becomes more established, the mentor can become more challenging if clear objectives have been set regarding the mentee's development needs, linked to the needs of the organisation (if appropriate). These should be in the form of 'SMART' (specific, measurable, attainable, realistic, timely) objectives, which should be monitored and reviewed regularly. Typically these might include:

- acting on the decisions agreed with the mentor as part of the development plan
- introductions to other departments to find out about other career opportunities.

The mentor should consider the key areas in which the mentee needs to develop to enhance their goals.

Recording learning

It is important to keep a mentoring/learning log, as this will help both sides to review and monitor progress. A checklist such as that shown in Box 26.4 for reviewing the mentoring meetings will ensure that the process and the relationship is working effectively. This log and checklist can be agreed jointly by the mentor and the mentee in the initial meeting.

Dissolving the relationship

The mentoring contract will have set an initial period after which the relationship should be reviewed. This review should be encouraged on a regular (perhaps 6-monthly) basis to ensure that it continues to meet the mentee's development needs and that the mentor can still provide the commitment. If it is no longer achieving its intended purpose, it becomes important that the relationship should be dissolved without blame or fault so that the mentee can develop increasing independence.

Confidentiality

The mentee's right to confidentiality is fundamental because the mentoring relationship has to be based on trust in order to be successful. Most mentees are likely to divulge information about their situation, their past and their innermost feelings in the belief that they are sharing confidences, because this is necessary if help is to be obtained. They trust the mentor with such information, assuming that it will remain confidential. The following guidelines may help to clarify matters:

- the issue of confidentiality should be discussed early in the mentoring relationship

Box 26.4 Sample checklist for ongoing mentoring

Contact
- Have we got a good rapport?
- Are we able to discuss issues openly?
- Do we feel able to challenge each other when appropriate?
- Does the relationship enable self-disclosure and sharing of feelings?

Contract (quality of contracting process rather than specific content of contract)
- Do we have clear agendas for each session and for the overall mentoring relationship?
- Have we reviewed the different levels of the contract – procedural, professional and psychological?
- Are the contracts enabling the mentee to learn?
- Have we taken into account the impact of our contract on other people?

Content (way in which content is being dealt with rather than detail of content)
- Is the content of the discussion relevant to the learning agenda?
- Are we focusing on content that relates to the mentee and not the mentor?
- How satisfied are we that we understand each other's mind maps?
- Is the mentee obtaining necessary information, organising coaching from specialists, and arranging training or other activities when these are needed?

Contrast
- How are our similarities strengthening or weakening the mentoring process?
- How are differences strengthening or weakening the mentoring process?
- How do we handle differences in beliefs and values?
- Is there an effective balance between support and challenge from the mentor?

Personal
- How well do we get on together?
- How do our psychological* styles affect the mentoring process?
- How do our personal* styles affect the mentoring process?
- How do our working* styles affect the mentoring process?
- What is our time management like during the mentoring sessions?
- How do the mentee's learning* styles affect the process?
- Are we both growing as a result of the relationship?

*Or substitute whatever frameworks you prefer to use for analysing your styles.

Psychological
- Are there dynamics affecting us at an unspoken level?
- Are we being completely open and honest with each other?
- What happens when we disagree?
- Are we avoiding getting into dependency mode?
- Is the mentor pleased when the mentee makes his or her own decisions?
- Are we able to handle this review comfortably and honestly?

Professional
- What did the mentor do that was helpful?
- How did the mentee respond?
- What did the mentor do that was not helpful?
- How well is the mentor using listening, questioning, reflecting, feedback, etc.?
- What additional skills might the mentor develop for the future?
- Are we using models and frameworks that we both understand?

cont'd

Box 26.4 *cont'd*

Parallels
- Are there any similarities in the way we are interacting and the way in which the mentee interacts with others?
- Are there any similarities in the way we are interacting and the way in which the mentor interacts with others?
- Are we creating parallels by inadvertently repeating these patterns with each other?
- Are we getting into conflicts with each other that really relate to people outside the mentoring relationship?

Aim (process of clarifying the aim, not detail of the aim itself)
- Does the mentor recognise the aims of the mentee rather than imposing what they think is best?
- Are we consistently working towards the goals of the mentee?
- Is the mentee being helped to develop a clear vision for their future direction?
- Are we using information related to the mentee appropriately?

Alternatives
- Have we identified some alternative ways of interacting with each other?
- Are suggestions from the mentor presented tentatively so that the mentee is the decision maker?
- Are we consciously seeking alternative viewpoints and perspectives?

And when the mentoring has been in effect for some time:
- Does the mentee have genuine new ways of viewing their own situation?
- Have they been helped to identify alternative options?
- Do they have more strategies for achieving their aspirations?

Action (how has mentoring enabled the mentee to draw up action plans?)
- Has the mentoring included discussion of short-term actions?
- Has the mentee been helped to plan action that they will be taking?
- Are the actions carefully thought through?
- Does the action plan take account of possible barriers?
- Does the action plan include ways to reinforce and celebrate successes?

And when the mentoring has been in effect for some time:
- Repeat the same questions but with a long-term focus.

Autonomy
- Has the mentoring enabled the mentee to become more independent?
- Does the mentee accept responsibility for his or her own development?
- Is the mentee confident about aiming for what they really want?
- Is the mentee able to ask appropriately for what they want?

And when the mentoring has been in effect for some time:
- Have we celebrated achievements to date?
- Do we need to plan for the ending of the mentoring relationship yet?

- it is likely to form part of the mentoring contract
- if referral to another person or consultation with another member of staff seems appropriate, the mentee's prior permission should be sought
- when a mentee specifically requests confidentiality regarding a particular disclosure, this must be respected
- where confidentiality has to be broken because of organisational or legal implications, this should be discussed with the mentee as soon as possible.

Effective communication as a mentor

Active listening

Listening is fundamental to all mentoring discussions. It requires that the mentor be silent most of the time and use all their senses to get the total message. Active, accurate listening is vital throughout a mentoring discussion but especially at the beginning, when the mentor usually takes a less verbally active part. Mentors need to listen carefully to what mentees are saying both verbally and non-verbally.

Active listening is not as easy as it sounds (Box 26.5). Obstacles and distractions abound. Active listening requires the ability to focus almost exclusively on another person while forgetting oneself and other concerns.

Challenging and questioning

One of the aims of the mentor is to challenge the mentees but this must be carried out correctly: confrontation is not challenge. The mentor should challenge whenever necessary, but with due consideration to the mentee and avoiding challenges that are driven more by the mentor's own agenda. Typical goals of challenging include:

- helping mentees to become aware of their blind spots in thinking and acting, and helping them to develop new perspectives

---

Box 26.5 Active listening checklist

Mentors should be asking themselves:

- What am I doing to read the mentee's non-verbal behaviours?
- What am I doing to listen to what the mentee is actually saying?
- What am I doing to challenge the mentee's point of view?
- What am I doing to identify the core messages being conveyed?
- What am I doing to manage any distractions?

- challenging mentees to find solutions to own their problems and draw on their unused potential
- helping mentees to state problems in solvable terms
- challenging mentees' distortions and excuses
- inviting mentees to explore the short- and long-term consequences of their behaviour and actions
- helping mentees to move beyond discussion to action.

Boxes 26.6 and 26.7 show checklists on challenging and on the related skills of prompting, probing and questioning.

Shadowing

Shadowing offers an excellent opportunity to gain a broad overview of different management roles and understand the wider picture of an organisation. In the context of busy clinical commitments the opportunity of shadowing is under-utilised for gaining insight into the managerial paradigms within the NHS.

Box 26.6 Checklist on challenging

Mentors should be asking themselves:

- To which type of 'challenge' will the mentee respond most effectively?
- Am I getting the mentee to challenge themselves and act on their own values?
- Has the relationship developed and have I earned the right to challenge in a particular way?
- Is this challenging going to hit the mark and provide a development opportunity for the mentee?
- Am I focusing on challenging the strengths rather than the weaknesses of the mentee?
- Am I pressurising the mentee?

Box 26.7 Prompting, probing and questioning checklist

Mentors should be asking themselves:

- What am I trying to achieve from this – how will this benefit the mentee?
- Am I balancing the use of open and closed questions?
- Is this becoming a question and answer session – a 'grilling'?
- Am I dealing with this in an empathetic manner?
- How can I build on this session to help the mentee's development?

What is shadowing?

Shadowing is essentially work-based learning. It is an opportunity to observe a job holder and to discuss with them key aspects of their role and the environment in which they work. Shadowing means what it says, that is, an individual identifies a job that they want to know more about and arranges to spend time with the job holder, observing what they do and how they undertake the role. The observation maybe within or outside the individual's organisation.

To get the best from shadowing, preparation should be carried out beforehand. After getting agreement to shadow someone in a job role it would be helpful to review the job holder's responsibilities and key objectives. It would make the shadowing more productive if it were to take place on the days or occasions when the job holder is doing something that enables the 'shadower' to find out more about the role and there is time to ask questions and review learning. The permission of the job holder's colleagues may need to be sought for an observer to be present. During and after shadowing, the 'shadower' should also spend time reflecting on the learning experience. Shadowing is not just about acquiring new skills: it is an opportunity to develop learning in a particular organisation.

Shadowing need not be a long-term arrangement: it can be done over a short period of time.

Benefits of shadowing

There are many benefits to shadowing for a person who is seeking to move on in their career and who may not be sure of the direction to take, because of the choices open to them. Shadowing:

- provides the opportunity to see a job holder in action
- provides an opportunity to gain an overview about a role and the environment
- broadens knowledge about career opportunities
- identifies the skills, qualifications and experience needed for a job
- increases networking
- helps the individual to identify gaps in their skills and knowledge
- helps the individual to understand the ethos and culture of an organisation
- contributes to general learning in an organisation.

Planning to shadow

To get the best from an experience such as shadowing both the learning and the practical elements should be planned: for example, what happens during the time that an individual may be away from their current role. Individuals planning to shadow should:

- identify the benefits to themselves of shadowing

- identify who to shadow and for how long
- discuss and agree the plan with their manager if it is to be carried out during work time
- discuss the plan with their mentor
- decide with the person to be shadowed which aspects of their job would provide most benefit
- prepare for the shadowing by reviewing the organisation and the job role that will be shadowed
- keep a diary and note questions for a review meeting with the job holder
- review their learning after the shadowing
- share their learning with their manager and team
- apply their learning in their current role.

Options to consider

When deciding whom to shadow, individuals should consider a range of management/leadership roles. This will provide a broad overview of organisational roles and an opportunity to develop learning set networks. Learning sets provide confidential forums for experimenting with and clarifying ideas, sharing learning experiences and supporting members.

Conclusions

Mentoring adds value to both the individual and the organisation. It is an effective mechanism for promoting and supporting management development. In addition, shadowing provides a quick and effective means of enabling an individual to gain insight into management roles and responsibilities and an organisational environment.

References and further reading

Clutterbuck, D. (2004) *Everyone Needs a Mentor: Fostering Talent at Work* (3rd edn). Charted Institute of Personnel and Development.

Downey, M. (2001) *Effective Coaching: Lessons from the Coach's Coach*. Thomson Texere.

Hay, J. (1997) *Action Mentoring: Creating your own Developmental Alliance*. Sherwood Publishing.

Higgins, M. C. & Thomas, D. A. (2001) Constellations and careers: toward understanding the effects of multiple developmental relationships. *Journal of Organizational Behavior*, **22**, 223–247.

Kline, N. (1999) *Time to Think: Listening to Ignite the Human Mind*. Cassell Illustrated.

Raelin, J. A. (2000) *Work Based Learning: The New Frontier of Management Development*. Prentice Hall.

Shea, G. F. (1999) *Mentoring: A Guide to Basics*. Kogan Page.

Thomas, D. A. (1990) The impact of race on managers' experiences of developmental relationships. *Journal of Organizational Behaviour*, **2**, 479–492.

Thomas, D. A. (1993) Mentoring and irrationality: the role of racial taboos. In *The Psychodynamics of Organizations* (ed. L. Hirschorn & C. K. Barnett). Temple University Press.

Thomas, D. A. (1999a) Beyond the simple demography–power hypothesis: how blacks in power influence whites to mentors blacks. In *Mentoring Dilemmas: Developmental Relationships within Multicultural Organizations* (eds A. Murrell, F. Crosby & R. Ely). Lawrence Erlbaum Associations.

Thomas, D. A. (1999b) Mentoring and diversity in organizations: the importance of race and gender in work relationships. In *Diversity in the Workplace: Issues and Perspectives* (ed. A. Daly). National Association of Social Workers Press.

Thomas, D. A. (2001) The truth about mentoring minorities: race matters. *Harvard Business Review*, **79**, 98–112.

Thomas, D. A. & Gabarro, J. J. (1999) *Breaking Through: The Making of Minority Executives in Corporate America*. Harvard Business School Press.

Thomas, D. & Higgins, M. C. (1996) Mentoring and the boundaryless career: lessons from the minority experience. In *Boundaryless Careers: A New Employment Principle for a New Organizational Era* (eds M. B. Arthur & D. M. Rousseau). Oxford University Press.

Thomas, D. A., & Kram, K. E. (1988) Promoting career-enhancing relationships in organization: the role of the human resource professional. In *Career Growth and Human Resource Strategies* (eds M. London & E. Mone). Quorum Books.

Weinstein. K. (1995) *Action Learning: A Practical Guide for Managers* (2nd edn). Gower Publishing.

Whitmore. J., Kimsey-House, K., Kimsey-House, H., *et al* (1998) *Co-Active Coaching: New Skills for Coaching People Toward Success in Work and Life*. Davies-Black Publishing.

CHAPTER 27

The MRCPsych examinations

Stephen Tyrer and Femi Oyebode

The Royal College of Psychiatrists developed its Membership examinations, widely abbreviated to the MRCPsych examinations, shortly after the College was founded. In June 1971 Professor Trethowan, the then Chief Examiner, arranged for the first part I examination to take place in November 1971 and the first part II examination in February 1972. Previous to that time the only further specialty qualification in psychiatry available to psychiatric trainees was the Diploma in Psychological Medicine (DPM). This diploma was issued by the Royal College of Physicians and Surgeons in England and by a number of universities in the UK and Ireland. Although there are still a number of DPM examinations in existence, the MRCPsych is now the accepted standard for any psychiatrist working in the UK or Ireland who wishes to obtain a certificate of completion of training (CCT). It is salutary to note that when the MRCPsych examinations were first proposed the College organisation representing junior psychiatrists, the Association of Psychiatrists in Training (APIT), opposed the forthcoming test and advised their members against taking it. The exam is now fully supported by trainees.

The prime aim of the MRCPsych examinations was, and still is, to set a standard to determine whether candidates are suitable to progress to higher professional training at specialist registrar level. In addition, possession of the qualification is considered to be an indicator of professional competence in the clinical practice of psychiatry.

The first MRCPsych examinations emphasised the possession of factual knowledge of psychiatry and psychology. The exams tested this knowledge both in sciences basic to psychiatry and in the clinical field. There was less attention paid to fundamentals of history-taking, mental state examination and to assessment of clinical skills. It is relevant in this regard that the first examiners in the College examinations were largely academic psychiatrists with a reputation of knowledge and research experience in a specific area of psychiatry. Many of these senior people had profound wisdom but were not widely trained in assessment of the skills of clinical competence. Furthermore, many of the questions that these examiners asked in the exam were concerned with factual knowledge, which could have been assessed very adequately in written form. One of us (S.T.) remembers clearly his interrogation in the viva voce part of his part II MRCPsych examination (later called the 'patient management problems') by an esteemed professor of psychiatry at an august centre of excellence. The examiner asked the candidate to define what he meant by autism, and then quizzed him on the historical origins of this concept. There was no test of the candidate's ability to be able to assess and treat a person with childhood autism, nor to assess autistic thinking in psychosis.

Development of the MRCPsych examinations

Over the years, there has been much greater standardisation of all parts of the MRCPsych examinations. The theory papers now largely test factual knowledge and appraisal abilities, whereas other parts of the exam are focused on clinical skills and clinical competence.

Previously the examination was in two parts. Part I (originally called the 'preliminary test' – the designation was changed in 1986) was taken after 1 year of specialist training in psychiatry. The written part of this exam has for over 30 years comprised a multiple choice format. This was followed by a clinical exam, which until 2003 involved an assessment of the candidate's ability to take a complete history and mental state examination of an actual patient, followed by presentation of the salient features of the case concerned. In 2003 this part of the exam was replaced by an 'objective structured clinical examination' (OSCE). Candidates used to take both the written and the clinical exams, irrespective of performance in the written part. In 1998 the rules were changed so that only those candidates who had passed the multiple choice question (MCQ) part were able to go on to the clinical part of the exam. This change was made for pragmatic reasons – there seemed little point in candidates taking part in the clinical exam when they had already failed their MRCPsych part I because of an inadequate mark on the MCQ paper.

The part II examination, taken after at least 2½ years experience in psychiatry, consisted of five parts. These included three written papers, MCQ, essay and critical review papers, and two clinical sections – the individual patient assessment (IPA) and patient management problems (PMPs). Although the abilities and skills tested in this part of the examination are now largely not evaluated in a single examination setting, many of these abilities are assessed in other ways during training.

As a result of the changes to ensure standardisation of professional examinations a different examination programme is being brought into effect in Spring 2008. The new College examination and assessment programme now combines workplace-based assessments (WPBAs) with formal examinations. The structure of the examination is being simplified considerably.

Aims of the MRCPsych examinations

Possession of the MRCPsych qualification or its equivalent is a prerequisite for appointment to the specialist registrar grade and consequent receipt of a national training number (NTN), a guarantee of further specialist training. This enables the trainee to proceed to higher specialist training, completion of which leads to a CCT. This qualification enables the individual concerned to practise psychiatry in any country in the European Union, although in practice sufficient ability in the language of the country concerned would be considered essential for the person to contribute effectively as a senior mental health specialist.

The ultimate aim of the MRCPsych examinations is to ensure that those with sufficient ability pass the exam and, of even more importance, that candidates with inadequate skills do not. Because of its significance, the MRCPsych is termed, in educational parlance, a high stakes examination. This means that it must be highly reliable and valid in order to be defensible. There should also be evidence that the exam is testing appropriate skills and that only able candidates who reach a sufficient standard pass it. The MRCPsych examinations are, above all, a test of clinical competence. How can this be assessed?

Tests of clinical competence require assessment of factual knowledge, comprehension of subject matter, adequate critical analysis of the topic under enquiry, evaluation of clinical issues and application of all these elements in patient management. These were all evaluated in the old MRCPsych examinations and frequent refinements of the examination process have taken place over the past decade to ensure that candidates who pass the examination are clinically competent and that this assessment is reliable. However, the assessment of anything but knowledge of facts is difficult in a single examination. A correct response in an examination paper and ability to carry out a process when witnessed by others in an examination setting establishes what a candidate knows (e.g. in a multiple choice paper), what he or she can do (e.g. in an extended matching questions (EMQ) format) and what clinical skills he or she possesses (e.g. in an OSCE). These are clearly tests of competence but they are not assessments of day-to-day performance. They also do not, for instance, assess other attributes that all doctors must have to carry out their job successfully, for example team-working skills. It is for this reason that other methods of assessment have been introduced into the examinations.

These alternative methods involve assessments of doctors' longer-term performance during training. Most of these are assessed while working in post and largely comprise what are termed workplace-based assessments. These contribute significantly to the summative assessment in the new MRCPsych examinations and are discussed later in this chapter. The formal traditional ways of assessment will be covered first but a prerequisite before any appraisal of any discipline is made is the construction of a curriculum.

Curriculum

The knowledge and skills required to achieve a sufficient standard of ability need to be stated concisely in all examination procedures. A curriculum has been provided for the MRCPsych examinations since their development and this has recently been revised to take into account the more extensive assessments required from the modular aspect of the new system. The new curriculum can be accessed from the Royal College of Psychiatrists' website (http://www.rcpsych.ac.uk/training/curriculumpilotpack.aspx).

Safeguards are necessary to ensure that essential items in the MRCPsych curriculum are tested in the examinations. The competencies that are set out in the curriculum are evaluated in various parts of the MRCPsych examinations in what is known as a blueprint assessment (Table 27.1; Dauphinee, 1994). Such a blueprint ensures that the competencies that are considered to be core skills and abilities are assessed in at least one part of the exam or in a WPBA.

Recent changes to the MRCPsych examinations

From its inception the MRCPsych examinations comprised two parts. Success in part I permitted the trainee to advance to part II, and passing this part enabled the trainee to achieve specialist registrar status. The whole examination process was organised by the Royal College of Psychiatrists with little to no external control. However, concerns about the training of doctors in general led to the formation in 2005 of the Postgraduate Medical Education and Training Board (PMETB), in conjunction with

Table 27.1 Example of a blueprint for evaluation of depression

	MCQ	EMQ	OSCE	CRP	WPBA
History of concept of depression	✓	✓			
Assessment of depression	✓	✓	✓		✓
Course of depression			✓	✓	
Evaluation of research in depression				✓	
Treatment of depression	✓	✓	✓		✓

✓ refers to element of examination that is able to assess the ability of the candidate in the topic indicated. CRP, critical review paper.

the Modernising Medical Careers (MMC) group, and working under the auspices of the Chief Medical Officer of England. PMETB oversees and promotes the development of postgraduate medical education and training in all specialties, including general practice, across the UK.

The responsibilities of PMETB include:

- establishing standards and requirements for postgraduate medical education and training
- making sure these standards and requirements are met
- developing and promoting postgraduate medical education and training across the country.

PMETB has published a set of principles to which all assessments must adhere (Southgate & Grant, 2004). These form the basis of the changes that have been made to all postgraduate medical examinations in the UK, including the MRCPsych examinations, and they consist of the following:

- the assessment must be fit for the educational purpose selected
- the content must be based on curricula
- the methods of assessment must be based on the purpose of that component of the assessment
- the methods used for setting standards must be transparent
- assessments must provide relevant feedback
- examiners must be recruited using criteria for the tasks to be performed
- there must be lay involvement in the development of assessment measures
- documentation of assessments must be standardised and available nationally
- there must be resources sufficient to support the assessment.

These principles have been included in the new examination structure. From spring 2008 the candidate will be required to pass only four examinations. The four papers consist of three knowledge-based written papers and a final objective structured clinical examination (OSCE), taken only after defined training goals have been reached. Before progressing to each new part of the examination the candidate will need to have achieved certain competencies at agreed levels in their WPBAs. The standards of these tasks will be high and assessment of skills in these areas will be rigorous.

The three papers on which candidates will be tested comprise the following.

Paper 1

This paper covers the assessment of a patient, including history and mental state examination, leading to a diagnosis. Neurological and cognitive assessments are covered. Subsequent separate sections are concerned with basic psychopharmacology, psychological processes, human psychological development, social psychology and basic psychological treatments. Knowledge of descriptive psychopathology and measures to prevent psychiatric disorder is also required. The history of psychiatry, its ethics and philosophy and the issue of stigma complete the syllabus for this paper.

This paper can be taken after 1 year's training in general adult psychiatry or 6 months working in this discipline plus 6 months training in old age psychiatry.

Paper 2

This paper is concerned with more advanced knowledge of the principles of psychopharmacology, including pharmacokinetics, pharmacodynamics and information about psychotropic drugs, covering relevant adverse reactions and interactions. Neuropsychiatry, including the relevant branches of physiology, endocrinology, chemistry, anatomy and pathology, forms a large part of this paper. Finally, genetics, epidemiology, and statistics and basic research design are included. There is also a section on advanced psychological processes and treatments.

This paper can be taken after 18 months' training in psychiatry, including at least 1 year's experience in general adult psychiatry or 6 months working in this discipline plus 6 months training in old age psychiatry.

Paper 3

This final paper covers evidence-based psychiatric practice, research methods, more advanced statistics and critical appraisal. In critical appraisal, candidates are presented with a published scientific paper in psychiatry, about which they have to answer questions on the design of the study, appraisal of the methodology and the significance of the results to clinical practice. Much of the remainder of this paper covers knowledge of the clinical areas in psychiatry other than general adult psychiatry. Thus child and adolescent psychiatry, old age, liaison, forensic and addiction psychiatry, psychotherapy, learning disability and rehabilitation psychiatry are all included.

This paper can be taken after 24 months' training in psychiatry, including at least 1 year's experience in general adult psychiatry and 2 (or 3) periods of working in the sub-specialties of the disciplines indicated above.

Objective structured clinical examination (OSCE)

The final part of the exam is an adapted OSCE, named the clinical assessment of skills and competencies (CASC), in which candidates progress through a series of stations at which they have to interact with a role-player. The tasks may involve history-taking, mental state examination, physical examination and information-giving to patients, relatives or other professionals, including doctors. All stations in the MRCPsych adapted OSCE are concerned with clinical scenarios that require either communication or practical skills. The new clinical assessment will be more complex than the current clinical exam for the MRCPsych part I. Linked stations will be used and candidates will be required to perform at a higher level and to pass a minimum number of stations.

This paper can be taken after 30 months' training in psychiatry, including at least 1 year's experience in general adult psychiatry and 2 (or 3 or more) periods of working in the sub-specialties indicated above.

Essential knowledge, skills and competencies

The aims of those setting the MRCPsych examinations are to ensure that essential knowledge and skills are tested somewhere in the assessment. It is instructive to examine the core knowledge needed and the clinical skills required to practise safely and competently. These fall into the following categories:

- tests of knowledge
- tests of reasoning
- comprehension of clinical problems
- communication skills
- evaluation of research methodology
- application of retained knowledge.

Tests of knowledge

Factual knowledge can be tested well by means of an MCQ examination. Such questions were introduced in the MRCPsych examinations in 1974, at the time of Professor Martin Roth's presidency, and they are now included in the three written papers in the new examination. Originally, the true–false format was used, with a stem question followed by five branches, each of which could be true or false. This format has a number of weaknesses. The psychometric properties are poor, in that the candidate can guess correctly for each test item 50% of the time. Furthermore, for each question, the test designer has to write five branches, all of which must be grammatically consistent with the stem and must not be obviously false or trivial. The MCQ format was changed in 2003 to stand-alone questions, referred to as 'individual statements'. These have the advantage that they are unambiguous statements but continue to suffer from the disadvantage that the candidate can guess correctly 50% of the time. Examples of individual statements are:

'Acetylcholine binds to both nicotinic and muscarinic receptors'

'Significantly more normal females than males have problems with right–left orientation'

(both are true). Until recently, this test was marked using the negative marking technique, with all correct answers scoring +1 and incorrect answers scoring −1. Negative marking is no longer well regarded as it penalises candidates whose guesses are informed and intelligent. The marking procedure was therefore altered in 2001 to a system in which wrong answers were not scored negatively. This principle is still used.

Candidates' knowledge is tested to some degree in all other parts of the MRCPsych examinations but all other parts also test other skills.

Tests of reasoning

Reasoning skills are not evaluated by standard MCQs. To test clinical reasoning in a written format, a different type of test is used in the MRCPsych examinations. This uses the EMQ format. In this test, a particular clinical scenario is chosen, which may be in either the basic science or clinical field, a number of options are listed, and a specific problem is given for which the appropriate option should be selected (Case & Swanson, 1993). An example of an EMQ question is shown in Box 27.1.

Box 27.1   An example of an EMQ question

Theme: Drug treatment of depression

The group of questions below consists of lettered options followed by numbered items. For each numbered item, select one appropriate lettered option. Each option can be chosen once, more than once, or not at all.

Match each item with best treatment option.

List of options:

A.   Fluoxetine

B.   Flupenthixol

C.   Gabapentin

D.   Imipramine

E.   Lamotrigine

F.   Lithium

G.   L-tryptophan

H.   Sodium valproate

I.   Venlafaxine.

Items:

1.   A 45-year-old female patient has a history of bipolar mood disorder. She was first treated at 20 years of age. She has had five depressive episodes and one hypomanic episode since then. She is asking for advice about future treatment in order to prevent further recurrences.

2.   A 45-year-old male patient is presenting with a first episode of moderate depression. He has a history of coronary heart disease. What is the most appropriate treatment?

Analysis of EMQ questions shows that they discriminate better than MCQs between able and less able candidates. They also test reasoning capacity.

Comprehension of clinical problems

To accurately assess and understand clinical difficulties, trainee psychiatrists need a good knowledge of the illness in question, how it is manifest, its natural course and the prognosis. The accuracy of diagnostic labels applied and how far alternative treatment may be appropriate if the diagnosis is not completely accurate also needs assessment. Full clinical comprehension can only be adequately tested in a clinical situation. In the MRCPsych examinations there is some test of this skill in the OSCE exam. These skills will be tested more fully in work-based assessments.

Communication skills

The ability to communicate with patients empathically and relevantly is an essential ability for any psychiatrist. These elements are tested mainly in the WPBAs but are also tested in the OSCE examination. The OSCE tests the ability of a candidate to communicate adequately with a simulated patient, relative of a patient or other professionals, including doctors. The development of this test in psychiatry has been well described by Rao (2005).

Evaluation of research methodology

Until 1998 the written part of the MRCPsych examinations comprised three parts: an MCQ paper, an essay question and a short answer question (SAQ) paper. However, it was recognised that the SAQ paper was testing very similar abilities to the MCQ paper, the only difference being that the SAQs required recall of relevant facts whereas the MCQs, by their very nature, involved recognition of factual material. In any event, the correlation between SAQ scores and MCQ scores was high. The SAQ paper was therefore discontinued. It was replaced by the critical review paper (CRP), a paper that requires a very different skill that needed to be assessed – the ability to accurately appraise a scientific paper and determine its merits and relevance to the practice of psychiatry.

In the CRP a condensed version of a published paper is reproduced. The candidate has to examine the design of the study, identify problems in bias, determine whether the power of the study and statistical analysis are appropriate, and assess how far the authors' conclusions are valid from the results given. Evidence-based material is covered in this paper, including appraisal of research methodology, economic analysis, qualitative research, meta-analysis and systematic reviews. Paper 3 of the new examination assesses this ability.

It has been shown that such instruction is of benefit in improving the evidence-based medicine skills of both postgraduate and medical students

(Fritschke *et al*, 2002). Introduction of this paper has been shown to improve the standard of presentations at journal clubs and scientific meetings (Taylor & Warner, 2000).

Application of knowledge and information

The application of knowledge about psychiatric issues is tested to some extent in the theory papers but more extensively in the OSCE examination. It is more thoroughly examined in the WPBAs.

Examiners

Examiners are selected carefully. Advertisements are published twice yearly in the *Psychiatric Bulletin* inviting applications from consultants who wish to be considered for appointment as examiners. Each application must be supported by references from regional advisors and professors of psychiatry. All examiners attend a training day at the Royal College of Psychiatrists, where they receive instruction about marking and mark mock tapes.

Once examiners are appointed they normally serve for up to 7 years. All examiners are required to attend a Board of Examiners meeting at least once every 2 years for refresher training, which includes a standard-setting procedure similar to the initial training event. The aim is to reach consensus on what constitutes an adequate level of performance in the IPA and PMP. There is also feedback to examiners of their performance compared with that of other examiners. Examiners will also have to update their examining skills by marking a video of CASCs which have been standardised and submitting their marks for review.

The procedure of standardising the performance of examiners is carried out in a different way in the written parts of the MRCPsych examinations. The standard for the MCQ and EMQ parts of the examination is set using the modified Angoff technique, a criterion referenced method (Angoff, 1971; Searle, 2000). This ensures that the examination standard is determined by the examination paper rather than by the candidature. It also ensures that subsequent examinations can be calibrated so that they are of equal standard.

Work-placed based assessments

There have been major changes to the MRCPsych examinations over the past 5 years (Tyrer & Oyebode, 2004) and even more radical alterations have been made since. PMETB has advised that traditional formal assessments by examination should not be the main gateway to achievement of professional qualifications. Clinical skills should now be examined in more realistic clinical situations by means of workplace-based assessments. Workplace assessment aims to collect information on trainees' performance by witnessing their interactions with patients over time.

The aim is for these assessments to be 'authentic' (van der Vleuten & Schuwirth, 2005), i.e. to evaluate the performance of the trainee in all relevant areas at all times. This involves continuous educational assessment during training. Continuous assessment is said to evaluate better the capacity of candidates to carry out a competent skill. Although recently OSCEs have been developed to assess whether candidates can 'show how' to do something, they are insufficient on their own to assure teachers that the candidate actually 'does' this in practice. Tests of performance, in actual clinical settings, have therefore assumed more significance.

Types of WPBA

The mini-clinical evaluation exercise

The mini-clinical evaluation exercise (mini-CEX) has been adapted from the clinical evaluation exercise (CEX), an instrument designed by the American Board of Internal Medicine for assessing junior doctors at the bedside. This exercise involves an oral examination during which the trainee, under the observation of an examining psychiatrist, takes a full history and completes a full examination of a patient. Following this the candidate has to give a differential diagnosis and describe a management plan.

The standardised patient examination

A standardised patient is a person who is trained to take the role of a patient in a way that is similar and reproducible for each encounter with different trainees. Hence they present in an identical way to each trainee. The standardised patient may be an actor, an asymptomatic patient or a patient with stable, abnormal signs on examination. Standardised patients can be employed for teaching history-taking, examination, communication skills and interpersonal skills. They can also be used in the assessment of these skills. Only actors are used in the OSCE examinations but patients can be used in WPBAs.

Case-based discussion

Case-based discussion is also known as management simulation (Satish *et al*, 2001). The trainee discusses his or her cases with two trained assessors in a standardised and structured oral examination, the purpose of which is to evaluate the trainee's clinical decision-making, reasoning and application of medical knowledge with real patients. The assessors question the trainee about areas such as diagnosis, interpretation of findings, management, treatment and care plans (Southgate *et al*, 2001).

Directly observed procedures

Directly observed procedures (or objective structured assessment of technical skills) are similar to the mini-CEX. The process has been developed by the Royal College of Physicians to assess practical skills (Wilkinson *et al*, 2003). Two examiners observe the trainee carrying out a procedural task on a patient and independently grade the performance. This form of assessment lends itself well to medical specialties where the acquisition of practical skills is important. Examples include suturing a wound, taking an arterial blood sample and performing a lumbar puncture. At present it is less clear what procedures would be observed in psychiatry because psychiatrists are less involved with practical tasks. However, these may be adapted in areas such as risk assessment and assessment of consent and capacity.

Multisource feedback

Multisource feedback, which is commonly known as 360° assessment, consists of measurements completed by many people in a doctor's sphere of influence. Evaluators completing the forms are usually colleagues, other doctors and members of the multiprofessional team. A multisource assessment can be used to provide data on interpersonal skills such as integrity, compassion, responsibility to others and communication; on professional behaviours; and on aspects of patient care and team-working.

Portfolios

A portfolio is a collection of material, collated by the individual over time, used to demonstrate their chronological learning, performance and development. This record enables individuals to reflect on their abilities and highlight areas that could be improved to enhance the quality of their practice. There are numerous models for portfolio use. In medicine, portfolios tend to be used both formatively (to improve one's own practice) and summatively (for recertification and revalidation). These will be used for all trainees.

The assessment of other parts of the curriculum is based on the standards that have been laid down in the booklet produced by the General Medical Council (2006), *Good Medical Practice*. A large part of this is concerned with good clinical care of patients, but the candidate's ability to work with other colleagues will also be rated in these modules. The probity, i.e. the integrity and honesty, of the candidate will also be objectively rated.

Conclusions

Despite the radical changes to the assessment of candidates, the MRCPsych examinations will still be required as evidence of ability and competence at the end of a course of training. There remains considerable demand for this qualification. The examination is now taken by close to 2000 candidates every year, with almost two-thirds of these receiving their undergraduate medical education outside the UK (Tyrer *et al*, 2002).

The MRCPsych examinations are in the throes of a major change in emphasis. The programme of instruction is likely to be modified over the next few years and it is vital for all prospective candidates to determine the latest requirements on the College website at http://www.rcpsych.ac.uk/exams/newassessmentprogramme2008.aspx.

References

Angoff, W. H. (1971) Scales, norms and equivalent scores. In *Educational Measurement* (ed. R. L. Thorndike), pp. 508–600. American Council on Education.

Case, S. M. & Swanson, D. B. (1993) Extended matching items: a practical alternative to free response questions. *Teaching and Learning in Medicine*, **5**, 107–115.

Dauphinee, D. (1994) Determining the content of certification examinations. In *The Certification and Recertification of Doctors: Issues in the Assessment of Clinical Competence* (eds D. I. Newbie, B.C. Jolly & R.E. Wakeford), pp. 92–104. Cambridge University Press.

Fritschke, L., Greenhalgh, T., Falck-Ytter, Y., *et al* (2002) Do short courses in evidence-based medicine improve knowledge and skills? *BMJ*, **325**, 1338–1341.

General Medical Council (2006) *Good Medical Practice 2006*. GMC.

Rao, R. (2005) *OSCEs in Psychiatry*. Gaskell.

Satish, U., Streufert, S., Marshall, R., *et al* (2001) Strategic management simulations is a novel way to measure resident competencies. *American Journal of Surgery*, **181**, 557–561.

Searle, J. (2000) Defining competency – the role of standard setting. *Medical Education*, **34**, 363–366.

Southgate, L. & Grant, J. (2004) *Principles for an Assessment System for Postgraduate Medical Training: A Working Paper from the Postgraduate Medical Education Training Board*. PMETB. http://www.pmetb.org.uk/fileadmin/user/QA/Assessment/Principles_for_an_assessment_system_v3.pdf

Southgate, L., Cox, J., David, T., *et al* (2001) The General Medical Council's performance procedures: peer review of performance in the workplace. *Medical Education*, **35**, 9–19.

Taylor, P. & Warner, J. (2000) National survey of training needs for evidence-based practices. *Psychiatric Bulletin*, **24**, 272–273.

Tyrer, S. & Oyebode, F. (2004) Why does the MRCPsych examination need to change? *British Journal of Psychiatry*, **184**, 197–199.

Tyrer, S. P., Leung, W.-C., Smalls, J., *et al* (2002) The relationship between medical school of training, age, gender and success in the MRCPsych examinations. *Psychiatric Bulletin*, **26**, 257–263.

van der Vleuten, C. & Schuwirth, L. W. (2005) Assessing professional competence: from methods to programmes. *Medical Education*, **39**, 309–317.

Wilkinson, J., Benjamin, A. & Wade, W. (2003) Assessing the performance of doctors in training. *BMJ Career Focus*, **327**, s91–s92.

CHAPTER 28

Flexible training

Jane Marshall

Psychiatry has been at the forefront of flexible training since the introduction of the scheme to the National Health Service (NHS) in 1969. Indeed, the origins of flexible training in psychiatry pre-date the formal NHS scheme, as psychiatrists were training on a part-time basis in Oxford as early as 1966 (Department of Health, 1991). This chapter charts the historical background of flexible training in the UK. The roles of the postgraduate deaneries and the Royal College of Psychiatrists are discussed, and a 'rough guide' to flexible training is presented.

Historical background

1969–1991

Flexible training was introduced to the NHS in 1969 with the HM(69)6 notice, and aimed specifically at women with domestic commitments (Department of Health, 1969). It was not seen as a mainstream career pathway, and apart from some posts established in Oxford, the scheme was little used in other regions until 1979, when the PM(79)3 scheme was introduced, specifically focused on senior registrar grades (Department of Health, 1979). The 1979 Department of Health memorandum reflected the Equal Opportunities Act 1974, the increase in the number of women doctors graduating and the increase in the number of women in the workforce (Goldberg & Maingay, 1997). It also focused on the need for part-time trainees to be of similar calibre to full-time trainees and to ensure that the training posts they occupied had educational approval from the appropriate medical Royal College. Regions were allowed to set up flexible posts at other grades at their own discretion (Clay, 1998). Candidates had to show 'well-founded personal reasons' to train flexibly and senior registrars had to enter a national competition to get 'manpower approval' (Clay, 1998). Successful candidates then had to find a local post with educational approval, obtain funding and finally satisfy a local appointments committee (Department of Health, 1991). Funding was not readily available and there was an average delay of 18 months between application and taking up a post (NHS Management Executive, 1993). Although bureaucratic and slow, this scheme allowed more doctors to complete higher specialist training (Scriven, 1996). The report of the Joint Working Party on women doctors and their careers commented on the cumbersome nature of the scheme and called for a review of procedures (Department of Health, 1991).

In 1991 EL(91)5 introduced a new scheme for career registrars. Manpower approval and funding for the posts were provided centrally and the interviews carried out locally. This scheme increased the numbers of flexible trainees. Further administrative changes made postgraduate deans responsible for flexible training. No specific scheme was introduced for senior house officers (SHOs) but deaneries were able to make local provision for SHOs and pre-registration house officers (PRHOs). However, flexible training opportunities for PRHOs and SHOs were rarely implemented, owing to perceived lack of demand, views of postgraduate deans that flexible training should be reserved for higher training only, restricted training budgets and lack of support from the medical Royal Colleges (Rees & van Someren, 1984). Flexible training at SHO level was therefore sporadic, with some successful job-sharing where posts were split 50/50 (5 sessions each). However, after 1993, the 50/50 split was not acceptable for training in general practice, because of the European Union (EU) requirement that a minimum training commitment be 60% that of full-time workers.

1992–1998

In April 1993 the report of the Joint Working Party on Flexible Training was published (NHS Management Executive, 1993). This report reviewed the operation of flexible training at both SHO and senior registrar level, and identified action for the Department of Health, the medical Royal Colleges and health authorities. It proposed that the term 'flexible training' be used to describe part-time working arrangements, because of the 'unhelpful connotation' of the term part-time. The report also recommended that flexible training should be provided for at least 5% of doctors in training by the year 2000.

The NHS regions began to appoint associate deans with specific responsibility for flexible training. It was at this point that the unmet demand for flexible training at the SHO level became apparent, and this was noted by the Joint Working Party (NHS Management Executive, 1993) and by the Conference of Postgraduate Medical Deans (COPMeD) (Conference of Postgraduate Medical Deans, 1995).

In 1993, the European Union directive 93/16/EEC consolidated various European directives concerning medical education. Its purpose was to facilitate the free movement of doctors and the mutual recognition of their diplomas, certificates and other formal qualifications (Goldberg & Maingay, 1997). Article 235 of this directive permitted part-time specialist training 'when training on a full-time basis would not be practicable for well-founded reasons'. This was a broader interpretation than the previous

British requirements. This support and the devolution of decision-making to regional postgraduate deaneries changed the way in which decisions were made.

Following the report of the Joint Working Party on Flexible Training (NHS Management Executive, 1993), two flexible training schemes were introduced. One replaced the scheme for senior registrars and the second formally extended flexible training to career registrars. This was backed by central funding and became very successful (Scriven, 1996). One drawback of this success was that flexible training became very popular in some specialties (anaesthetics, obstetrics and gynaecology, paediatrics and psychiatry in particular) to the extent that waiting lists were created because there were limited places in each specialty (Scriven, 1996). In 1995 the waiting lists for staffing approvals were removed, but this coincided with a shortage of funding, and some regions were unable to fund all their flexible trainees.

The next important change was the transition to 'Calman training' and the introduction of the unified training grade (NHS Executive, 1996). With the introduction of the specialist registrar grade, appointments for flexible training were, for the first time, integrated into the appointments systems in each deanery, allowing part-time trainees to be assessed equally alongside full-time counterparts (Goldberg & Maingay, 1997; Clay, 1998).

After 1995 flexible training achieved much wider recognition, with more uniform opportunities throughout England and Wales (Clay, 1998). The Conference of Postgraduate Medical Deans established a Flexible Training Working Group to advise it about the specific issues. Opportunities developed in Scotland and Northern Ireland, and the Scottish deaneries were represented as full members on COPMeD (Clay, 1998). (A centrally funded flexible training scheme was introduced in Scotland in 1993. The organisation of the scheme and the appointment of trainees was carried out at local level. Trainees were only able to work five sessions per week under this scheme until 2003, when this was increased to six.)

Demand for flexible training posts continued to grow, with a reported increase of 30% across grades and specialties by 1997 (Goldberg, 1997). Although no national scheme existed for SHOs, posts began to be made available by local postgraduate deans, and the numbers of SHOs applying to train flexibly began to increase (Redfern & Scriven, 1998).

A comparison of flexible training opportunities in the European Union found that few other countries in the EU had begun to implement flexible training in the same way as the UK (Maingay & Goldberg, 1998). This was explained in part by the differences in training patterns across the EU. Higher levels of flexible training in the UK were due to a combination of health authority need and trainee demand.

1999–2005

In 1999 the British Medical Association's Junior Doctors Committee published a survey of flexible trainees (Norcliffe & Finlan, 1999). At the time the Junior Doctors Committee was seeking greater availability of flexible training, competency-based assessment rather than a time-served approach, and standard rates of pay for flexible trainees for the first 40 contracted hours. A 70% response rate was achieved ($n = 797$, of whom 22 were men). Most trainees (75%) were in higher specialist training, although a sizeable minority of respondents were from the SHO grade. Most respondents were in their mid-30s and the most common reason for training flexibly was responsibility for children (89%). The profile of the 'average flexible trainee' was that of 'a 34.6 year old woman with children and a partner who is in the specialist registrar grade'. Respondents reported that they regularly worked more than their contracted hours, and that the intensity of their on-call work was greater than for their full-time counterparts. The overwhelming impression was of a working environment that was not family friendly. Respondents, however, were reasonably satisfied with the clinical and teaching aspects of their flexible training experience. They were less satisfied with opportunities for study and for undertaking and completing research. Other issues that emerged were problems of continuity and 'handing over', and a perception that they were regarded as 'lesser' members of the department. Finally, pay was a particular problem, with respondents commenting about the unfairness of not being paid for hours routinely worked.

Nationally, the numbers of doctors training flexibly continued to rise from 719 in 1994 to 2413 in 2005 (Fig. 28.1). The overall percentage of flexible trainees in the UK remains fairly stable at 6% (Flexible Training Committee of COPMeD, 2005).

Flexible trainees are mainly women. Overall 78% of flexible trainees are at specialist registrar level (72% are women and 6% men), 11% are at SHO level (10% are women and 1% men) and 1% are at PRHO level (all

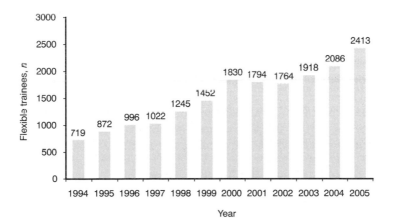

Fig. 28.1 Total number of flexible trainees for all deaneries in the UK for the period 1994–2005.

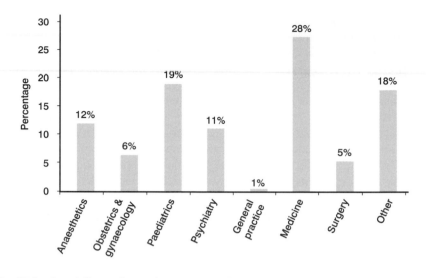

Fig. 28.2 Specialist registrars by most popular specialties across all deaneries in the UK for the period 1994–2005.

women). (At the time of the 2005 survey, the total number of trainees in the 18 UK deaneries was 39 097). Psychiatry is still a popular specialty for both specialist registrars and SHOs (Figs 28.2 and 28.3).

Women doctors and their careers

The proportion of women medical students remained between 20% and 25% until 1968, when it increased steadily, reaching 50% in 1990 and exceeding 50% in 1991 (McManus & Sprotson, 1999). The proportion of women being admitted to UK medical and dental schools has continued to rise steadily: 35% in 1975; 45% in 1985; 54% in 1996; 57% in 2000; 58% in 2001; and 60.8% in 2002 (4797 women and 3088 men) (Allen, 2005). The numbers and percentages of women consultants have also increased steadily, doubling from 12% in 1983 to 24% in 2003. The specialties with the largest numbers of women consultants in 1983 were psychiatry, pathology and paediatrics. By 2003, 40% of consultant paediatricians were women. Women were also well represented in community and public health and in psychiatry, although overall numbers in these groups were low compared with numbers in general medicine (Royal College of Physicians, 2004). The proportion of women working in general practice had doubled, from 19% in 1983 to 38% in 2003. Surgery, however, remains a male preserve, having only 7% of women consultants in 2003 (Allen, 2005). In 2003 the percentage of men and women consultants working full-time was 55%. Only 9.8% of men worked part-time, compared with 30% of women. Current numbers of women consultants reflect numbers of women entering

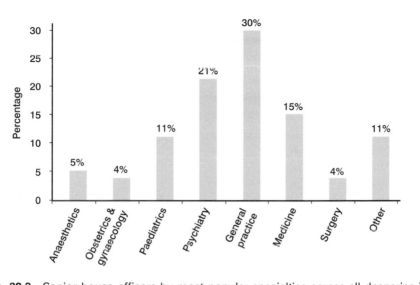

Fig. 28.3 Senior house officers by most popular specialties across all deaneries in the UK for the period 1994–2005.

medical schools in the 1970s and 1980s, prior to the early 1990s when the gender intake equalised. Women account for 39% of specialist registrars and for 44% of SHOs in hospital medicine. However, significant numbers of doctors in training qualified overseas. Taking UK qualifiers, women account for 44% of specialist registrars and 50% of SHOs (Department of Health, 2004).

Isobel Allen's study on doctors and their careers (Allen, 1988) found that the lack of opportunity for flexible training was a significant factor affecting women doctors' choice of specialty. The level of flexible training declined in the mid- to late 1980s, and there was criticism of the arrangements then in force. However, 87% of the women doctors interviewed for this study thought that there should be greater provision for flexible training. Allen's follow-up research found that men and women were experiencing similar problems in their careers, mainly related to the rigid medical career structure (Allen, 1994).

In 1995 a survey found that 73% of female doctors and 10% of male doctors wished to work part-time at some stage in their careers (Department of Health, 1995). In the following year Allen highlighted the need for the NHS to make a 'radical assessment' of how to

'make use of the talents of the brightest and best of successive generations of young people who enter medicine. Assumptions still predicated on a medical workforce made up of men working full-time in one specialty for 40 years are hopelessly misguided, and it is time that the medical profession woke up to this fact. A strategic overview is urgently required of what we need from tomorrow's doctors and how we should plane to achieve it' (Allen, 1996).

291

A more recent survey of work–life balance in a sample of London-based women hospital consultants highlighted the importance of time management and role models (Allen *et al*, 1999). Proximity to the workplace was considered crucial. The view that women may have different career paths from men was emphasised. The years in employment of women are more likely to have an M-shaped distribution, with a peak in the early years, a dip in the middle and a potential peak in the later years (Allen, 2005). The issue of supporting women in academic medicine was also raised (Reichenbach & Brown, 2004).

Women in medicine have come of age. Work patterns have changed in recent years and the shorter hours worked by junior doctors have helped to keep women in the system. There has been a culture change in British medicine and today's medical students and young doctors no longer want to work 'all hours'. They increasingly want a better work–life balance, i.e. a personal and family life.

Flexible training and psychiatry

It has been estimated that, nationally, 14% of psychiatrists train flexibly, but with regional uptake ranging from 3.5 to 26% (NHS Management Executive, 1993). This figure may be an underestimate because a more recent survey of consultant psychiatrists over the age of 50 indicated that 16% had trained flexibly, of which 76% were women (Mears *et al*, 2004*a*).

Flexibly trained psychiatrists have been shown to out-perform their full-time counterparts in terms of how quickly they gain Membership of the Royal College of Psychiatrists (assessed by number of examination attempts) and they also gain experience in other specialties before entering psychiatry (Herzberg & Goldberg, 1999). A survey of flexible trainees in the Thames region found that they largely considered part-time training satisfactory, although acknowledging that it was not without its difficulties (Etchegoyen *et al*, 2001).

A national retrospective survey of 300 female consultant psychiatrists who had trained flexibly indicated that respondents were satisfied with their training and that their clinical progress had not been hindered (Mears *et al*, 2002, 2004*b*). However, there was a perception that flexible training had had a negative influence on their academic progress, an important finding, given the under-representation of women in academic psychiatry (Killaspy *et al*, 2003). Family reasons were cited as central to the decision to train flexibly.

A rough guide to flexible training

The role of the postgraduate deaneries

Flexible training is available for all doctors in training grades who, for well-founded individual reasons, cannot work full-time. Most postgraduate

---

Box 28.1 Websites

Postgraduate deanery websites have a wealth of information on flexible training and about the steps involved. In particular the London Deanery website (http://www.londondeanery.ac.uk) and the West Midland Deanery flexible training website (http://www.wmdeanery.org) are recommended.

You should contact your associate dean if you think flexible training may be a possibility. Setting up posts often takes time.

Other websites

Medical Women's Federation: http://www.medicalwomensfederation.co.uk

BMA's Flexible Training Forum: http://www.bma.org.uk

The Department of Health's Improving Working Lives website has information for all healthcare workers: http://www.dh.gov.uk/iwl

The Doctors Forum: http://www.nhsemployers.org/kb/kb-628.cfm

---

deans have an associate dean to manage the flexible training scheme in their area. Information on flexible training can be obtained from the local postgraduate dean's office or deanery website (Box 28.1). At the local level, clinical and postgraduate tutors and educational supervisors may be aware of flexible training. The Royal College of Psychiatrists currently has two co-directors of flexible training, appointed in 2004.

Flexible training in medical disciplines is defined by European Law (EC directive 93/16/EEC) as being part-time training that involves a limitation in participation in medical activities for at least half the time of a full-time trainee. It can be undertaken at any stage during training. All trainees, both men and women, are eligible to apply for flexible training. Those wishing to do so must show that training on a full-time basis would not be practical for them, for well-founded individual reasons. The main reasons include pregnancy and the need to care for young children, ill or disabled dependants, or their own ill-health or disability. Others reasons have been accepted in the past, for example an international athlete needed to keep up a fitness schedule and a former full-time researcher wished to return to clinical practice and needed to update clinical skills while continuing to write up research (Clay, 1998).

Doctors wishing to train flexibly should in the first instance make an appointment to see their local postgraduate dean or the associate dean for flexible training, who will decide whether they are eligible. They will usually have to attend a formal interview, where their eligibility will be assessed and the mechanism for arranging a suitable programme discussed. Trainees who do not meet the eligibility criteria are usually encouraged to discuss alternative career pathways with their postgraduate clinical tutor.

293

As already mentioned, the only formal requirement to be permitted to train flexibly is a well-founded individual reason. In practice, COPMeD has drawn up two main categories of reasons for needing to train on a flexible basis, and these are used by deaneries to assess eligibility. It should be noted that these categories are not exhaustive: other well-founded reasons may be considered but acceptance would be dependent on the particular situation and the needs of the specialty in which the individual was training.

Category 1

Doctors in training who have:

- disability or ill health (this may include those on *in vitro* fertility programmes)
- responsibility for caring (men and women) for children
- responsibility for caring for an ill or disabled partner, relative or other dependant.

These result in the individual doctor being professionally disadvantaged by circumstances, and less able to fulfil their potential if training on a full-time basis.

Category 2

Doctors in training who have:

- unique opportunities for their own personal or professional development, for example training for national/international sporting events, or short-term extraordinary responsibility, for example sitting on a national committee
- religious commitment, involving training for a particular religious role that requires a specific amount of time commitment
- non-medical professional development such as management, law or fine arts courses or a diploma in complementary therapies.

Category 1 applicants have priority and deaneries will support all applicants in this category. In general, non-medical interests will be treated on their individual merits. Access to Category 2 is dependent on individual circumstances and the availability of funding. Where an application is refused by the deanery the applicant has a right of appeal.

Number of sessions and out-of hours work

European Community directive EC75/636 requires that part-time training shall be for a minimum of 50% of a full-time post, i.e. a standard 20 hours (or five sessions) per week. In some regions flexible trainees are required to work for a minimum of six sessions. The maximum permissible number of sessions is eight. Although most would agree that the amount of actual training and learning acquired by a flexible trainee exceeds these percentages in terms of experience, the directive insists that the precise duration of training should be *pro rata* that of full-time trainees, including out-of-hours experience.

The majority of trainees must do some out-of-hours work, for which they are paid a full basic salary and a supplement. Trainees who do not do any out-of-hours work are paid the basic pay, usually calculated *pro rata* for the number of sessions they work.

Many postgraduate deans allow flexible trainees the same study leave entitlement as for full-timers.

Funding

In most postgraduate deaneries in England, all the basic salary of flexible trainees is paid by the deanery, whereas the out-of-hours supplement is the responsibility of the local NHS trust. Many deaneries will fund only a five- or six-session post (50% or 60% of a full-time post) because of the demands on their budget. In Wales the out-of-hours payment is also funded by the postgraduate deaneries. It is important to be aware that local trusts may be involved in paying a portion of the salaries of flexible trainees and that this will require local negotiation.

Pay has two basic components – basic salary and supplement. Basic salary is determined by the actual hours worked by the flexible trainee. This needs to be no more than the appropriate proportion of the actual hours worked by full-time trainees on the same rota. The supplement is determined on the basis of frequency and proportion of out-of-hours duties. It is paid as a proportion of the basic salary determined by the actual hours worked.

The new pay arrangements introduced in 2005 are complex, but they bring rates of pay for flexible trainees into line with rates for their full-time counterparts(NHS Employers, 2005).

Appointments process

Trainees applying for their first specialist training post are not required to disclose to anyone their intentions to train flexibly. Even if they are applying from a flexible training post, and their intention may be obvious, the advisory appointment committee is not allowed to make any assumptions and should not ask questions about intentions to train flexibly at interview.

Candidates are considered on exactly equal terms and ranked in order of merit. When an appointment is offered, the candidate can then disclose their eligibility and wish to train flexibly. If they have already discussed their situation with the postgraduate dean, it is likely that funding will already be available.

Candidates are advised to give postgraduate deans (or associate deans) as much notice as possible of any planned change between flexible and full-time status. Flexible trainees will need to continue in training for longer than full-timers to be eligible for certificate of completion of specialist training (CCT). For instance, those working 50% of full-time will be in training for twice as long. Those working more that 50% could qualify for a CCT in a shorter time *pro rata*.

It is not unusual for flexible trainees in psychiatry to tailor their training to their needs, for instance moving from 50% to 60% and perhaps 70%. Such changes can be arranged with the help of the postgraduate dean and the College, provided enough time is allowed for the administration involved.

Ways of working

Supernumerary posts

Flexible trainees have historically worked in supernumerary posts, which were funded by the deanery flexible training budget. These posts were separate and different from mainstream posts: there was a separate quota governing the overall number, different appointment procedures, a different mechanism for getting approval from the medical Royal Colleges, a separate budget supporting them and different expectations as to outcome (Goldberg, 2002). Unfortunately, flexible trainees perceived that they were viewed by their consultants and peers as being of lower status than full-timers.

Funding problems emerged following the 2000 pay deal, which was favourable to flexible trainees, entitling them to receive a full-time salary plus a supplement if they did out-of hours work. Initially some deaneries were able to pay the 'top-up' from the *pro rata* salary (50–80%) to a full-time salary (100%) using non-recurrent funding from the Department of Health. However, this funding ceased at the end of the financial year 2003/04. The trusts were expected to pay the supplement, which was equivalent to 0.05, 0.25 or 0.5 of the full-time salary, depending on the flexible training band to which the trainees had been allocated. After April 2004 trusts were expected to pay the 'top-up' as well as the supplement, which created cost pressures. Many trusts were not prepared to fund supernumerary trainees. This situation continues to date, even after the introduction of the 2005 flexible training pay deal.

Slot sharing

Two flexible trainees can slot-share a full-time post, and each work between 6 and 8 sessions. The trust already has funding for 100% of the full-time basic pay from the full-time budget, and the flexible budget adds another 100% of basic pay. The trust pays only for the banding supplements. Although this format is cost-effective, it is difficult to implement, except on large rotations with a high proportion of flexible trainees (e.g. paediatrics rotations).

Reduced sessions in a full-time post

Reduced sessions in a full-time post require no contribution from the flexible training budget, because the post is already funded for full-time training.

Flexible training and Modernising Medical Careers

The *Guide to Postgraduate Specialty Training in the UK: The Gold Guide* (Modernising Medical Careers, 2007) provides the framework for the new postgraduate specialty training programmes which commenced in August 2007. It is very positive towards flexible training ('less than full-time training' or LTFT), and clearly sets out the categories for prioritising requests and / or eligibility agreed by COPMeD. The guide specifically notes that, during the application process, trainees are able to tick a box indicating that they wish to train flexibly. However, this information remains confidential and trainees are appointed on merit. The ultimate aim is to integrate flexible training (LTFT) into the mainstream by using slot shares, job shares and full-time posts where possible, and also by developing permanent flexible training posts. Supernumerary posts will continue to exist, but are likely to be affected by funding issues.

Trainees applying for LTFT will be required to undertake at least 50% of a normal working week (some deaneries require 60%), to move between posts within rotations on the same basis as full-time trainees and not to engage in any other paid employment while in LTFT.

Flexible training and PMETB

The Postgraduate Medical Education and Training Board (PMETB) became the official body for approving psychiatric training on 30 September 2005. All supernumerary posts that began after that date were required to have PMETB approval, irrespective of whether or not they had College approval. This approval had to be prospective, i.e. obtained before the post is started, as PMETB is unable to grant retrospective approval of training.

Special guidance applied to flexible training programmes/posts that were running between 30 September 2005 and 31 July 2006. Where a trainee had documentary evidence of approval of flexible training by the deanery and the Royal College of Psychiatrists, PMETB agreed to accept that recognition and consider the training approved. This training could contribute to a CCT. Any existing training that took place before 30 September 2005 that had College approval was recognised and deemed approved by PMETB.

Applications for approval of flexible training made between 1 August 2006 and 30 November 2007 were processed under PMETB guidance published in April and November 2006. This guidance required that applications came from the deanery with a covering letter giving its support and a completed PMETB Form B obtained from the PMETB website. Form B had to be accompanied by a description of the learning objectives of the flexible training, a timetable and a copy of the trainee's CV. Applications had to be sent prospectively. Any flexible training that took place between 1 August 2006 and 30 November 2007 without prospective PMETB approval could not contribute to a CCT, and trainees were required to apply to have this training counted towards a certificate of specialist registration (CEFR).

New PMETB requirements for flexible training from 1 December 2007 were published on the PMETB website (http://www.pmetb.org.uk/fileadmin/user/QA/Post_and_programme_approval/Flexible_training.doc) in November 2007. The requirement to complete a PMETB Form B for every new flexible training placement/slot/course was discontinued from 1 December 2007. Under the November guidance the deaneries, in conjunction with the medical Royal Colleges, take responsibility for ensuring that all flexible training of any kind is undertaken in prospectively approved posts and programmes, and that it meets the statutory requirements of the General and Specialist Medical Practice (Education, Training and Qualifications) Order 2003. Thus, the deanery is not required to send a separate set of individual approval applications for flexible training if it is within the approved maximum capacity of the specialty training programme. Full guidance is available on the PMETB website (http://www.pmetb.org.uk).

Individual Colleges are allowed to have their own processes for ensuring that flexible training meets the required standards, and the Royal College of Psychiatrists will be putting these standards in place. It is up to the Colleges to set the amended CCT date, and they will require prospective evidence of flexible training in order to recommend the award of the CCT to PMETB. Thus, although PMETB remains the only body that can approve such training, it lays responsibility for quality management at the deanery level, in conjunction with the Colleges.

Conclusions

Flexibility in working hours is now part of mainstream thinking. As more women with dependent children remain in employment, so will the demand for flexible working continue to increase. The medical profession has pioneered flexible working among medical trainees and this has evolved over the past 35 years in response to the needs of trainees, demands of the service and budgetary constraints. Supernumerary flexible training posts have existed for many years and have been very successful. With women now making up more than half of new medical graduates, a culture change and review of the system is needed, with a focus on career planning and development. It is essential that more opportunities for flexible training are implemented in order to improve the working lives of doctors and to retain them in the NHS workforce. Extending and integrating the flexible training scheme, and flexible working in general, may be popular with men and women who wish to work less than full-time but who do not have children.

Flexible working should not be the preserve of trainees. The new consultant contract should make it easier to design flexible working patterns for them too. However, a cultural change is needed to enable the establishment of stand-alone part-time consultant posts (Gray *et al*, 2005).

References and further reading

Allen, I. (1988) *Doctors and their Careers*. Policy Studies Institute.

Allen, I. (1994) *Doctors and their Careers: A New Generation*. Policy Studies Institute.

Allen, I. (1996) Career preferences of doctors. *BMJ*, **313**, 2.

Allen, I. (2005) Women doctors and their careers: what now? *BMJ*, **331**, 569–572.

Allen, I., Paice, E., Hale, R., *et al* (1999) *Stress among Consultants in North Thames*. Policy Studies Institute & North Thames Department of Postgraduate Medical and Dental Education.

Bowen-Simpkins, P., Mellows, H. & Dhillon, C. (2004) Royal College of Obstetricians and Gynaecologists mentoring scheme. *BMJ Career Focus*, **328**, 56.

Chambers, R., Mohanna, K. & Thornett, A. (2003) Changing the culture to support doctors' careers. *BMJ Career Focus*, **326**, s193–s194.

Clay, B. (1998) Flexible training? What are the opportunities? *BMJ Career Focus*, **316**, 2.

Conference of Postgraduate Medical Deans (1995) *SHO Training: Tackling the Issues, Raising the Standards. Report of Conference of Postgraduate Medical Deans (COPMeD) Working Party*. COPMeD.

Davidson, J. M., Lambert, T. W., Goldacre, M., *et al* (2002) UK senior doctors' career destinations, job satisfaction, and future intentions: questionnaire survey. *BMJ*, **325**, 685–686.

Dean, A., El Abd, A. & York, A. (1999) Flexible higher training in psychiatry: attitudes and perceptions of flexible trainees. *Psychiatric Bulletin*, **23**, 613–615.

Department of Health (1969) *Re-employment of Women Doctors* (HM(69)6). Department of Health.

Department of Health (1979) *Opportunities for Part-Time Training in the NHS for Doctors and Dentists with Domestic Commitments, Disability or Ill-health*. Department of Health, (PM(79)3). Department of Health.

Department of Health (1991) *Women Doctors and their Careers*. Department of Health.

Department of Health (1995) *Planning the Medical Workforce. Second Report of the Medical Workforce Standing Advisory Committee*. Department of Health.

Department of Health (2002) *Improving Working Lives For Doctors*. Department of Health.

Department of Health (2004) *Hospital, Public Health, Medicine and Community Health Services Medical and Dental Staff in England: 1993–2003*. Department of Health.

Dornhurst, A., Cripps, J., Goodyear, H., *et al* (2005) Improving hospital doctors' working lives: online questionnaire survey of all grades. *Postgraduate Medical Journal*, **81**, 49–54.

Dosani, S. (2003*a*) Flexible training: moving on and up. *BMJ Career Focus*, **326**, S85.

Dosani, S. (2003*b*) Implications of the gender revolution in medicine. *BMJ Career Focus*, **326**, S159.

Etchegoyen, A., Stormont, F. & Goldberg, I. (2001) Career success after flexible training. A survey of former flexible trainees in the Thames Region. *British Journal of Hospital Medicine*, **62**, 355–357.

Evans, J., Goldacre, M. J. & Lambert, T.W. (2000). Views of medical students about flexible and part-time working in medicine: a qualitative study. *Medical Education*, **34**, 355–362.

Firth-Cozens, J. (1994) The five years after qualification. *BMJ*, **309**, 1524–1525.

Flexible Training Committee of COPMeD (2005) *Annual Survey of Flexible Trainees*. COPMeD.

Gibson, H. (1997*a*) Are part-time doctors better doctors? *BMJ Careers Focus*, **315**, 2–3.

Gibson, H. (1997*b*) The system must change. Personal view. *BMJ*, **314**, 1286–1287.

Goldberg, I. (1997) Flexible training in psychiatry. *Psychiatric Bulletin*, **21**, 387–388.

Goldberg, I. (2002) *Review of Established Flexible Training Posts at SHO Grade in the Thames Regions*. London Department of Postgraduate Medical and Dental Education.

Goldberg, I. & Hornung, R. (1998) Doctors need flexible training and flexible jobs. *BMJ*, **316**, 1169.

Goldberg, I. & Maingay, J. (1997) Eligible for flexible training? *BMJ*, **315**, 2–3.

Goldberg, I. & Paice, E. (1999) Flexible training compared with full-time training. *Hospital Medicine*, **60**, 286–290.

Goldberg, I. & Paice, E. (2000) Job sharing in medical training: an evaluation of a 3-year project. *Hospital Medicine*, **61**, 125–128.

Gray, S., Finlay, I. & Black, C. (2005) Women doctors and their careers: what now? *BMJ*, **331**, 696.

Haine, L. & Rogers, M. (2005) A flexible career – making it work. *BMJ Career Focus*, **330**, 116–117.

Heath, I. (2004) Women in medicine. *BMJ*, **329**, 412–413.

Herzberg, J. & Goldberg, I. (1999) A survey of flexible trainees in psychiatry in the North and South Thames Regions. *Psychiatric Bulletin*, **23**, 616–618.

Jones, R. & Cawley, H. (1997) Job sharing. *BMJ*, **314**, 2.

Kapadia, L. H. (1996) Women at work. *BMJ*, **313**, 1073–1076.

Killaspy, H., Johnson, S., Livingston, G., *et al* (2003) Women in academic psychiatry in the United Kingdom. *Psychiatric Bulletin*, **27**, 323–326.

Klemperer, F. & Ramsay, R. (2000) Working part time as a consultant. *BMJ Career Focus*, **321**, 2–3. doi:10.1136/bmj.321.7272.S2-7272.

Kvaerner, K., Aasland, O. G. & Botten, G. S. (1999) Female medical leadership: cross sectional study. *BMJ*, **318**, 91–94.

Leaman, C. & Lyle, S. (2002) Training late – from branch to mainline at 40. *Psychiatric Bulletin*, **26**, 233–234.

Maingay, J. & Goldberg, I. (1998) Flexible training opportunities in the European Union. *Medical Education*, **32**, 543–548.

Mather, H. M. (2001) Specialists registrars' plans for working part time as consultants in medical specialties: questionnaire study. *BMJ*, **322**, 1578–1579.

McDonald, R. (2003*a*) Flexible and family friendly working in the NHS. *BMJ Career Focus*, **326**, s59–s60.

McDonald, R. (2003*b*) Informing choices: the inside story. *BMJ Career Focus*, **326**, s191.

McManus, C. & Sprotson, K. A. (1999) Women in hospital medicine in the United Kingdom: glass ceiling, prejudice or cohort effect? *Journal of Epidemiology and Community Health*, **54**, 10–16.

McNally, S. (1999) Having a baby as a surgical trainee. *BMJ Career Focus*, **319**, S2–S3.

Mears, A., Kendall, T., Katona, C., *et al* (2002) *Career Intentions of Psychiatric Trainees and Consultants*. Department of Health.

Mears, A., Kendall, T., Katona, C., *et al* (2004*a*) Retirement intentions of older consultant psychiatrists. *Psychiatric Bulletin*, **28**, 130–132.

Mears, A., Etchegoyen, A., Stormont, F., *et al* (2004*b*) Female psychiatrists' career development after flexible training. *Psychiatric Bulletin*, **28**, 201–203.

Modernising Medical Careers (2007) *A Guide to Postgraduate Specialty Training in the UK: The Gold Guide*. Department of Health. http://www.mmc.nhs.uk/download_files/Gold_Guide_290607.doc

Morrell, J. E. & Roberts, A. J. (1992) Making an application for part-time senior registrar training. *BMJ*, **305**, 1411–1413.

NHS Employers (2005) *Doctors in Flexible Training: Principles Underpinning the New Arrangements for Flexible Training*. NHS Employers.

NHS Executive (1996) *A Guide to Specialist Training*. NHS Executive.

NHS Management Executive (1993) *Flexible Training: Report of the Joint Working Party*. NHS Management Executive.

Norcliffe, G. & Finlan, C. (1999) Attitudes to flexible training. *BMJ*, **318** (7185), 2.

Peters, E., Flett, A., Challis, M., *et al* (2000) Perceptions of flexible training in medicine. *Hospital Medicine*, **61**, 129–132.

Ramsay, R. (2004) Women in Psychiatry Special Interest Group. *BMJ Career Focus*, **328**, 116.

Redfern, N. & Scriven, P. (1998) Flexible training is possible as a senior house officer. *BMJ*, **316** (7128), 2.

Rees, L. & Van Someren, V. (1984) Personal view. *BMJ*, 289.

Reichenbach, L. & Brown, H. (2004) Gender and academic medicine: impacts on health workforce. *BMJ*, **329**, 792–795.

Roberts, J. H. (2005) The feminisation of medicine. *BMJ Career Focus*, **330**, 13–15.

Royal College of Physicians (2004) *Briefing on Women in Medicine*. Royal College of Physicians.

Schofield, C. & Schofield, Z. (2005) Flexible training for men and women – is this the way forward? *BMJ*, **331**, 1211.

Scriven, P. (1996) Flexible training as a specialist registrar. *BMJ*, **313**, (7055), 2.

Showalter, E. (1999) Improving the position of women in medicine. *BMJ*, **318**, 71–72.

Sinha, A. & Cook, A. (1997) What do medical students think of flexible training. *BMJ*, **315** (7121), 2.

Sundaram, R. (2003) An insider's guide to flexible training. *BMJ Career Focus*, **327**, 61.

Valentine, J. P. & Martin, C. J. (1996) Job sharing at a children's hospital: evaluation by medical staff. *BMJ*, **312**, 115–116.

Warren, V. J. & Wakeford, R. E. (1989) 'We'd like to have a family' – young women doctors' opinions of maternity leave and part-time training. *Journal of the Royal Society of Medicine*, **82**, 528–531.

CHAPTER 29

UK training for overseas doctors and opportunities for UK doctors to train outside the EEC

Nick Rose

The National Health Service (NHS) is by far the largest postgraduate medical training organisation in Europe, with about a third of its 21 000 senior house officer junior doctors having an overseas medical degree. At present, the NHS is a monopoly provider of specialist training in the UK, although this may change as the government increasingly buys services from the private sector. Standards for training are set by the Postgraduate Medical Education and Training Board (PMETB) in collaboration with the medical Royal Colleges, and involve professional examinations and inspection of training posts and schemes.

The General Medical Council (GMC) is the regulator of the medical profession in the UK, and is there to protect the interests of patients. All doctors wishing to practise in the UK must be registered and given a licence to practise. This licence must be revalidated on a regular basis, and for this individual doctors must satisfy the GMC that they are up to date and fit to practise.

Postgraduate training arrangements brought in by the government-created Modernising Medical Careers (Box 29.1) initiative during 2006/7

Box 29.1 Abbreviations and acronyms

Although I have used abbreviations and acronyms sparingly in this chapter, those below are common in the discussion of medical training in the UK

CASS   Consultant Assisted Sponsorship Scheme
IELTS   International English Language Testing System
IMG   international medical graduate
ITF   international training fellowship
MMC   Modernising Medical Careers
PLAB   Professional and Linguistics Assessment Board
PMETB   Postgraduate Medical Education and Training Board

---

proved unworkable, and following a highly critical inquiry by Sir John Tooke (Tooke, 2007), further changes are planned from 2008. These are likely to include retaining the pre-registration Foundation year 1; incorporating Foundation year 2 as the first of a 3-year core training programme for psychiatry; abandoning the concept of a 6-year 'run through' specialty training programme; and basing entry into higher psychiatric specialty training on marks obtained in national assessment centres, with each deanery undertaking structured interviews for shortlisted candidates selected on the basis of curricula vitae (CVs).

Other changes introduced by Modernising Medical Careers and in the process of being implemented by the Royal College of Psychiatrists will remain in place. These include the programme of workplace assessments, the new competency-based curriculum and the impending changes in the MRCPsych examinations (see Chapter 27, this volume). Existing non-training junior posts such as trust doctors and staff-grade doctors will remain for the present, but are likely to be developed into a new cadre of competency-defined service posts in due course.

How can an overseas doctor obtain specialty training in the UK?

Competition for UK specialist training posts in all specialties is likely to increase over the next few years. This is partly because UK medical schools have increased their output by over 50% in the past 10 years, and partly because government investment in the NHS and in new medical posts is planned to slow over the next 5 years. This has meant that the large-scale employment of doctors from outside the European Economic Area (EEA) is no longer needed to run the NHS. In a controversial move in mid-2006, the government therefore introduced a Home Office work permit requirement for all individuals who are not European Economic Community (EEC) nationals – non-EEC nationals – wanting to train in the UK. Work permits would normally be issued only when a UK or EEC national could not be appointed to a vacancy. European Economic Community nationals were not affected by these new requirements.

In October 2007, the GMC introduced a new registration framework for all doctors no matter where they qualify. The main changes were the abolition of limited registration, the introduction of approved medical settings for all medical graduates and the introduction of a new framework of provisional and full registration. The implication for non-EEC nationals is that although they will need to satisfy rigorous criteria before they are registered, they no longer need an offer of employment; although if they wish to work or train in the UK, they will still need a Home Office work permit. Provisional registration is given for doctors who have not completed a pre-registration post. All new full registrants taking up new jobs (including UK graduates) and doctors returning to the register after a prolonged period out of UK practice will be required to work initially in GMC-approved practice settings.

Doctors who are not UK or EEC nationals, sometimes known as international medical graduates, therefore currently have reduced access to training in the UK because of the combined effect of work permit requirements and the lack of unfilled training posts. However, they are still able to compete for jobs in the UK, and to do so they need to obtain GMC registration. This requires them to pass both parts of the Professional and Linguistics Assessment Board (PLAB) test as well as provide evidence of a good standard of spoken and written English on the International English Language Testing System (IELTS). Part 1 of the PLAB can be taken at one of about 120 overseas centres run by the British Council, whereas part 2 must be taken in the UK. The IELTS can also be taken overseas, although doctors are exempt if they have obtained their primary medical qualification from a university where the language of instruction and examination is English and if they have practised for 2 years preceding registration in a country in which the principal working language is English.

For some years, the Royal College of Psychiatrists has been involved in sponsoring international medical graduates of exceptional ability to train in the UK, most recently under a Consultant Assisted Sponsorship Scheme (CASS). However, sponsorship arrangements were revised in 2007 to bring them into line with new government requirements. As a result, CASS was suspended and new sponsorship arrangements are to be introduced during 2008. These are likely to be in the form of international training fellowships.

The Home Office recently introduced international training fellowships as part of the Medical Training Initiative, which allows international medical graduates to be sponsored for up to 2 years for advanced training in the UK. They would not normally be sponsored for core or basic training. Individuals with international training fellowships would be exempt from PLAB and work permit requirements, but would still have to pass the IELTS, unless they were able to meet the language criteria given earlier. They would be required to leave the UK at the end of their training period, and the period of training would not count towards the award of a certificate of completion of training needed for inclusion on the GMC's specialist register, although it could be considered as part of an application under article 14.

It is envisaged that the overseas sponsor would be a senior doctor at a postgraduate institution, and the UK sponsor would be the head of a deanery school of psychiatry supported by the postgraduate dean. The number of placements is likely to be relatively small, and in more specialist fields such as child or forensic psychiatry. However, because national training arrangements remained in a state of flux as this book went to press, international medical graduate doctors are strongly advised to get up-to-date information on training opportunities before coming to the UK. Information on sponsorship will be available on the Royal College of Psychiatrists website (http://www.rcpsych.ac.uk).

Doctors trained in the EEC are free to compete for training posts in the UK provided that the GMC recognises the training institute where they obtained their primary medical qualification. They would then be exempt from the PLAB test, would not need to be sponsored, would not need a work permit, and would not be required to take the IELTS. The onus would be on the employer to ensure that the candidate's linguistic skills were fit for the job. To enter specialist psychiatric training beyond year 1, they would need to demonstrate that they had the equivalent level of competency to UK trainees for the year they planned to join. This would normally include evidence of formal assessment results and confirmation of accredited specialist training experience.

Training in the UK: why bother?

By any standard the NHS is an extraordinary organisation. As a nationalised industry under tight central control, it provides over 99% of specialist psychiatric care to the people of UK. And although it is poorly sensitive to market forces that might otherwise shape it, it is very sensitive to populist political agendas. From 2001, as a result of public demand and political prioritisation, it has benefited from unprecedented investment. At present it is building more new large hospitals than all the other G7 countries put together, although this building bonanza will slow from 2008, when investment in the NHS is set to decline.

As a single system with a budget of £76 billion for England alone in 2005–2006, the NHS can respond on a national scale to central command. This means that new initiatives can be rolled out across the country with speed. For example, recently imported Australian and American innovatory models of community care have been quickly replicated nationwide as a result of political will and targeted new investment. The most important of these models are 'crisis teams' to intensively support people at home who would otherwise be in hospital, and 'assertive outreach teams' to work with people who have severe mental health problems but are hard to engage with once they leave hospital. These changes have completely altered the way psychiatric services are delivered, and have opened up many new and exciting training opportunities unavailable in most other Western countries. In addition, recent major investment in renewing the NHS estate has meant that most psychiatric services are now delivered from relatively new and purpose-built units. The often remote and hard to adapt 19th-century hospitals inherited from the Victorians and replicated worldwide have now been pretty much confined to history.

Psychiatric training in the UK is overseen by the Royal College of Psychiatrists, which has a long track record of ensuring that trainees have regular access to good-quality academic and clinical support, wherever they are working. For example, all trainees must be able to attend an academic day-release course, and receive an hour of professional development supervision each week, in addition to having regular clinical supervision. The College is also developing a new competency-oriented psychiatric curriculum and assessment system that, along with similar developments in Canada and the USA, promises to be a world leader. These changes started in August 2007 and are aimed at further improving UK specialist training.

Two further changes are also worthy of note. The NHS has for some years adopted an evidenced-based approach to clinical decision-making and to the design of patient services. This way of thinking is now firmly embedded in psychiatric culture and integrated into training at every level. The second change is more of a lifestyle issue. Since August 2007, the European Working Time Directive has limited the working hours of junior doctors to 56 hours a week, and by August 2009 the limit will be further reduced to 48 hours. This means that trainees are reasonably protected from working excessive hours, allowing them to achieve a better work–home balance.

Why training in the UK may not be for you

Training, like psychiatry, is to some extent culture bound. What is appropriate for one sociocultural context may be out of place in another. In the UK, training is influenced by many factors, including the College curriculum, the UK economy, the demands of the NHS, and (in the post-Shipman era) the need to meet politically inspired national agendas about what society requires of doctors.

How does this play out for doctors coming to train in the UK? On the positive side, there is ample opportunity for much valued sub-specialty experience in areas such as child psychiatry, psychotherapy and forensic psychiatry, which can provide training simply not available in many countries. But this has to be set against the fact that many skills learnt in the UK may not be relevant in the trainees' country of origin, either because of resource constraints (for example, providing intensive community care), or because of cultural inappropriateness (for example, some forms of psychotherapy). Likewise, particularly useful skills for working in less rich countries, such as those in clinical service development and public health, including the prioritisation of fixed resources, are generally not well covered in UK training.

It is therefore important to ask yourself how useful it would be to train in one economic and sociocultural setting in order to work in an entirely different one. How would the experience help you to provide a better service for your patients and trainees in the future?

How to prepare for training in the UK

Most importantly, you should check the job market before committing yourself to coming. This is because it is in a constant state of change. Before 2006, for example, there were too few doctors chasing too many jobs, many newly created with increased NHS funding. The combined effect of boosting local medical student numbers by 50%, substantial migration of EEC and international doctors to the UK, a slowing down in the creation of newly funded jobs, and the early effects of devolving some medical skills to others has caused the situation to flip. As a result, in 2005–2006 there was an unprecedented level of unemployment among junior doctors. Competition for places on UK training schemes is likely to intensify, making it harder for international medical graduates to obtain the newly required work permits. It is also possible that the GMC may restrict the number of applicants allowed to take the PLAB test. Under such conditions, it would be important to consider coming to the UK only if you had a job offer.

Adjusting to NHS life in the UK

Daily living

Living overseas can be tough. Housing, being away from family and friends, finances, schools, driving, isolation, tax, food, weather (lots of it) and all the countless minutiae of taken-for-granted everyday things can all mount up. The College produces a helpful leaflet on getting by, and the organisation that employs you should also be an important source of information.

Expectations

Experienced overseas trainees can find it quite difficult adjusting to the fact that the status of doctors may be more challenged by other disciplines than might have been the case back home. In addition, clinical placements may be miles away from the main training centre. And all the while, the expectations of those back in the home country may create a constant pressure to succeed.

NHS culture

At a local level, team-working skills are not only important in delivering care, but are now a key learning objective for all medical postgraduates, and are assessed accordingly. Working closely with colleagues from nursing, social work, psychology and occupational health is especially important. Also, at a local level it is important to be familiar with the considerable number of local and national protocols and standards that have become part of NHS care delivery. Examples include the care programme approach (CPA), National Institute for Health and Clinical Excellence (NICE) guidelines, and the National Service Framework (NSF) for Mental Health.

Nationally, the NHS quite rightly puts meeting the needs of patients and carers, together with patient choice, firmly at the top of its agenda. Within mental health, it has prioritised services for people with severe illnesses, and in particular has invested heavily in forensic and assertive outreach services following a number of high-profile homicides by mentally ill people. There is also a national target to reduce suicides. Given that the government runs the NHS, and given that the NHS is a potential election winner (or loser), it is not surprising that the British media have become fascinated by bad medical outcomes, which in turn has resulted in the service becoming more risk sensitive in an already litigious culture. Adjusting to working in this value system, which emphasises individual accountability, tight clinical governance and adherence to set procedures, is crucial for anyone wanting to train in the NHS.

Patients and their carers

Probably the biggest single difference a trainee from a less financially well-off country would notice is the way Western culture positions the individual rather than the family at the centre of things. In many subtle ways this serves the interests of consumer culture, but means that many people live alone and carers may have little support from extended families.

Real or perceived discrimination

Generally, the UK is reasonably successful at being a multicultural society. One recent milestone was the highly publicised conclusion of the MacPherson Inquiry in 1999 that the police were guilty of 'institutional racism', as shown by the way they had investigated the murder of Stephen Lawrence, a man of African–Caribbean ethnicity. Soon afterwards, the NHS was required by law to provide its services in a way that was non-discriminatory, even in an unintended way, and to monitor its performance. These changes have been accompanied by a policy of zero tolerance of racial harassment against NHS staff. Importantly, the NHS itself is very much a multicultural workforce, nearly a half of the doctors it employs having trained overseas.

This is not to say that discrimination or harassment never takes place. There is certainly ongoing debate in the medical press about a perceived glass ceiling to promotion in some specialties, although psychiatry has good representation from ethnic minorities, both among the consultant workforce and on the main College committees and examination boards.

What may help you settle in once you arrive

Some tips to help you settle in professionally

Get an induction pack for overseas doctors from the College and enlist on the next induction day. Make the most of any clinical attachment by getting to know how the health system works, talking with patients, using the dictaphone, searching databases and being generally curious about how things are made to happen.

When you start paid work, make sure you attend a local induction programme which, apart from giving you essential information and training, will also give you a chance to meet other trainees together with key people in the organisation. See your nominated trainer regularly, always asking when you are not sure. Get your trainer or supervisor to give you regular feedback, some of it based on direct observations of your clinical performance. Establish close links with junior doctor colleagues, who can give you tips on the local system and on how to survive in the UK. Some training schemes have a mentoring scheme, where you team up with a more experienced junior doctor; do this if you have the opportunity or set it up on your own.

It is well worth joining the College as a psychiatric trainee member. You will then be sent information on College educational meetings, including the international forum at the annual general meeting, at which overseas doctors' training issues are discussed. Your employer will give you study leave and a study budget, which normally covers fees and expenses for courses and meetings. And, finally, remember that good psychiatric care stands or falls on that hard to pin down skill, the quality of your thinking. As Einstein is reported to have said, imagination is more important than knowledge. So use every opportunity to discuss cases and issues in depth and with imagination, so as to improve this cross-cultural skill, which should then stay with you wherever you choose to work in future.

UK trainees wanting experience overseas

Trainee psychiatrists on UK schemes can have an overseas training post counted towards eligibility to take MRCPsych part 2, but not part 1. Such overseas training posts must be for a minimum of 6 months' duration and are approved on an individual basis by the Examinations Sub-Dean in the College. There are also four overseas schemes fully approved by the College (Bermuda, Cairo, Hong Kong, Malta) for MRCPsych training. Some UK training schemes also have links with overseas programmes.

In 2005 the College developed a volunteer programme that allows those doing higher training to arrange an 'out-of-programme' placement approved by the College towards requirements for the certificate of completion of training. This scheme is for individuals in their fifth or sixth year of specialist training, and is aimed at creating opportunities for UK psychiatrists to work in less well off countries in ways that are mutually beneficial to all involved. Such overseas placements need to have an affiliation or formal attachment to a university department, a hospital or the ministry of health in the host country, as well as a local mentor, usually either a Member or Fellow of the College or an individually approved senior psychiatrist. In addition, the trainee needs to have a mentor in the UK, usually an approved trainer, who has knowledge of the country of placement. Provided that these conditions are met, and approval is sought prospectively, up to 1 year of an overseas placement can be approved.

Although the changes introduced by modernising medical careers initially appeared to make it harder for UK trainees to work overseas, the Tooke inquiry (Tooke, 2007) has recommended that doctors undertaking core training should be able to spend up to 12 months working abroad while still retaining their UK training place, and this flexibility should also apply to advanced specialty training.

Conclusions

Although setting up a period of overseas training can be time-consuming, the stimulation of practising psychiatry in a completely different setting, and of seeing your specialty from an entirely new perspective, is immensely refreshing and may well become an experience that makes a lasting difference to your professional development.

Reference

Tooke, J. (2007) *Aspiring to Excellence: Findings and Recommendations of the Independent Inquiry into Modernising Medical Careers*. MMC Inquiry.

CHAPTER 30

Academic careers

Anne Farmer

Deciding that you want to be a clinical academic psychiatrist in the UK is not a career choice for the faint-hearted. Although combining academic and clinical interests is stimulating and fulfilling, none the less it involves many additional stresses that do not affect those who work entirely in a clinical setting.

First, as a clinical academic psychiatrist you serve two masters: the NHS trust for which you do your clinical work and the university for which you do your academic work. The number of programmed activities belonging to each will be carefully detailed in your job plan. At the time of writing, the majority of clinical academic psychiatrists spend 50% of their time working in the NHS and 50% for the university. The latter will be committed either to undergraduate and postgraduate teaching or to research. Clinical academics whose university time is spent on research are being increasingly pressured to obtain research funding, carry out the research and publish the results in high-impact journals (a journal whose papers are widely cited by others); the greater the number of citations an 'average' paper receives, the higher the impact score of the journal. This is due to the demands of the research assessment exercise (RAE), a regular (currently 5-yearly) peer review of all university academic departments' research activity. Each university and academic department is ranked according to the international standing of its academic staff. Those with the highest ranking (currently a score of 6) receive the most financial support from the government. Consequently, like football teams, some major universities engage in headhunting 'star players', that is, individuals with the best track record of obtaining research grants and whose publications appear in high-impact international journals. From 2010, the RAE will be replaced by a 'metrics'-based assessment for university academics. In addition to publications and grant income, this will include other measures of esteem in its evaluation.

Not all universities seek to engage in the RAE rounds of assessment. Instead, they focus on their teaching activities and in this respect academic departments are ranked on the teaching quality assessment (TQA). Although the ranking in the TQA is not as directly linked as the RAE to a university department's income, having a good reputation for teaching attracts more students, and more students means more fee income for the department. Hence, departments of psychiatry that do not participate in the RAE and that designate themselves as teaching departments will wish to employ clinical academics whose excellence is in undergraduate and postgraduate teaching and whose research is (arguably) less important. However, in practice most clinical academics do both research and teaching, as well as participate in service delivery.

Whether your career ambitions to become a clinical academic psychiatrist lie in research or teaching, your training will take longer to complete than that of doctors whose ambitions are to become entirely clinical consultant psychiatrists. This is largely because of the difficulty in completing both the clinical and academic requirements of training. Although in the past it was just possible to undergo higher clinical training while simultaneously studying for a Doctor of Medicine (MD) or Doctor of Philosophy (PhD) qualification, this has become increasingly difficult. For the majority of aspiring academic clinicians it is necessary to take time out of clinical training to obtain a doctorate.

Getting started

Graduate-entry medical training schemes enable students to obtain some research experience before starting their clinical studies. Similarly, undertaking an intercalated Bachelor of Science (BSc) or PhD programme while at medical school is a good first step on the ladder. Spending one or more years engaged in full-time academic enquiry provides an opportunity to see whether you are fired with enthusiasm for a particular area of research. Undertaking research of sufficient quality to get a paper published at this stage in your career is extremely helpful too. Obtaining a PhD before you start foundation jobs can also make your career path less arduous at a later stage. However, this is not always possible, neither is it necessary.

After completing foundation training it is important to choose a runthrough grade training scheme that allows the opportunity for you to develop your academic ideas and interests. Alternatively, a training scheme that offers opportunities for regular undergraduate teaching and/or interactions with other students would be important for those whose talents lie in teaching. Although it is not usually possible to work for a postgraduate teaching qualification while still in the early stages of training, obtaining lots of experience of teaching in different settings may be possible if you select the right scheme.

Pre-Membership training

During your years of training before you are awarded Membership of the Royal College of Psychiatrists (MRCPsych), you will need to concentrate on obtaining your clinical experience, undertaking sufficient on-call work and on passing parts I and II of the MRCPsych examination (or equivalent following the implementation of the current changes to training and examination). However talented you may be as a researcher or teacher, you will not be able to become a clinical academic without completing your psychiatric training and passing the appropriate exams. Consequently, concentrating on these examinations and passing them at the earliest opportunity allows you to move swiftly on in your training, where it is much easier to build up a research portfolio or take time out of training to complete work for a PhD. Certainly, you would need to obtain a PhD or MD before you could be appointed to a permanent post in a research-oriented university department.

Some deaneries annually advertise academic foundation programmes that include a 4-month research or teaching post. Although it is probably not possible to undertake a major research project in such a short time, it does, none the less, provide an opportunity to participate in an ongoing project.

Post-Membership training

Half or one day a week for research

Once the MRCPsych examination is behind you, you will have moved on to an ST4 clinical appointment. At the time of writing, such posts still include one-half or a full day a week to undertake research or obtain a postgraduate teaching qualification (usually at master's level). However, it is unlikely that this will be sufficient to do the work necessary to complete a doctorate. However, if you are highly motivated and single-minded there is plenty of time to do smaller-scale projects that result in publication. You will need to find the academic psychiatrists locally who can help you with your area of interest, whose research teams you can join and who can provide you with supervision and mentoring. It is very important that you use your research time effectively and do not allow clinical work to encroach into your study time. It is so much easier to use a 'free' day to catch up on clinic letters, see a relative or for other sundry bits of undone clinical business. However, it is important that you do not allow this to happen, and that you use the whole study time to think, plan, read and write.

Full-time research within specialty training

Academic research fellowships provide integrated clinical and research training and enable post-Membership trainees to undertake full-time research to obtain a PhD or MD, apply for an Medical Research Council (MRC) or Wellcome Trust training fellowship, and continue their clinical experience. Such posts involve full-time research, working on a specific project, for example running a research team, recruiting trial participants, or carrying out clinical assessments or other laboratory-based or imaging procedures. There is usually time within such posts for trainees to do work on their own projects or to undertake a doctorate. It would clearly help if your own project were in the same area of research as that on which you are employed. Most posts include a session or two a week for limited clinical work.

Obtaining a full-time research post means that you will give up your salary on a substantive specialist training scheme and you will become an employee of a university department. Although your basic salary will remain the same, you may not have the same opportunity to undertake on-call work and you may also forfeit your right to any study-leave payments.

Undertaking a doctorate (MD or PhD)

The equivalent consultant-level post for an aspiring clinical academic is that of senior lecturer, and for appointment as a senior lecturer most university departments would require that you have completed your clinical training and that you are eligible to go on the specialist register, i.e. that you can perform the duties of a consultant psychiatrist. In addition, you should have obtained your doctorate and have a number of publications in peer-reviewed journals. Ideally, for the RAE, academic departments want their staff to have publications that have arisen from hypothesis-driven research rather than reviews or book chapters. To date, the RAE panels that assess the worth of each academic department review the four 'best' publications from each 'returned' staff member. Hence, in appointing a senior lecturer, academic departments are looking for at least four such publications.

A PhD or MD is a substantial piece of research work, usually requiring a period of 2 or 3 years for data collection and analysis and the writing of the thesis (see chapter 31, this volume). Most university libraries keep copies of PhD and MD theses and these can provide you with some idea as to the scale of the work required. Much research these days requires the efforts of a whole team of individuals, sometimes in more than one department or even one country. Therefore, provided that the greatest part of your thesis is your own work, reliance on others for some part of it is acceptable provided that this is acknowledged.

Once your thesis has been written, checked for the umpteenth time, reviewed by your supervisor in careful detail and undergone its final revision, it is time to submit it and prepare for the *viva voce*, your 'defence' of your thesis. Known for short as the viva, this is an intense 2–3 h discussion with two experts in your research area. Usually, one of your examiners will be from your own department and the other will be an external examiner who can be nominated by your supervisor. In the viva your examiners will undertake a careful review of your methodology, statistics, results, conclusions, etc. They will decide whether your thesis is acceptable for the award of a PhD or MD or whether you need to undertake any corrections to your text or even any further analyses. By the time you get to your viva it is unlikely that you will fail, but having to undertake further work on your thesis can be arduous.

Medical Research Council (MRC) and Wellcome Trust training fellowships

Academic research fellowships are expected to lead not only to a higher degree but also to an application for one of the prestigious training fellowships. These highly prized and highly competitive awards allow you to undertake your own research by paying your salary for 3 years. These post-doctoral fellowships are equivalent to the old-style clinical lecturer position.

Postgraduate teaching qualifications

The half or full day a week for research that is available in specialist training gives individuals who wish to become university teachers an opportunity to study for postgraduate qualifications in teaching. Many universities offer part-time postgraduate diplomas or master's courses in medical education.

Is it all worth it?

After you have succeeded in obtaining your PhD, publishing some adequate papers in high-impact peer-reviewed journals and are starting to embark on presenting your research at national and international conferences you are finally beginning to establish your clinical academic career. It is now that the hard work and commitment really begin. Both of your employers, the NHS trust and the university, will expect more than 50% of your time. Inevitably, you will spend long hours after you have completed a busy out-patient clinic, preparing your presentation for tomorrow's conference. You will then rise early in the morning, to make your way through rush-hour traffic to the local airport. After several hours' travelling to some remote location, you give your presentation and then you travel back, just in time for your ward round, Care Programme Approach (CPA) meetings and so on. The travel may sound exotic, but it is hard work and there is little opportunity for sightseeing. Achieving the right balance between work and personal life can be hard, especially in the early years when you are trying to develop an international reputation. However, it is a necessary part of the job since the only way to establish your academic credibility among your peers is by meeting them at conferences, hearing what research they are doing while they hear about yours.

However, there are also a great many rewards. Undertaking original research gives many of us quite a buzz and the job is never boring. There are constant intellectual challenges. The clinical work keeps your feet on the ground and the contact with patients means that you remain in tune with their difficulties and concerns. This provides a constant reminder of why you do what you do.

Postscript

Many of the brightest medical graduates who have academic ambitions are women, so having read this chapter many of you will want to know whether it is possible to do all this and find time for a family. What about working part time and becoming a clinical academic? The short answer is yes, it is possible but careful planning and an understanding, supportive partner, family or hired help who can take over childcare while you are away at conferences are essential. Some academic work, such as data analysis and writing, can be done quite flexibly, and working from home for some of your academic time is possible. Working at home can be very productive, as many of the usual interruptions to the working day can be filtered or deferred. Indeed, many senior academics choose to work from home 1 day a week, to be free from interruptions to thinking and writing.

For further advice, it is helpful to talk to those who have managed to combine a clinical academic career with taking time out to have a family, and there are now senior female clinical academics in all specialties of psychiatry in the UK. Such role models may be willing to provide mentoring and advice.

CHAPTER 31

Higher degrees

Sube Banerjee

In this brief chapter, I consider what role, if any, a higher degree plays in psychiatric training in the UK. It is written from the viewpoint of a chair of a local PhD committee. It is worthwhile taking a little time to consider this, since undertaking a PhD essentially means that you will spend 3 years full time (or 6 years part time) writing a 60 000-word book that perhaps only two people ever really read: and one of those will be you, but more of this later.

First, we need to define what we mean by a higher degree. If there are 'higher' degrees, then there are presumably 'lower' degrees, and in medicine there are none lower than the basic medical qualifications Bachelor of Medicine and Bachelor of Surgery (abbreviated as MB BS, MB BChir, etc). These are not higher degrees but they do deliver one of the only tangible benefits and incentives of completing a higher degree, in that they confer the (honorary) title of 'doctor'. In Germany you can use the title 'Dr Dr' if you are a medical doctor with a higher degree, but in the UK you do not get an extra title and the only use of 'Doctor Doctor' is as a start to a set of some of the very worst jokes ever composed.

Next there are master's degrees such as Master of Science (MSc), Master of Arts (MA) and Master of Medical Sciences (MMedSci). In the UK these are most commonly 1-year full-time (or 2-year part-time) taught degrees, involving lectures, examination and the completion of a short dissertation, which may well involve a small amount of (usually pointless) original research. Some Scottish Universities give an MA as their basic degree, while Oxford and Cambridge will sell you one for a very reasonable price if you just make it through their undergraduate courses. Taught MScs are often an excellent way of gaining a greater depth of understanding of a specific subject and can help to differentiate a candidate from a crowd at interview, but they are also not 'higher degrees' in the sense we mean it here.

Finally, there are 'higher degrees proper'. There are doctorates available across the academic spectrum, and the PhD (*Philosophiæ Doctor* or Doctor of Philosophy) is the general research doctorate available throughout arts and sciences, including medicine. In addition, specific doctorates are available for specific (often professional) subjects (e.g. MD for medicine, MS for surgery, LLD for law, and DD for divinity). The two higher degrees that may be of relevance to the psychiatric trainee are the PhD (or DPhil at some universities, including Oxford and Sussex) or the MD (from *Medicinæ Doctor* or Doctor of Medicine). Doctor in this sense has the meaning of teacher and the thing that sets these degrees apart is that they are research degrees, the output is a thesis that reports and discusses a substantial piece of independent research, which should make an original contribution to an academic area or discipline.

PhD or MD?

A PhD is generally an individually structured programme of training in how to do research, along with the (simultaneous) completion and writing up of a substantial piece of research. Completing a PhD will therefore generally require some specific technical training supplemented by modelling and learning from two supervisors, who guide the work. The process of carrying out a PhD is increasingly well monitored by universities in an attempt to assure the quality of the experience and to maximise completion rates within stipulated time frames (this is a marker of the effectiveness of the university on which funding depends). Hitherto the main differences between an MD and PhD have been that the elements of training, monitoring and supervision required in a PhD have not been necessary for those completing an MD.

The MD has therefore been considered a more self-directed piece of study with fewer stipulations for study period and supervision. However, there have been concerns raised about the quality of research completed by MD students and the lack of supervision provided. Regulations for MDs and their status relative to PhDs vary markedly between universities: in some MDs are regarded as inferior doctorates, whereas in others (e.g. London and Cambridge) they have a higher status because they are not supervised.

Anderson & Jankowski (2001) compared MDs and PhDs on 15 criteria and found MDs to be superior in two (completion rate and part-time study), PhDs to be superior in eight (supervision, recognition, funding, examination, kudos, scientific training, progress reporting and examiner anonymisation) and for there to be only subjective differences in four (time scale, content, entry criteria and clinical sessions workable). In practice, the ability to do an MD quickly, flexibly, with minimal extra paperwork and while carrying on with higher training has meant that MDs have been more popular than PhDs with doctors of all specialties.

However, things are changing and the motivation for this (quality aside) is university funding. Universities receive much more kudos and funding for PhD students than they do for MDs. The PhD fees are higher for individuals and universities receive further funding for each student enrolled. These funds are also available over a 6-year period if a student is part time. These issues taken together have led universities (and those medical academics employed by them whose budgets are being squeezed) increasingly to tighten up MD regulations and to steer individual students towards the PhD path.

A final consideration is that the MD is the basic medical qualification in the USA and in some other jurisdictions. The higher degree of choice for medics in the USA is the PhD. Therefore there is less international reach in a UK MD, since Americans may not realise how well qualified you are. If you are concerned what Americans think this may be an issue for you.

What is a PhD?

The regulations of the university I work for, King's College London, state that a PhD must:

'form a distinct contribution to the knowledge of the subject and afford evidence of originality by the discovery of new facts and/or by the exercise of independent critical power' (http://www.iop.kcl.ac.uk/virtual/?path=/studying/research/what-is-a-phd).

As noted above, a PhD is also a research training. The PhD student in the course of their study should learn how to develop and investigate scientific theories, how to critically synthesise previous research and develop a new scientific enquiry and how to evaluate the impact of the new data they have generated. Students learn from their supervisors, their own studies and from being in an academic research environment through contacts with other students and researchers.

However, there is only one absolute answer to the question 'What is a PhD?': the PhD is an entry-level qualification into an academic career. As such, it is vital only to that small proportion of psychiatric trainees who wish to pursue (or keep open the possibility of) an academic career.

A PhD can be done on a full-time or a part-time basis. A full-time PhD means doing nothing other than the work for the PhD. It may be possible to do a day's clinical work a week but any more than that will bring into question the full-time status, as well as get in the way of completing the very large amount of work needed.

A PhD involves 3 years' full-time or 6 years' part-time very hard work. It is expensive in time, energy and also in money if work or opportunities for advancement are foregone to complete the degree. Many who start a PhD find the process lonely (you may be a sole researcher with little direct contact with supervisors), anxiety-provoking (Is what I am doing right? Is it enough?) and eventually a waste of time (What have I learned? What good has this done me?).

For psychiatric trainees the costs can be minimised by completing the PhD as part of a training fellowship, or by being employed as a researcher on a grant where the data for the PhD is obtained. In a training fellowship the Medical Research Council, the Wellcome Trust or the Department of Health pay you for 3 or 4 years study. This may start with an MSc or other period of training, followed by 2 or 3 years of full-time supervised research, during which you generate the data for your PhD and also write the thing up. Applications for such fellowships have at their core a high-quality, well-designed scientific protocol for research and the desire to invest in the development of individuals who will be the next generation of lead researchers. Unsurprisingly, these fellowships are few and very highly sought after. In the three mentioned above, you as a psychiatrist will be measured against doctors in training from any specialty and in the case of the Department of Health fellowships also with everyone else in the NHS who wants a PhD.

Why do a higher degree?

The only absolute indication for doing a higher degree is a desire to pursue a formal academic career. Although there are likely to be many examples of distinguished senior lecturers, readers and professors of psychiatry who have risen to eminence without a higher degree, they did so under a different system with different rules. Now it is almost impossible to become a senior academic without a higher degree and it is almost certainly not worth trying. So if you want to be employed by a reputable university as a senior lecturer or above (and therefore have a consultant's salary) you will need to have an MD or a PhD, with the PhD increasingly valued over the MD.

No other psychiatric trainee needs to do a higher degree. Reasons cited for doing one anyway include the following (in parentheses I show why these reasons are potentially silly):

- wanting to keep the academic option open (at high cost and, if you are not absolutely committed to being an academic, it probably will not work out anyway)
- interest in a particular subject (nothing is guaranteed to make you heartily sick of a subject than being tied to it for 3–6 years and having to write a thesis on it)
- having it recommended by an academic (not all that glisters is altruism: the academic may be being pressured into finding PhD students to increase income, they may be looking to get some research done cheaply and, even if well-motivated, they may not understand your career needs)
- to improve employability (this has never really applied in psychiatry and matters less and less in medicine and surgery as new posts are created; a higher degree will make your CV look different and may help to get you shortlisted in some posts, but it may work against you if you are going for a 'normal' consultant job and you are perceived really to

be interested in being an academic who will therefore be sneaking off to do research, leaving colleagues with the clinical work)

- raise your earning potential (this is a motivation for non-clinical researchers but should not be for psychiatric trainees: you will earn no more if you have a higher degree, and if you pursue an academic career you are likely to become a consultant later and have lower earnings, for example via private practice, than your clinical peers)
- to gain a prestigious qualification (those who have not got one will not notice that you have one and those that have will not care)
- as a personal challenge, to prove that you can do it, as a voyage of personal development (there are a lot of other better, quicker and cheaper ways of finding yourself or proving that you are bright than doing a higher degree).

Still want to do a higher degree?

If you have worked through all the reasons why you should not do an MD or a PhD and you still want to do one then you should prepare yourself for a different experience. As discussed above, doing a PhD is not an easy task and is very different from the rest of medical education, which is essentially an apprenticeship with lots of rote learning thrown in. To complete a PhD successfully you need to be bright, highly motivated, enthusiastic and capable of working very hard for no discernible return (so there are ways in which the life of a psychiatric trainee may have prepared you for this). Whether you are looking for a career in academic psychiatry, personal development or just a change, the demands are the same.

Nothing, including your own commitment, is more important to success at a higher degree than your supervisor. You will probably be required to have two supervisors, but the primary supervisor is the all-important one with the second supervisor often providing highly specific input. The formal nature of PhD supervision means that you will be better protected doing a PhD than doing an MD. Your research question and project may come entirely from the supervisor(s) or they may hone it with you, but it is their skills that will generate something that is researchable and generates data that can be fashioned into a thesis. Here past form predicts future performance: find out how many higher degrees they have supervised successfully (best answer: lots) and how many failures (best answer: none). It is absolutely vital to talk to current students: is the supervisor a tyrant and a bully? Are they never there? Do they actually provide any supervision? Is the laboratory or department a happy place or a den of bullying woe? What is the publication record like? Sometimes when an individual is limited to a geographical area or a very specific subject there may not be a wide choice of supervisors. However, if you are not stuck in that way you should consider yourself a commodity and find the best place to sell yourself to for the life of the PhD.

What do you get from a higher degree?

As discussed above, a PhD is a research training as well as research in its own right, whereas an MD does not necessarily contain the training. From a higher degree, in addition to the letters after your name, you should expect to walk away with specific expertise in three areas:

- research skills and techniques (e.g. critical thinking, analysis and evaluation; specific laboratory or fieldwork techniques; and general scientific communication, writing and presentation)
- research management skills (e.g. computer skills; project management; budgeting; making grant applications; keeping records of experiments; health and safety management; and managing supervisors)
- individual effectiveness (flexibility; self-motivation; task completion; a mood of enquiry, taking the initiative; self-directed learning; debating skills; and problem-solving).

However, the bottom line is that both the PhD and the MD study generates a thesis. The exact configuration of this beast varies between universities, but it is a book presenting a substantial piece of independent research that makes an original contribution to an academic area or discipline and that is generally between 50 000 and 100 000 words in length.

It is the thesis along with yourself that is examined. At the end of 3–6 years your supervisor will identify an external and an internal examiner and there will be a *viva voce* (except for MDs in some universities) during which you will be called on to 'defend' your thesis, the book that you have written. The only people you can expect ever to read your thesis are yourself, your supervisors and, with luck, the two examiners. You should therefore have sympathy for them, they are your audience. At the end of a 1–4-hour viva the options are that:

- you will be told that you have passed
- you have passed but need to make a few very minor corrections that the examiners do not need to see
- you need to make some revisions and these must be seen again by the examiners before they will agree that you have passed
- you need to make some revisions and need to be seen again by the examiners before they decide whether you have passed
- you have only performed to a master's level and so they are awarding an MPhil
- you have failed.

So at the end of all this there remains the possibility that you will fail. This will be a failure for your supervisors as well as yourself, but it is you that will have mostly wasted an appreciable part of your life.

A very large number of students drop out before completing their thesis and the final examination. It is therefore very important to think carefully before committing to completing a higher degree. Be choosy and ask a lot of questions before making the decision, as this will maximise your chances of a positive outcome all round. To paraphrase the wartime poster campaign aimed at saving petrol, before you set out you should ask yourself: 'Is my higher degree really necessary?'

Reference

Anderson, M. & Jankowski, J. (2001) Higher research degrees: making the right choice. *BMJ Careers*, **322** (7277).

Index

Compiled by Caroline Sheard